AF323820

AAOS
Symposium on
Upper extremity injuries
in athletes

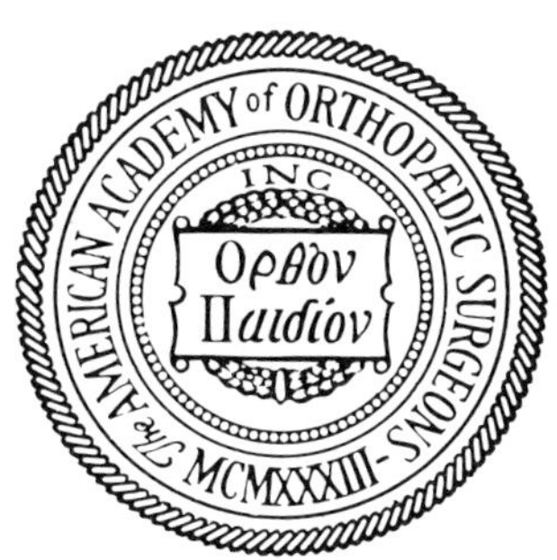

American Academy
of
Orthopaedic Surgeons

Symposium on
Upper extremity injuries in athletes

Washington, D.C.
June 1984

Edited by

Frank A. Pettrone, M.D.
Assistant Clinical Professor of Orthopaedic Surgery,
Georgetown University Medical School,
Washington, D.C.;
Staff, Arlington Medical Center,
Arlington, Virginia

with 382 illustrations

The C. V. Mosby Company
ST. LOUIS • TORONTO • PRINCETON   1986

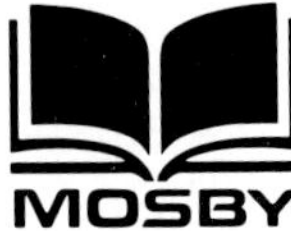

MOSBY

A TRADITION OF PUBLISHING EXCELLENCE

Acquisition editor: Eugenia A. Klein
Assistant editor: Jean Carey-Brendle
Manuscript editor: Carl Masthay
Design: Staff
Production: Barbara Merritt, Jeanne Gulledge

Printed in the United States of America

The C.V. Mosby Company
11830 Westline Industrial Drive, St. Louis, Missouri 63146

Library of Congress Cataloging-in-Publication Data

Symposium on Upper Extremity Injuries in Athletes
    (1984: Washington, D.C.)
    Symposium on Upper Extremity Injuries in Athletes.

    At head of title: American Academy of Orthopaedic
Surgeons.
    Includes index.
    1. Extremities, Upper—Wounds and injuries—
Congresses. 2. Sports—Accidents and injuries—
Congresses. I. Pettrone, Frank A. II. American
Academy of Orthopaedic Surgeons. III. Title.
[DNLM: 1. Athletic Injuries—congresses. 2. Extremities
—injuries—congresses. WE 805 S9898s 1984]
RD776.S96   1984   617'.57044   85-18875
ISBN 0-8016-0026-X

TS/MV/MV 9 8 7 6 5 4 3 2 1   03/B/355

Contributors

James R. Andrews, M.D.

Clinical Professor, Section of Sports Medicine, Department of Orthopaedic Surgery, Tulane University School of Medicine, New Orleans, Louisiana; Director of Orthopaedic Training, Hughston Orthopaedic Clinic, Columbus, Georgia

George P. Bogumill, Ph.D., M.D.

Professor of Orthopaedic Surgery, Department of Surgery, Georgetown University, Washington, D.C.

Jay S. Cox, M.D.

Associate Clinical Professor of Surgery, Uniformed Services University of Health Services, Bethesda, Maryland; Consultant in Sports Medicine, U.S. Naval Academy, Annapolis, Maryland

James H. Dobyns, M.D.

Professor of Orthopedic Surgery, Mayo Medical School; Consultant in Orthopedics and Surgery of the Hand, Mayo Clinic, Rochester, Minnesota

Rod Dulany

Director of Tennis, Washington Golf and Country Club; Vice President, U.S. Professional Tennis Association, Arlington, Virginia

Charles H. Epps, Jr., M.D.

Professor and Chief, Division of Orthopaedic Surgery, Howard University Medical Center, Washington, D.C.

Joe H. Gieck, Ed.D., A.T.C., R.P.T.

Assistant Professor, School of Education; Assistant Professor, Orthopaedics and Rehabilitation; Curriculum Director, Head Athletic Trainer, Division of Sports Medicine and Athletic Training, Department of Athletics, University of Virginia, Charlottesville, Virginia

Scott D. Gillogly, M.D.

Captain, Medical Corps, United States Army, Walter Reed Army Medical Center, Washington, D.C.; Resident in Sports Medicine, Hughston Orthopaedic Clinic, Columbus, Georgia

Joel B. Grad, M.D.

Assistant Professor of Orthopaedic Surgery, Department of Orthopaedics, New York University Medical Center; Attending Surgeon, Department of Orthopaedics, St. Vincent's Hospital and Medical Center, New York, New York

Jack L. Groppel, Ph.D.

Associate Professor of Physical Education and of Bioengineering, Department of Physical Education and Department of Bioengineering, University of Illinois at Urbana-Champaign, Urbana, Illinois

David C. Johnson, M.D.

Clinical Instructor in Orthopaedic Surgery, Department of Surgery, Georgetown University Medical Center; Team Physician, U.S. National Swimming Team; Medical Consultant to the President's Council on Physical Fitness and Sports, Washington, D.C.

Donald M. Knowlan, M.D., F.A.C.P.

Associate Professor of Medicine, Georgetown University School of Medicine, Washington, D.C.; Director, Georgetown Affiliated Program, Arlington Hospital, Arlington, Virginia; Team Physician, Washington Redskins and George Mason University Patriots

Vi A. Mayer, O.T.R.

Instructor in Orthopaedics and Rehabilitation, Department of Orthopaedics and Rehabilitation, University of Virginia, Charlottesville, Virginia

Frank C. McCue III, M.D.

Alfred R. Shands Professor of Orthopaedic Surgery and Plastic Surgery of the Hand; Director, Division of Sports Medicine and Hand Surgery; Team Physician, Department of Athletics, Department of Orthopaedics and Rehabilitation, University of Virginia, Charlottesville, Virginia

Charles P. Melone, Jr., M.D., F.A.C.S.

Associate Professor of Orthopaedic Surgery, Department of Orthopaedics, New York University Medical Center; Director, Hand Surgery Service, Department of Surgery, Cabrini Medical Center; Attending Surgeon, Department of Orthopaedics, St. Vincent's Hospital and Medical Center, New York, New York

Gary A. Miller, M.D.

Hand and Sports Medicine Fellow, Department of Orthopaedic Surgery, University of Virginia, Charlottesville, Virginia

John F. Mosher, Jr., M.D.

Associate Professor, Orthopaedic Surgery, Department of Orthopaedics, State University Hospital, Syracuse, New York

Robert J. Neviaser, M.D.

Professor of Orthopaedic Surgery, George Washington University School of Medicine; Director of Hand and Upper Extremity Service, Department of Orthopaedic Surgery, George Washington University Medical Center, Washington, D.C.

Robert P. Nirschl, M.S., M.D.

Assistant Clinical Professor of Orthopaedic Surgery, Georgetown University; Orthopedic Consultant, President's Council on Physical Fitness and Sports, Washington, D.C.; Attending Orthopedic Surgeon, Arlington Hospital; Medical Director, Viriginia Sportsmedicine Rehabilitation Institute, Arlington, Virginia

Eric L. Radin, M.D.

Professor and Chairman of Department of Orthopedic Surgery, West Virginia University School of Medicine, Morgantown, West Virginia

Edward Ricciardelli

University of Virginia Medical School, Charlottesville, Virginia

Janet Sobel, R.P.T.

Director of Rehabilitation, Virginia Sportsmedicine Rehabilitation Institute, Arlington, Virginia

Russell F. Warren, M.D.

Associate Professor of Orthopedic Surgery, Cornell Medical College; Director of Sports Medicine, The Hospital for Special Surgery, New York, New York

Bertram Zarins, M.D.

Assistant Clinical Professor, Department of Orthopaedic Surgery, Harvard Medical School; Chief of Sports Medicine Unit, Massachusetts General Hospital, Boston, Massachusetts

Preface

Our society has experienced an increased awareness of the values of personal physical fitness. This has contributed to the boom in recreational and competitive sports participation. The recent Olympic Games in Los Angeles further enthused Americans. With increased participation has come an awareness of injury potential. Much is known and has been said about knee and lower extremity problems in athletes. There is relatively little information on upper extremity injuries. In sports such as baseball, tennis, gymnastics, and swimming, upper extremity problems predominate.

The American Academy of Orthopaedic Surgeons held a Symposium on Upper Extremity Injuries in Athletes in Washington, D.C., on June 7-9, 1984. Two hundred health professionals met to learn about these problems. Orthopaedic surgeons, trainers, physical therapists, orthotists, and professional coaches all contributed. Material was presented on anatomy, fractures, biomechanics, mechanisms of injury, diagnosis, treatment (conservative as well as surgical), and rehabilitation. Demonstration clinics were held on proper and, importantly, improper technique as a predisposition for injury in throwing, swimming, and tennis. Emphasis was given to proper diagnosis, prompt recognition, proper treatment, preventive steps, and rehabilitation to allow safe return to sports participation.

The concept of the course was to disseminate information on a topic of growing sports medicine significance for the benefit of all practitioners.

As chairman of the course, I wish to thank the authors both for their work at the meeting and for their superb efforts and clear presentation of new material in this text.

Frank A. Pettrone, M.D.

Contents

PART ONE

General principles

1 Biomechanical applications in the upper extremity, 3
Eric L. Radin

2 Medico-legal aspects of treating athletes, 11
Charles H. Epps, Jr.

3 Upper extremity pain: medical aspects, 16
Donald M. Knowlan

4 Biomechanical precursors to upper extremity trauma, 26
Jack L. Groppel

5 The utilization of proper racket sport mechanics to avoid upper extremity injury, 30
Jack L. Groppel

6 The upper extremity in swimming, 36
David C. Johnson

7 Tennis strokes, 47
Rod Dulany

8 The pitching motion, 59
Frank A. Pettrone

PART TWO

Hand, forearm, and wrist

9 Functional anatomy of the forearm and hand, 67
George P. Bogumill

10 Soft-tissue injuries to the hand, 79
Frank C. McCue III and Gary A. Miller

11 Fractures of the distal ends of radius and ulna, 95
Charles P. Melone, Jr., and Joel B. Grad

12 Flexor and extensor tendon injuries, 114
John F. Mosher

13 Carpal injuries, 122
Robert J. Neviaser

14 Ligament injuries about the wrist, 134
James H. Dobyns

15 Complex joint injuries of the hand, 142
Charles P. Melone, Jr.

16 Short-shrift problems: a grab bag of athletic injuries, 170
James H. Dobyns

17 Peripheral nerve injuries and entrapments of the forearm and wrist, 174
John F. Mosher

18 Upper extremity splinting and bracing (hand), 182
Frank C. McCue III, Vi A. Mayer, and Joe H. Gieck

PART THREE

Elbow and shoulder

19 Functional anatomy of the shoulder and elbow, 193
George P. Bogumill

20 The adolescent elbow, 211

Frank A. Pettrone

21 Bony injuries about the elbow in the throwing athlete, 221

James R. Andrews

22 Tennis elbow (epicondylitis), 233

Epidemiology and conservative treatment, 233

Russell F. Warren

Surgery and rehabilitation of the professional athlete, 244

Robert P. Nirschl

23 Fractures of the proximal humerus, clavicle, and scapula, 266

Robert J. Neviaser

24 Acromioclavicular joint injuries in athletes, 284

Jay S. Cox

25 Anterior subluxation and dislocation of the shoulder, 290

Bertram Zarins

26 Shoulder arthroscopy, 300

Frank A. Pettrone

27 Shoulder examination and diagnosis in the throwing athlete, 306

James R. Andrews and Scott D. Gillogly

28 Shoulder tendinitis, 322

Robert P. Nirschl

29 Shoulder rehabilitation: rotator cuff tendinitis, strength training, and return to play, 338

Janet Sobel

30 Supplemental exercise program for throwing, swimming, and gymnastics, 348

Janet Sobel

xii *Contents*

PART FOUR

Other injuries

31 Gymnastic injuries: the Virginia experience, 359

Edward Ricciardelli and Frank A. Pettrone

General principles

1. Biomechanical applications in the upper extremity

Eric L. Radin

THE SHOULDER

The shoulder in sports is primarily used to achieve acceleration and power. Once one understands this, it should be no surprise that the anatomy has to be so complicated. The shoulder is the most mobile joint complex in the body. It is very useful to be able to work with the upper extremity over one's head. In order to be maximally useful, though, it is also necessary to achieve power in the upper extremity, even when it is over the head.

What is meant by power is force over time: one has to move an extremity quickly to get power. Many shoulder injuries occur because of attempts to move the upper extremity with tremendous force, at speeds that are really quite incredible. Consider the force required to throw a baseball 100 miles per hour. The relationship between relative motion of the humerus and scapula (Fig. 1-1) is not a simple one of 1 to 2 or 2 to 3 but is a more complex arrangement. The major provider of the acceleration of the humerus is the deltoid. The design specifications mandate power in the deltoid whether the arm is over the head or it is positioned at the side. There is a relationship between the force generated in the contraction of a muscle and its length. This is called Blix's curve after the Swedish physiologist. A muscle must be contracted down to a certain length in order to get maximum force. If the muscle is stretched out too much, it will rip apart. So muscle length is critical.

The deltoid muscle is pennate shaped for power (Fig. 1-2). The fibers are arranged in such a way that minimal contraction results in maximal power. How is it then that the deltoid can be as powerful above the shoulder as below, since it would have to have a huge excursion? The secret is that it is mounted on a movable platform, the scapula (Fig. 1-3). If one appreciates that in order to achieve power there must be a movable base for origination of the major shoulder motors, then the scapula makes sense. Of course, since the scapula is movable, there is a multiplicity of muscles attached to its periphery to move it in all directions.

The final factor involving power in the shoulder is that it is designed to take advantage of the relationship between force and leverage. The torques that can be

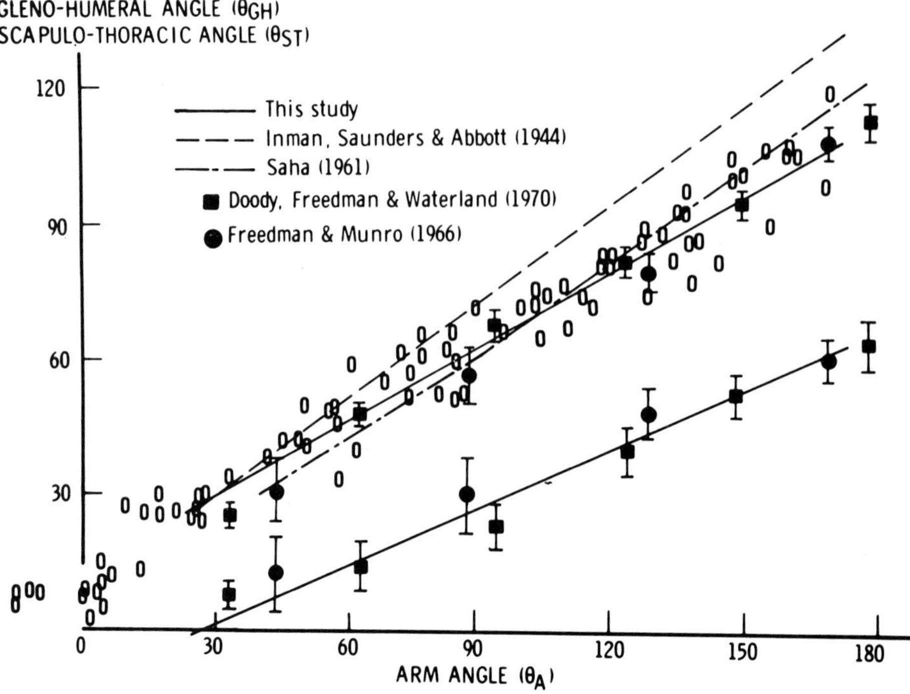

Fig. 1-1. Relationship between glenohumeral angle (θ_{GH}) and arm angle (θ_A) and between scapulothoracic angle (θ_{ST}) and arm angle. (From Poppen, N.K., and Walker, P.S.: J. Bone Joint Surg. **58A:**195-201, 1976.

generated with a big lever arm would be much higher with a given force than they would be with a small lever arm. To get leverage then from the center of rotation, muscles must be placed at some distance from the center of rotation. The deltoid inserts at some distance from the center of humeral head rotation (Fig. 1-4). There are several major muscles that insert out on the humerus, that is, at some distance from the rotation center of the joint; obviously they have to originate from somewhere. They originate on the thoracic cage. If one were to sit down and figure out what was needed to move the humerus through its possible motions, one would almost have to devise the latissimus dorsi and pectoralis major (Fig. 1-5).

The next consideration is the shape of the scapula. Why a spine? The answer is to have a place to originate muscle. The strength of the muscle is related to its cross-sectional area. If pulled too hard, a muscle could be pulled out of the bone. That is a very common sports injury. Ideally, powerful muscles should have a very broad bony origin. A nice, bony prominence is a terrific place from which to originate muscles. There is also the problem of rotation of the humerus. The rotator cuff, which does rotate, has to originate somewhere. It would be difficult to come up with a design in which the rotator cuff originated somewhere other than on the scapular platform. So

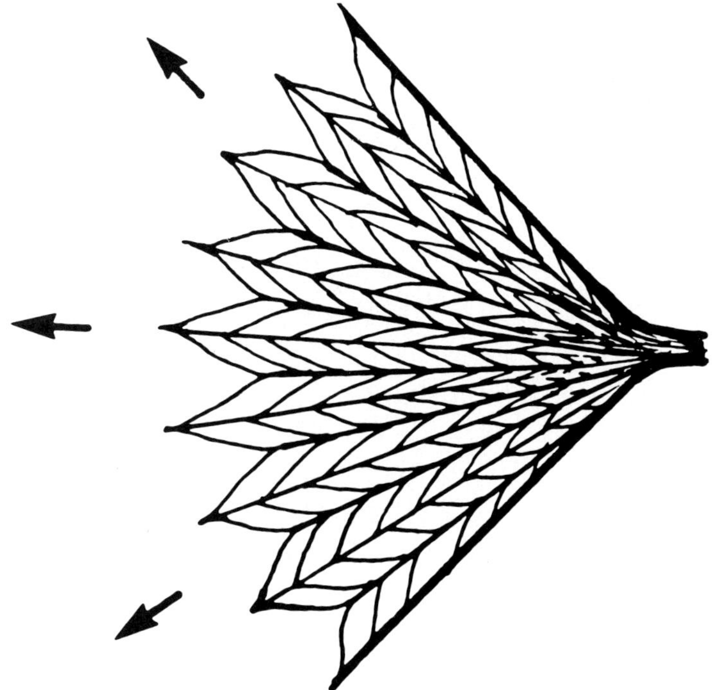

Fig. 1-2. Multipennate stucture of deltoid muscle provides for great power relative to its excursion. (From Radin, E.L.: Biomechanics and functional anatomy. In Post, M., editor: The shoulder: surgical and nonsurgical management, Philadelphia, 1978, Lea & Febiger.)

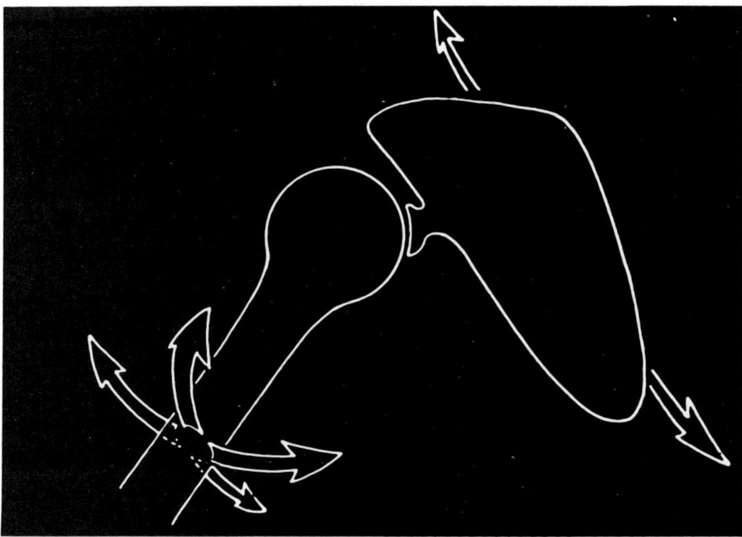

Fig. 1-3. Deltoid is mounted on a movable platform, the scapula, and thus allows the upper extremity to function above and below shoulder level.

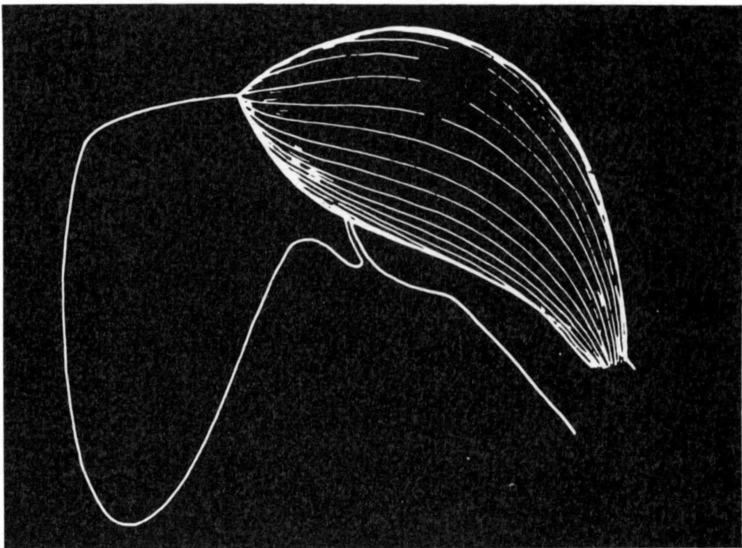

Fig. 1-4. Deltoid inserts at some distance from the center of rotation of the humeral head, thus allowing the humerus to have greater torque.

obviously there must be a place for that. The scapular spine makes very good sense.

A few words about the clavicle: the clavicle is used to fix the scapulothoracic joint. It connects the base of the platform and the thoracic wall. As the arm is raised over the head, the distance from the acromioclavicular joint to the sternoclavicular joint shortens. Since there can be no collapsing bone, as in one tube inside the other, how is the problem of changing clavicle length solved? The answer is an S-shaped bone that rotates.

What about the long head of the biceps? As it rotates, a different segment of the S presents itself and thus it is shorter. It is very efficient to combine elbow flexion and abduction, two joints working at once. The combination of elbow flexion and shoulder elevation with strength is really a pulling motion. In this activity both of the biceps heads will be used. Having muscles that span both joints is, from an energy point of view, very efficient. It is a very clever design having the long head of the biceps cross the glenohumeral joint.

THE ELBOW

The biomechanics of the elbow has not been well understood until just a few years ago. We are now beginning to understand the forces and stress distribution of the elbow. It really is two joints. There is a flexion-extension joint, the olecranotrochlear, and a rotatory joint, the radiocapitellar. It is very important in analyzing the elbow to remember that it is two joints. Although the combined flexion-extension and rotatory motions provide for a wide variety of motions, they do not create a stable joint, and

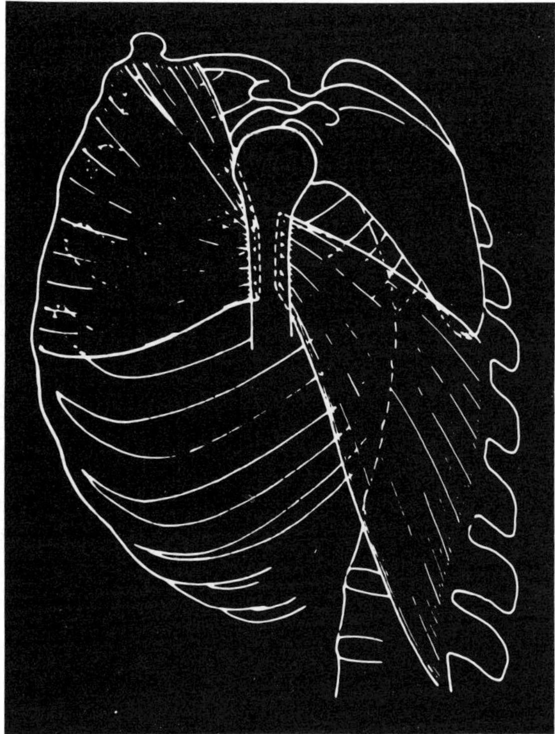

Fig. 1-5. Pectoralis major and latissimus dorsi insert on the humerus and attach to the thoracic cage, allowing the humerus to have a variety of motions.

hence a dislocated elbow is not an uncommon injury. The instability results from a lack of bony stability because there are two joints. The elbow relies upon a complicated ligamentous structure for stability. In comparison to the knee, being a hinged joint with less rotation, the elbow has a greater range of motion, which is less stable and has a greater likelihood of certain injuries.

The stability of the elbow is augmented by the origin of the long motors of the wrist and finger, which to some extent begins on the distal humerus. Attempts to use the wrist for power, particularly in dorsiflection, instead of the whole extremity, can tear the origin of the wrist extensors. As explained in detail by Dr. Nirschl in Chapter 28, this injury is called "tennis elbow." This chronic tendinitis can be relieved when the pressure is taken off the common extensor origin. The use of tight Velcro straps, applied just distal to the humeral upper epicondyle, is effective because it moves the origin of the common extensor tendons distal to the lateral epicondyle. Doing so rests that part of the origin and the muscle and therefore relieves the tendinitis. Another treatment is surgical release of the common extensor tendon. The only way one can have a failure operating on a tennis elbow is by misdiagnosing the problem.

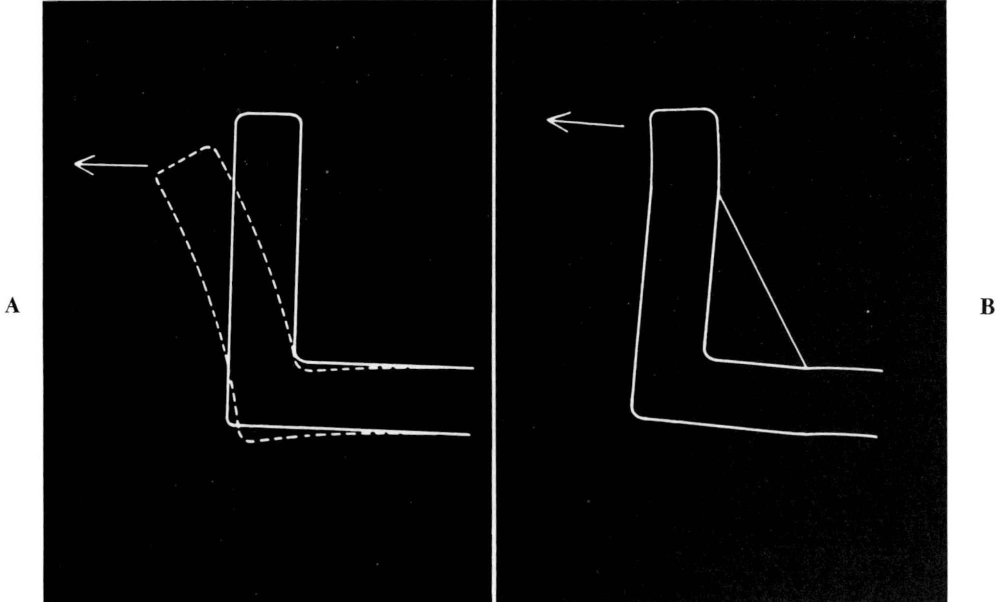

Fig. 1-6. Muscles reduce propensity for fracture of a bone, **A**, similar to a guy wire or strut attached to a standard, **B**.

Why are there so many muscles in the forearm and in the arm? It appears as if there are several muscles available for each job. The answer is that there is a very important job that muscles do that is frequently not considered. The job of muscles to move and accelerate the segments of the extremities is obvious. Consider, though, the need to reduce some of the bending stress on the bones. Fractures of bones can occur because of bending from activities of sports, a phenomenon familiar to practitioners of sports medicine. It is not just collisions that cause fractures. A bone subjected to bending stress can be protected if a guy wire or strut is attached to the end of the bone, which will reduce the bending stress by diminishing the tensile force. The muscle, analogous to a guy wire or strut, reduces the bone's propensity for fracture (Fig. 1-6). Because of the manner in which muscles protect bone from fracture, fatigued muscles cannot adequately play this role. Continuing to do an activity while being fatigued greatly increases the likelihood of sustaining stress fractures. One of the major ways to avoid repetitive stress fractures in athletes is to train the muscles. The advantage of so many muscles in the upper extremity is evident when one considers this second very important function. It is advantageous to have parallel fast-twitch and slow-twitch fiber muscles, one for each function, to prevent broken bones. Fewer stress fractures occur in the upper extremity when there is less repetitive bending stress because of these structural features.

The upper extremity, besides being a tremendous source of power, is also used for

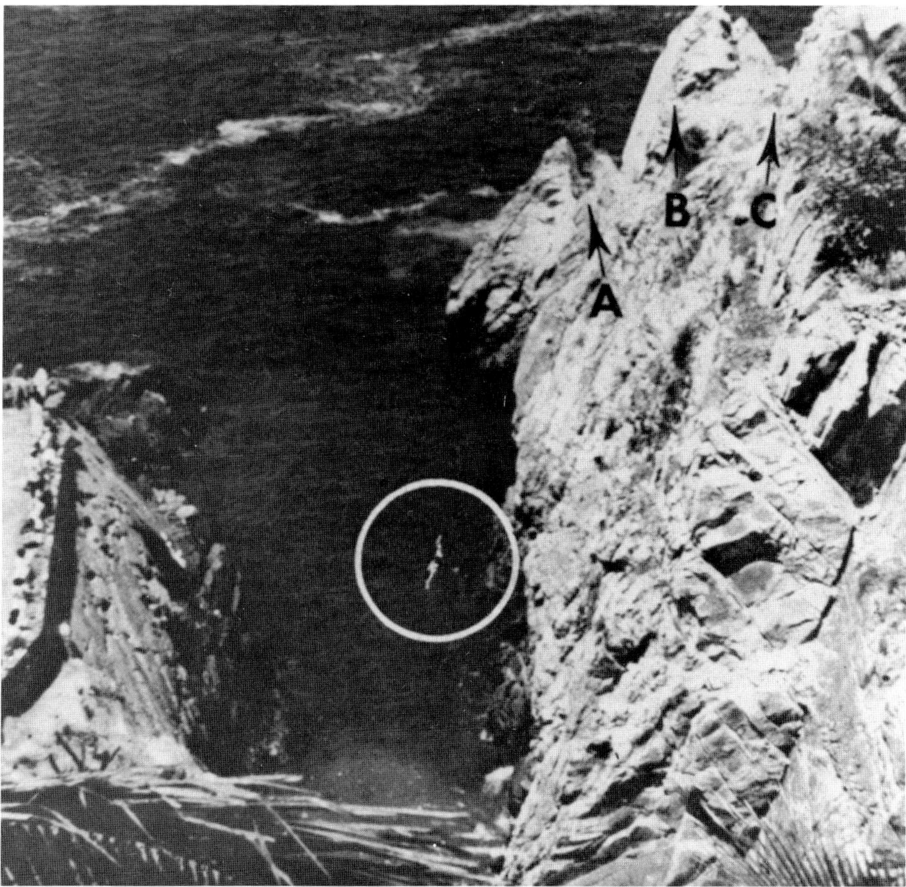

Fig. 1-7. *A*, *B*, and *C* indicate diving points from the Acapulco cliffs; the diver is shown midway through his dive. (From Schneider, R.C., Papo, M., and Alvarez, C.S.: J. Bone Joint Surg. **44A:**648-656, 1962.)

protection. A classic example of this is with the Acapulco cliff divers. The people who dived with their hands over their heads had no cervical fractures, whereas those who did not effectively protect their heads sustained cervical stress fractures, as evidenced by roentgenograms (Fig. 1-7). The divers who did not protect their heads could be selected from the whole group based on the roentgenographic evidence alone. It is not difficult to believe that these divers sustained stress fractures because dives of 150 feet cause tremendous force to be exerted as the person hits the water.

The upper extremity is highly complex in its functional anatomy, but this complexity is necessary to provide the upper extremity the ability to achieve power over the tremendous range of flexibility that humans, as upright animals, have. So we should celebrate the human upper extremity. It's really very cleverly designed.

SUMMARY

The shoulder allows for powerful movement of the upper extremity above and below shoulder level because of the multipennate structure of the deltoid, its attachment to a movable platform, the scapula, and its insertion to the humerus a distance away from the center of rotation of the humeral head. Other structural features of the shoulder allow for a wide variety of movements of the upper extremity. The elbow, actually two joints, allows for movement in many directions but as a result is not a particularly stable joint. Muscles associated with the elbow help to protect the bones of the upper extremity from bending stress by diminishing applied tensile force.

2. Medico-legal aspects of treating athletes

Charles H. Epps, Jr.

Treating athletes at all levels of competition can present situations that have important medico-legal considerations. The problems arise largely from new forces that are acting in our society today.

First is the fact that people of all ages have become increasingly interested in physical conditioning and athletic activities. As a natural consequence of increased numbers and activity, there are more injuries. The second is the fact that our country has become extremely litigous. People wish to be compensated for injuries whether there is liability or not. If one is treating professional athletes who are high earners making several hundred thousand dollars a year, a missed diagnosis or fracture that does not heal optimally can have devastating financial consequences. Whereas such injuries may be covered to some extent by workers' compensation and other contractural arrangements, the player may also look to the surgeon for additional compensation through malpractice action.

OBLIGATION OF PHYSICIAN

The physician who treats a patient, of course, whether he is an athlete or not, has as his prime responsibility a duty to protect the health of his patient. Despite the fact that the physician may be employed by a professional team or may be a volunteer for the high school team, as a treating physician he is obligated to his patient. There has been some concern in the legal arena as to what a team physician is and what his duties are. The obligations result from the conceptual nature of the physician-patient relationship, regardless as to who may have hired him.

Obviously, when physicians who are not trained to take care of injuries assume this responsibility, for example, the pediatrician team physician, arrangements should be made for an orthopaedist to provide back-up services. By the same token, an orthopaedist who is caring for a team should arrange to have another physician do the necessary cardiopulmonary evaluations.

ROLE OF TEAM PHYSICIAN

The team physician has been defined as one who undertakes to render professional medical services to athletic participants whose services are either arranged for or paid for, at least, in part by an institution or entity other than the patient, the patient's family, or some surrogate. That means that even the volunteer legally falls into this category. The scope of the services rendered by the physician may be limited, but he has to give the team timely notice of the limitations. There should also be provisions to get a player who is injured during a game to a proper emergency facility, and these arrangements should be made well in advance. There are other significant decisions, for example, whether the athlete will be acquired by a team, or when he can participate in a game after an injury. Such decisions can be very important ones for a professional team. This is especially true in the case of the quarterback or the punter or the running halfback or any player whose participation is crucial to the team's potential if he is unable to play.

The surgeon should not permit himself to be put in the position that allows the coach to dictate who shall play and who shall not play if the decision has to be made on medical facts. There may be conflicts with the coach or with the team owner if either is disposed to intervene or with the athlete himself if he decides that he is well enough to play and medical consideration determines that he is not. At other times the physician may have to deal with parents if the athletes are little leaguers or in the minor age group. The determination that the athlete is fit to play, when he is not, may also present a problem. The physician must make a careful assessment of previous injuries. If a prospective player is trying out for a team, the examining physician should review the past records and make a careful and thorough examination to determine whether the player is physically sound to be hired or given a trial. You want to make sure that there are proper measures to prevent new injuries. The team physician must be concerned that there are measures and programs to prevent injury. At the same time, if a team member has had a previous injury, you would need to protect him so that he does not aggravate this injury. You should be aware of the complications of an injury, which need to be explained to the patient in detail. You should also arrange to see that proper rehabilitaton is available for the patient after routine care has been given. Prevention may also relate to conditioning and to proper equipment. Even though the trainer and the coach are responsible directly, as the team physician you should have some knowledge of the situation and some duty of observation over training.

STANDARD OF CARE

A national standard of care is emerging as the legal standard. The orthopaedist who undertakes the care of a team will be judged by a standard higher than a physician who is dealing with nonathletes.[3]

Negligence legally has been defined as conduct that falls below the standard established by law for the protection of others against unreasonable risk or harm. In other words, as an orthopaedic surgeon, you must meet that standard of care. I believe that there are at least two standards of care. One would apply to surgeons who practice general orthopaedics, and the other would apply to that group of men who have made sports medicine a subspecialty. These surgeons are expected to perform at a level of sophistication and a level of efficiency and skill higher than the regular orthopaedists.

Some of the compounding factors are workers' compensation laws and special provisions in player contracts. Good samaritan statutes relate to the situation where the surgeon who has no contractual obligation provides emergency assistance. In some states, if one provides first aid, under such circumstances the surgeon is covered by the good samaritan law. However, in other states the surgeon, after making contact with that patient, has an obligation to follow through. He actually has to take care of the patient until the patient is turned over to someone else and that may be until the patient gets to the hospital or until some other arrangements are made for his definitive care.

Breach of confidence is an issue that will probably not be encountered except in a professional situation. This has to do with revealing facts about the condition of your athlete-patient who, for example, may be the star quarterback for the team. Under these circumstances, as you know, there will be public curiosity and great media interest in his ability to play. Gamblers may set the odds upon whether he is going to play, and the point spread becomes a factor. The press may pursue you as the treating physician to learn about the player's condition. You cannot divulge facts about your athlete-patient without his permission any more than you can discuss the condition of the ordinary patient who comes to your office.

The sports physician should not allow either financial considerations or his personal enthusiasm for the sport or the athlete's toughness or desire to play to prevent the best medical judgment and proper treatment. In other words, judgment should prevail even though the individual athlete-patient's playing might make a great difference to the particular game. If the player stands a risk of causing further injury to himself or compounding the physical problem, your obligation is to see that he does not play. Too often there is the injured athlete who wants to play before full recovery from an injury has been obtained. Even in high school and college, this attitude has become acceptable and admired behavior. Young athletes see the professionals playing the game with casts and special splints, and the commentators admiringly refer to the fact that the star is "playing hurt." As a physician, your primary responsibility is to the patient. If you believe that it is in his best interests not to play, he should not, despite the financial considerations for the team or the institution. The pressure can be substantial because even college teams that win the important games, tournaments, and especially national titles have significant financial impact on their institutions. Athletes will sometimes hide their injuries from the physician because they know that they will be benched if the true extent of the injury is known. The team physician must have a high index of suspicion in these matters.

PREPARTICIPATION EXAMINATION

At all levels of competition, the preparticipation athletic physical examination has become a requirement. The quality of the examination process is affected by many factors such as time, cost, and expertise of the examiner. Orthopaedic screening may be expected to uncover significant preexisting conditions that require treatment before participation in a sport is allowed. There are additional athletes who are predisposed to injury or overuse syndromes. The identification of these two groups should reduce significantly the number of serious injuries.[2,5] The preparticipation or qualifying physical examination is a duty that has great importance for the physician who is responsible for a professional team. Your medical opinion about the athlete-patient will influence the team's decision to draft or trade and even discontinue the player. This decision has significant financial consequences for the player and the team as well.

DRUG ABUSE PROBLEM

There have been highly publicized accounts of drug abuse among athletes on both the college and professional levels. In the last year, several National Collegiate Athletic Association (NCAA) schools have started drug testing. Most programs are aimed at education, prevention, and rehabilitation, not punishment, and concentrate on the performance-enhancing drugs such as anabolic steroids and stimulants. A 1981 study in the Big Ten Conference revealed that between 80% and 85% of male athletes and the general student body used alcohol and between 20% and 22% of both groups used marijuana. Two percent of the athletes used steroids, whereas almost no nonathletes used them.[1] The NCAA Special Drug Testing Committee has developed plans for random, on-campus drug testing at championship events for the 1985-1986 season.[1]

In the professional ranks, the National Basketball Association has taken a tough stand. Conviction of or pleading guilty to a crime involving the use, possession, or distribution of cocaine or heroin will disquality permanently a player from playing. Random testing of players is permitted under certain conditions. On the other hand, random testing is not permitted for professional football players or baseball players, and this remains a point of major contention between management and the respective professional players associations.[1]

The team physician must be alert to the problem and watch for signs of a drug problem, lack of energy, bloodshot eyes, depression, and missed practices.

TEAM PHYSICIAN—THE FUTURE

It is possible that in the case of professional sports, the team physician as we know him today may change in the not-too-distant future. Professional sports have become an industry that is big business with enormous pressures on teams to win and a new role for the professional athlete. Lawrence Fleisher,[4] general legal counsel of the National Basketball Players Association, has cited the conflict that develops among the athlete, the team physician, and the team. Recent legal reviews and medical tradition that put the physician's prime responsibility with the patient instead of the employer or team give rise to a number of problems involving confidentiality, conflicts of interest, and standard of care. Fleisher suggests that a player joining a team be examined solely for the benefit of the team and not for the benefit of the individual player. Furthermore, he opines that a team doctor should continue to be available at a sporting event to provide emergency care, but it should be the responsibility of the player to obtain his own doctor's services.

The winds of change are blowing hard and fast around the sports physician and the athlete in the medicolegal climate. The physician must remain alert to these changes.

REFERENCES

1. Duda, M.: Drug testing challenges college and pro athletes, Physician and Sports Med. **12:**109, 1984.
2. Elkstrand, J., Gillquist, J., and Liljedahl, S.: Prevention of soccer injuries, Am. J. Sports Med. **11:**116, 1983.
3. King, J.H.: The duty and standard of care for team physicians, Houston Law Rev. **18:**657, 1981.
4. NBPA Lawyer: Eliminate the team physician, Orthopaedics Today **4:**6, Nov. 1984.
5. Raskin, R., and Rebecca, G.S.: Post-traumatic sports related musculoskeletal abnormalities: prevalence in a normal population, Am. J. Sports Med. **11:**336, 1983.

3. Upper extremity pain: medical aspects

Donald M. Knowlan

There is a cliché popular among rheumatologists: "Shoulder pain is rarely caused by arthritis!" This serves as a warning to the physician-specialist that he not take too narrow a diagnostic view when considering the causes of upper extremity pain. This advice can apply to a general variety of specialists who, when confronted with a patient who presents with upper extremity pain, should consider a broad range of diagnostic possibilities before attaching their favorite diagnosis to the problem.

I would like to share with you a general survey of the common causes of upper extremity pain (see the following outline) and then present several case histories that illustrate certain helpful clinical points in the differential diagnosis.

Medical causes of upper extremity pain
1. Local
    a. Tendinitis
    b. Injury-tear
2. Referred from local structures
    a. Spinal cord
        (1) Tumor
        (2) Disc
        (3) Arthritis
    b. Compression syndromes and thoracic outlet syndromes
        (1) Anterior scalene
        (2) Costoclavicular
        (3) Brachial plexus
        (4) Cervical rib
    c. Shoulder-hand syndrome
    (3) General problem—systemic
    a. Rheumatoid arthritis
    b. Osteoarthritis
    c. Gout-pseudogout
    d. Collagen vascular diseases—polymyalgia rheumatica
    e. Carpal tunnel syndrome

16

    4. Referred from internal organs
       a. Cardiac
          (1) Coronary artery disease—angina
          (2) Pericarditis—rub
          (3) Aortic aneurysm
       b. Pulmonary
          (1) Upper lobe lesion (Pancoast's syndrome)
          (2) Diaphragmatic irritation—pneumonia, emboli, tumor, effusion, etc.
       c. Gastrointestinal
          (1) Liver
          (2) Gallbladder
          (3) Ruptured viscus
       d. Spleen (Kehr's sign)

As outlined above, upper extremity pain may be secondary to a local problem or may be part of a general systemic condition. It may be referred either from adjacent local structures or even from somewhat distant internal organs.

LOCAL CAUSES

Upper extremity pain may be secondary to a local problem with a variety of causes—calcific tendinitis, various musculoskeletal injuries, overuse syndrome, and so on. These causes are the main focus of this symposium and are well addressed elsewhere.

UPPER EXTREMITY PAIN REFERRED FROM LOCAL STRUCTURES

The cervical spine when involved with disease such as a tumor, disc, or an arthritic condition may refer the pain through C4-C5 or C5-C6 dermatomes to the appropriate area of the upper extremity. Knowledge of the dermatome distribution of the upper extremity sensory nerves is helpful in directing us toward a specific diagnosis.

Compression syndromes and various thoracic outlet problems are appropriately reviewed elsewhere in this symposium. Certainly the cervical rib is a leading culprit in upper extremity pain.

The shoulder-hand syndrome should be considered by all in evaluating pain in the upper extremity. This is particularly true in patients recovering from a stroke or a myocardial infarction. It is far less common today than it was a decade ago.

UPPER EXTREMITY PAIN AS A PART OF GENERALIZED DISORDER

The collagen vascular diseases, particularly polymyositis and polymyalgia rheumatica, are among the systemic disorders that may present with upper extremity pain. The arthritides, especially osteoarthritis and rheumatoid arthritis, present with upper extremity signs and symptoms that are characteristically familiar. Although gout is more commonly a lower extremity monoarticular arthritis, it may present with upper extremity involvement and thus lead to confusion and delay in diagnosis.

The many diagnostic possibilities indicated by the carpal tunnel syndrome are often overlooked when the symptoms present. Consideration of its various causes, such as hypothyroidism, may uncover a systemic disorder.

UPPER EXTREMITY PAIN REFERRED FROM INTERNAL ORGANS

Upper extremity pain may represent pain referred from deeper internal thoracic and abdominal structures. The heart and lungs, and even the esophagus and the organs of the upper abdominal area, where structures are adjacent to the diaphragm with its phrenic nerve innervation, may all refer pain to the upper extremity and confuse the clinical picture.

Certainly we are aware of the referred pain of coronary artery disease and its radiation to the upper extremity, but the pain of pericarditis and aortic aneurysm may present in a similar manner.

Pulmonary disorders may cause upper extremity pain. Pancoast's tumor in the lung apex, which invades local vessels and nerves, can cause severe pain. Lower lobe tumors and pleural effusions with diaphragmatic irritation may present with upper extremity pain as the presenting symptom. Pulmonary emboli, mentioned later, may do the same.

Elevation of the liver with disease or its acute distension may irritate the diaphragm and refer pain to the shoulder and upper extremity.

Gallbladder pain usually radiates subcostally to the right and at times around posteriorly to the scapular tip, or through the abdomen to the scapular area, but it may less frequently present as right shoulder or upper extremity pain.

A ruptured viscus, particularly of the stomach, duodenum, and the colon, may cause subdiaphragmatic irritation and refer pain to the shoulder and upper extremity causing a confusing clinical picture.

The value of Kehr's sign (pain in the left shoulder with rupture of the spleen) has been disputed to be of value by many, but not by Lowenfels,[2] who modified its use with elevation of the foot of the bed, combining this with gentle pressure to stimulate the phrenic nerve to produce the positive sign in nine of ten patients with confirmed ruptured spleens. In several cases presenting at our hospital over the years, persons have presented with severe left shoulder pain 1 to 2 weeks after an apparent minor trauma and alert house officers suspected the diagnosis of rupture based upon this finding among others.

THE PHYSICAL EXAMINATION

As important as the history is in uncovering the cause of upper extremity pain, a careful and thorough physical examination can be most informative, especially when one is confronted with unusual diagnostic possibilities. Previously in this symposium, there has been emphasis on a complete joint examination, which includes inspection, palpation, and proper range-of-motion evaluation of the various joint and neuromuscular structures.

The examination would be incomplete if one did not include a careful examination of the neck, including its range of motion and percussion (by percussion hammer) of the cervical vertebrae. The neurologic examination should include a sensory and motor examination and an examination for upper motor neuron signs, including reflex responses that might separate a distal from a central neurologic disorder.

The carpal tunnel syndrome should be considered and evaluated by use of the provocative tests of Tinel and Phalen.

The blood vessels should be palpated and compared. Allen's sign, which roughly evaluates fillings of the ulnar and radial vessels, may be helpful.

A careful search for lymph nodes in the neck, especially in the supraclavicular fossae, and the axillary and epitrochlear areas take but a moment but may be specifically diagnostically rewarding.

There is a need to inspect and palpate for muscle tenderness and atrophy. One should examine arthritic hands and observe if the changes are proximal or distal, monoarticular or polyarticular, and whether the findings are in the joint or in the periarticular area. The interesting finding of Dupuytren's contracture may open a whole new area of general diagnostic possibilities.

There is an unending variety of physical findings that are seen in the upper extremity that may be suggestive of systemic disease. Just consider the fingernails alone, which may subtly reveal diseases of the liver, kidney, heart, or even systemic blood vessels.

What I would like to do next, rather than discuss all the possibilities is share with you a series of special cases that may help in defining for you certain of the more common causes of referred or systemic causes of upper extremity pain.

CORONARY ARTERY PAIN

CASE 1

A 46-year-old, physically active executive in good health jogged regularly 3 to 4 miles per day. In November 1982, while jogging, he developed burning and aching pain in the left shoulder and left upper arm. The pain occurred during a cold and windy day.

A stress test was strongly positive, and despite medical efforts to control the pain, the pain continued, and a year later he underwent quadruple bypass surgery for coronary artery disease.

The key to the clinical diagnosis of coronary artery disease still lies in an accurate history and an understanding of the significance of that history.

I would like to review the clinical presentation of coronary pain with emphasis on certain features that I have found most helpful in distinguishing it from noncardiac causes of chest pain.

The pain of coronary artery disease (whether angina, coronary insufficiency, or infarction) is substernal in 90% of the cases. It is usually lower substernal, less frequently upper substernal, and rarely if ever epigastric. It is rarely located outside the midclavicular line. The quality of the pain is variable and seems to be related to a patient's previous experiences or common use of certain words. It may be a "pressure," "indigestion," "heartburn," or "tightness," but rarely is it sharp or jabbing.

It is amazing how often patients with previous duodenal ulcer disease will use the same quality description of "burning" or "indigestion" to describe new onset angina. I find the location much more valuable than the quality of the pain in deciding on a coronary cause.

Coronary pain commonly radiates to the jaw, teeth, shoulder, ear, elbow, wrist, down the arm (usually inner aspect at C8). In 5% to 10% of the cases, the radiation area is reported as the only source of coronary pain. With careful questioning, half these patients admit a vague, ill-defined substernal component.

The pain of coronary artery disease is commonly precipitated by the *E*'s, that is, *e*xercise, *e*ating (quantity, not type of food), *e*nvironment (wind and cold), and *e*motions. If these are the precipitating factors, certain factors that relieve the pain are of diagnostic note. The pain commonly ceases when exercise is stopped, the environment altered, and the diet quantity changed.

Nitroglycerin placed sublingually is extremely helpful therapeutically in relieving the pain of coronary disease. It has also been extremely helpful diagnostically. It can be used as a diagnostic tool. Sublingually administered nitroglycerin is rapidly absorbed into the bloodstream. It may cause tachycardia, flushing, and a headache. The presence of a headache after its use means that it has retained its potency. Nitroglycerin should relieve the pain of angina in 1 to 3 minutes, and this response is diagnostic. Any longer period of pain relief (5 to 15 minutes) means that the diagnosis is incorrect, the nitroglycerin is not effective (with a headache, this is ruled out), or the patient has more prolonged coronary pain than angina and has either coronary insufficiency or an impending infarction. Nitroglycerin is an excellent diagnostic tool!

Another helpful clue in the evaluation of coronary artery pain is to assess accurately the time involved. It may be helpful to have the patient time the length of the pain directly with a timepiece. Coronary artery pain commonly lasts minutes or hours but never seconds or days.

The more common, sharp, quick, stabbing pains in the chest that last moments to seconds and are located laterally often are musculoskeletal in origin and not attributable to coronary artery disease.

The heavy pressure in the chest that lasts several days seen in depressed patients is a manifestation of their depression and not of coronary disease.

The best points in the diagnosis of coronary pain are the location (substernal), radiation, precipitating factors, relief by nitroglycerin, and particularly its length in terms of minutes (angina) to hours (infarction). The quality of the pain has little bearing on the specific diagnosis and may represent previous illness experience, a form of denial, or even confusion and can be more misleading than diagnostic. The following outline may be helpful.

As was mentioned previously, in a small percentage (5% to 10%) of patients, coronary artery disease may present only as upper extremity pain, especially left sided, though it may less commonly be bilateral and is rarely right sided alone.

In the patient in case 1 the pain presents as shoulder and upper arm pain after vigorous exercise on a cold and windy day. Another patient, I recall, presented at the emergency room repeatedly with intense left wrist pain, and an electrocardiogram on this third visit revealed ST-segment changes of subendocardial ischemia.

A final point: an electrocardiogram obtained during the pain may show characteristic ST- or T-wave changes that may further help in pointing toward a diagnosis of coronary artery disease. An electrocardiogram between pains that is normal and one that is normal during pain are not very helpful in ruling out the diagnosis.

The history is the key!

Pearl 1. Upper extremity pain precipitated by exertion (especially when the upper extremity is not being used and the physical examination is normal) and is relieved by rest should make one highly suspicious of coronary artery disease.

PLEURAL EFFUSION
CASE 2

A 41-year-old white married female presented in August 1983 complaining of pain in the left shoulder. A roentgenogram of the shoulder was negative, a diagnosis of tendinitis was made, and treatment began.

A month later the pain intensified, and she developed an associated pain, less severe in the left posterior thoracic area. In October 1983 she developed numbness in the left arm. In November 1983 a roentgenogram revealed pleural effusion in the area of the left lower lobe.

A pleural tap revealed an exudate and a pleural biopsy specimen revealed an adenocarcinoma with the primary undetermined. The primary was still undetermined 4 months later.

This middle-aged woman illustrates the confusion that can arise when a primary pulmonary problem presents with referred pain to the shoulder or upper extremity. The more common pulmonary causes of referred pain are an upper lobe lesion (Pancoast's syndrome) and a diaphragmatic irritation such as pneumonia, emboli, tumor, or effusion.

Apical tumors of the lung (Pancoast's tumor) may invade directly into adjacent tissue, blood vessels, and nerves (even the brachial plexes) causing pain in the shoulder and upper arm.

Lower lobe involvement, secondary to pneumonia, pulmonary emboli, or pleural effusion (multiple causes) may cause diaphragmatic irritation, stimulate the phrenic nerve, and cause the patient to present with referred pain to the shoulder and upper arm.

Recently a 65-year-old white male, visiting in our community from the Midwest, was seen in the emergency room. He was 6 weeks postoperative from an open repair of a lower extremity fracture, and he presented with severe left shoulder pain but no local physical findings. A chest film revealed a left pleural effusion, which upon examination was observed to be a bloody transudate. Subsequent studies revealed a pulmonary embolus.

There are many cases like this in which referred pain from intrathoracic structures present only as upper extremity pain and lead to diagnostic confusion.

Pearl 2. In any case where the diagnosis of shoulder or upper extremity pain is not clear cut, taking a chest film is *mandatory*.

GOUT AND MONOARTICULAR ARTHRITIS
CASE 3

A 35-year-old white male professional baseball player developed sudden acute pain and swelling in the throwing arm, especially the elbow. It was his third attack in 2 years. An astute orthopedist tapped the joint and examined it for crystals and found urate crystals. He was treated for acute gout and later given medicine to lower his uric acid level to prevent further attacks.

This case illustrates a treatable form of joint involvement. The clinical features of gout should be familiar to all of us (see the following outline). It is an illness of males (9:1) that presents with an acute onset beginning in hours or overnight. The acute episode lasts 10 to 14 days. It is not unusual to see gout first appear during the postoperative recovery phase on the surgical floors.

Gout—pertinent clinical features
1. Males (9:1)
2. Acute onset
3. Course—10 to 14 days and recurrent
4. Monoarticular
5. Joints involved—big toe, ankle, knee, elbow
6. Tap—urate crystals

The disease is characteristically an acute monoarticular arthritis that more commonly involves the joints of the lower extremity, especially the big toe, ankle, and knee, but can involve the upper extremity, especially the elbow.

The diagnosis is made specially when one demonstrates urate crystals in the synovial fluid under the polarizing light. The results of treatment with nonsteroidal anti-inflammatory agents or more traditionally with colchicine can be dramatic.

It is helpful to make another point about acute monoarticular arthritis. Several years ago, I heard a noted rheumatologist on rounds say that the most important basic fact to learn in rheumatology is this:

Pearl 3. An acute monoarticular arthritis means infection or gout.

Monoarticular arthritis
1. Infected joint
2. Gout
3. Pseudogout
4. Reactive arthritis

In this limited list the last two other diagnostic possibilities are pseudogout and occasionally reactive arthritis. Pseudogout is similar to gout but more commonly involves the knee, ankle, wrist, and elbow and may have a characteristic roentgenographic finding with calcium in the joint and yields calcium pyrophosphate crystals on examination of the synovial fluid.

One can see that a corollary to the above pearl is developing—in the presence of an acute monoarticular arthritis, a tap is indicated and a careful and thorough exam of the synovial fluid for cells, organisms, and crystals is essential for a diagnosis.

Recently I had the opportunity to see an interesting case that was so instructive to me that I would like to share the history with you now. This gentleman presented on several occasions with acute monoarticulate arthritis, but the diagnosis was not made until later in the course of the illness.

CASE 4

A 25-year-old white male who is a professional football player developed an acute diarrheal illness during summer camp. The illness presented acutely with fever, chills, myalgia, and at first nausea and vomiting, but within 24 hours he developed cramping abdominal pain and then explosive diarrheal stools, as many as 10 to 14 times a day. When he did not respond to outpatient treatment, he was hospitalized. He continued with the diarrhea for 24 hours, and the stools became bloody. Symptoms improved in 48 hours and cleared in 72 hours. *Campylobacter* was grown from the stool, and despite the fact that he was improving, he was given a course of erythromycin therapy.

One week later, he went to the dentist complaining of jaw pain. No specific diagnosis was made. Ten days later, he developed soreness and aching in the right elbow, and the trainer treated him locally for a "hyperextended" elbow. Two weeks later, three days after a football game in which he played but recalled no injury, he awoke in the morning with a swollen, tender, warm right knee. A tap of the joint was nonbloody, with a noninfectious (no organism) inflammatory exudate (150,000 WBC, monocytes predominant). Later a bone scan revealed an increased uptake in the jaw, the elbow, and the knee.

A blood test was positive for HLA-B27.

This represents a case of reactive arthritis in a person who has the HLA-B27 presenting after a *Campylobacter* gastroenteritis, despite treatment. The interpretation of his symptoms was confusing until a synovial fluid examination sent us in the proper diagnostic direction.

Pearl 4. Thorough analysis of the synovial fluid is essential in the patient with monoarticular arthritis.

POLYMYALGIA RHEUMATICA

CASE 5

A 72-year-old white male, previously in good health, suddenly awoke one morning, hardly able to move. He complained of severe stiffness about the neck, shoulders, and upper arm. He said, "I feel like I'm carrying a bag of cement on my shoulders!"

On physical examination there was tenderness about the shoulder and upper arm area, with limitation on motion because of the pain, but muscle strength was normal. There was tenderness about the course of the temporal artery. The results of the laboratory studies were normal except for a sedimentation rate of 72.

A diagnosis of polymyalgia rheumatica was made. He was given prednisone that evening. When he awoke the following morning, he had dramatically improved: "Doctor, it's a miracle; I'm cured!"

Polymyalgia rheumatica is a disease that affects the elderly, usually over 60 years of age, with a slight preponderance in woman (3:2). Involvement is common in the area of the shoulder girdle but may affect the hip girdle area as well. Although it may begin in a slow and insidious manner, in more than half the cases it is abrupt in onset.

In a significant number of cases (perhaps half) there is associated tenderness along the course of the temporal artery, and biopsy of that artery may reveal giant cell granulomas in the arterial wall. This is a patchy involvement, and numerous sections are necessary to uncover the diagnosis.

Although the disease is debilitating, the real danger is involvement of the ophthalmic artery. This may result in blindness. In one sad case in my experience this occurred in a hospitalized patient overnight while waiting for the biopsy to be done. The blindness is complete and irreversible.

Fortunately the disease is very responsive to steroids, and the response is often as dramatic as in this patient. When the temporal artery is involved, the dangers of ophthalmic artery involvement is greater, and steroid therapy is begun at high-dosage levels (60 to 80 mg of prednisone daily).

The clues that are helpful in the diagnosis is the presentation of shoulder-girdle or hip-girdle pain, or both types, in an elderly patient with a very high sedimentation rate (exceeding 100 at times!). The response to steroids is dramatic and can be helpful in the diagnosis. Steriods suppress the disease, control symptoms, and prevent the blindness of ophthalmic artery involvement.

One other important point in the management of this problem is its natural history. Polymyalgia rheumatica usually "burns out" in 2 to 5 years and rarely is there a recurrence. Steroids can be discontinued at this point.

A review of the pattern of the pain in polymyalgia rheumatica may be helpful in sorting out the diagnosis.

The onset may be abrupt (overnight) or insidious and involves the shoulder- or hip-girdle area. It is commonly symmetrical and debilitating. Common descriptive terms from patients include, "I feel like I was splitting wood all day yesterday," "someone must have mugged me," "I don't want to move because it's so painful," and "I feel glued together." The patient is often asymptomatic at rest.

In the differential diagnosis one has to consider polymyositis.

In polymyositis the age group is different, and the discomfort is far less than in polymyalgia rheumatica. In polymyositis the muscle weakness and tenderness is much greater and there is more muscle atropy. Further, in polymyositis muscle enzymes are increased, and there are often EMG and muscle biopsy changes.

HYPOTHYROIDISM
CASE 6

A 62-year-old female presents complaining of numbness and tingling of both hands and fingers of increasing severity lasting for several days. Her physical examination is unremarkable initially, but on later reexamination the subtleties of her illness become apparent.

The only laboratory finding that needs reporting is a T_4 of 1.1, normal range 5 to 13.4, though her TSH level is greatly elevated as well. She is hypothyroid.

Hypothyroid disease is an illness I'm always looking for because it is treatable. Yet paradoxically even though I'm always looking for it, I seem to fail frequently to diagnose it, at least at first presentation. Last-moment discovery often saves the day.

Hypothyroidism is a subtle illness. It is gradual and insidious in onset. It "sneaks" up on you. If you are a family member or a family physician, you can so easily miss it.

The dulling effects of the lack of hormone on the skin and the hair and even the heaviness of voice, often commented about by friends, are easily missed.

It is helpful then to know that 90% of patients with hypothyroidism have numbness and tingling of their hands or fingers, or both, when they come for diagnosis. In one third of the patients, it is the presenting complaint!

The median nerve passes through the carpal tunnel (a closed space), supplying motor and sensory fibers to the thenar eminence and four of the fingers. Symptoms suggestive of a carpal tunnel include numbness, tingling, burning, and other paraesthestic sensations of the hands, particularly occurring at night.

Tests to elicit Tinel's sign (tapping over the area of the nerve with a reflex hammer) or Phalen's sign (hyperflexing the wrist for 60 seconds) are helpful in the diagnosis. An EMG/NCV (electromyography and nerve conduction velocity) test may be diagnostic.

When a person presents with the carpal tunnel syndrome one should consider for a moment possible other causes. Beyond trauma, arthritis, and pregnancy, two medical conditions warrant consideration—one common, in my experience, and the other rare. The rarer one is amyloidosis. The common medical diagnostic consideration is hypothyroidism.

Pearl 5. In every patient presenting with the carpal tunnel syndrome consider the diagnosis of hypothyroidism. A T_4 is a good screening test.

SUMMARY

Upper extremity pain may be secondary to a wide variety of causes that can originate locally but often may be referred from adjacent structures or represent referred pain from the heart or lung or even intra-abdominal structures, particularly those that are adjacent to the diaphragm. Even general systemic disorders may present as upper extremity pain.

In the absence of a clear-cut cause for pain in the upper extremity it is prudent to perform a thorough history and physical examination. It is helpful to include in the diagnostic search a chest roentgenogram and electrocardiogram during pain and exercise. Certain blood tests should be reviewed carefully, particularly the sedimentation rate, T_4, and muscle enzymes. A diagnostic tap of an involved joint may be most revealing.

REFERENCE

1. Lowenfels, A.B.: Kehr's sign— a neglected aid in rupture of the spleen, N. Engl. J. Med. **274**(18):1019-1049, 1966.

SUGGESTED READINGS

Blacklow, R.S., editor: MacBryde's signs and symptoms, ed. 6, Philadelphia, 1983, J.B. Lippincott Co.
Hamilton, C.R., Jr., Shelly, W.M., and Tumulty, P.A.: Giant cell arteritis, including temporal arteritis and polymyalgia rheumatica, Medicine **50**:1, 1971.
Williams, R.H.: Textbook of endocrinology, ed. 6, Philadelphia, 1981, W.B. Saunders Co.

4. Biomechanical precursors to upper extremity trauma

Jack L. Groppel

Biomechanics is defined as the study of the structure and function of biological systems by means of the methods of mechanics.[2] Within the field of biomechanics, one can study three areas involved in sport: (1) technique, (2) physical stress from performance, and (3) equipment design. Characteristically, biomechanics has been concerned with the study of the internal and external forces that cause motion. However, it also deals with the forces that can cause injury, either acute or chronic. With regard to technique, efficiency of movement can be defined as the attainment of an optimal outcome in sport using few moving parts in an economical fashion. Through the utilization of sport biomechanics, it is anticipated that the most efficient forms of motion can be achieved if one always bears in mind that the athlete wishes to be as effective as possible. In dealing with an athlete with regard to efficiency and effectiveness of motion, the sport scientist can reach a desired trade-off between optimal technique and the prevention of injury.

Most human action can be simply explained using Newton's three basic laws of motion. Newton's first law, or the law of inertia, is defined as follows: a body will stay at rest or in motion until acted upon by an outside force. For example, the rebounder in basketball who obtains possession of the ball and turns quickly to throw an outlet pass to a fast-breaking guard develops a great deal of angular velocity at his or her shoulder. One potential trauma is that as the player begins to release the ball, an opposing team member grabs the ball suddenly stopping the forward motion of the hand and the angular motion of the shoulder. The result of this action is a potential anterior humeral dislocation. The upper arm wanted to keep rotating in its angular fashion, but the motion was altered by an outside force.

Newton's second law is defined as follows: force equals mass times acceleration. Since mass is always held constant during any performance, this implies that force is directly proportional to acceleration. Therefore the more force you apply during a performance, the more acceleration you will create. However, many sport practitioners do not realize that this acts as a two-way street; that is, the more the athlete accelerates, the more the force must be accommodated by the bones, joints, and

26

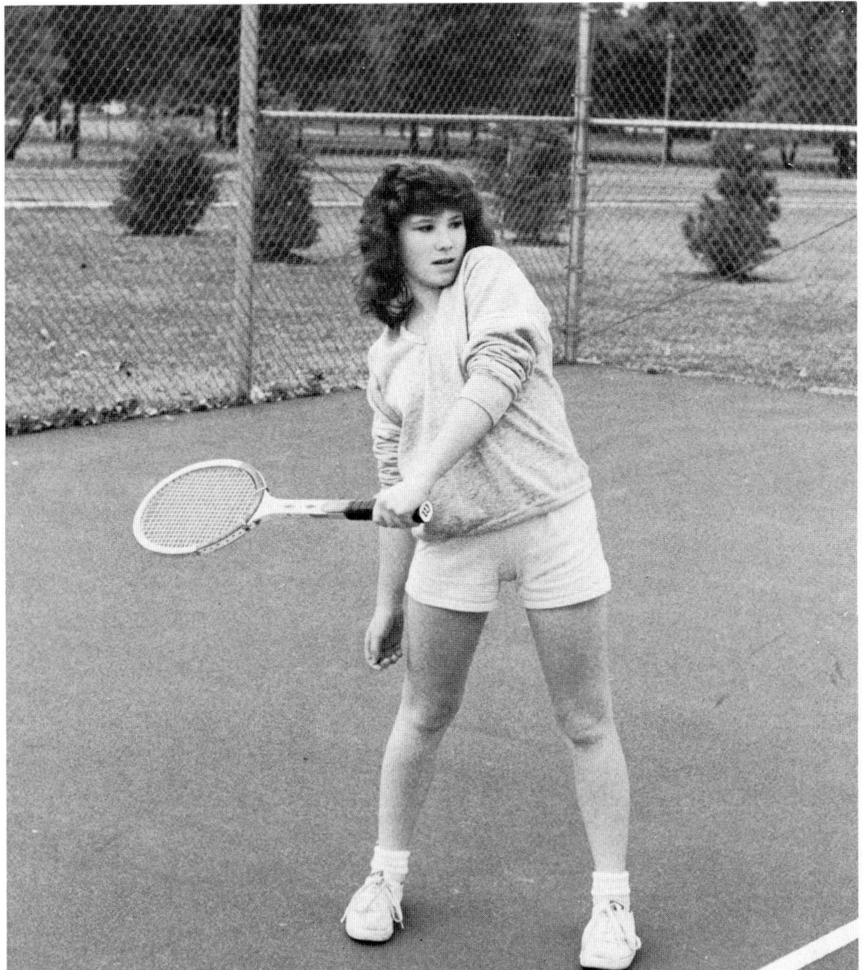

Fig. 4-1. Notice how this person has difficulty in swinging the implement.

supporting connective tissue and musculature. This merely emphasizes the need for improved warm-up and conditioning techniques for the athlete.

Newton's third law is the law of action and reaction. It states that for every action there is an equal and opposite reaction. Good examples of the effects of Newton's third law in the human body can be detailed through various impact forces. For example, did you realize that when a golf club hits a golf ball both deform? Everyone knows that the club hits the ball with a certain force, but they usually do not realize that the ball hits the club with the same force and that force is transmitted through the shaft of the club into the hand and upper extremity. In tennis impact, we very seldom realize that the tennis ball, if hit with a high velocity, almost flattens out like a pancake on the racket face.[1] But we all think of hitting the ball, not of the ball returning an equal and opposite force to the racket. During and after impact the strings deform, the racket head deforms, and then the racket shaft deforms. All this is transmitted into the hand. Therefore, as a tennis player accelerates maximally to hit an overhead smash, the faster the racket is swung, the harder the ball will be hit. However, most players don't realize that the harder the ball is hit the greater the force loads that are transmitted through the racket into the hand, wrist, forearm, and elbow. Following Newton's third law, it states that although the racket imparts a great amount of force to the ball the ball imparts an equal and opposite force to the racket. Similar examples can be derived through the various sport activities that deal with any type of impact.

Most impact forces encountered by the upper extremity are magnified by the use of sport implements. One physical principle that dictates how these sport implements can be manipulated by the human body is the moment of inertia. The moment of inertia of an object is defined as its mass times its radius squared ($I = m \times r^2$). Often a player using a sport implement such as a baseball bat or a tennis racket selects one that is either too massive for him or her or one that is too long. Fig. 4-1 depicts a player's actions when trying to swing a tennis racket that is simply too massive for her physique. Since the moment of inertia is verbally defined as a body's resistance to rotation, the more massive or lengthy an implement is, the more difficult it is to swing or rotate it into position for impact. For example, any time a baseball player has two strikes, the coach always advises the athlete to choke up on the bat. Obviously the rationale behind this is that the bat will be easier to swing, since the functional radius of the bat is lessened by choking up.

The moment of inertia of a sport implement can readily dictate any trauma that might occur to an athlete using a certain implement. Usually an athlete will not change implements to make the moment of inertia smaller to perform with more ease but will accommodate the use of an implement that is already owned. This merely enhances the potential for upper extremity trauma when one tries to swing or rotate a cumbersome implement at a high velocity and then accommodate the forces of impact.

Another mechanical concept that plays an important role in determining how injury might occur to an athlete's upper extremity would be torque. Torque is a rotational force that is determined when one multiplies the moment of inertia of a system times its angular acceleration. For example, the pitcher in baseball generates a high amount of torque at the shoulder to externally and internally rotate for a high pitching velocity. The tennis player will utilize a great deal of hip and trunk acceleration and transfer that torque to the upper limb. Since the human body is basically a third-class lever design, the amount of torque created to rotate a body segment is extremely high, especially when one considers the high velocities attained in some sporting activities. We might backtrack to Newton's third law and realize that for every torque created, an equal and opposite torque occurs.

The generation of high amounts of force in athletic endeavors is severe. This seems to further indicate the extreme need for warm-up and conditioning techniques. The biomechanics of a sport and how it relates to injury can help us understand prevention of injury. Educating the athletes on not only how to produce force but also how to accommodate force through warm-ups and conditioning is essential to their performance. In addition, once an injury occurs and a physician treats the problem, the biomechanics of rehabilitation can be utilized to enable the athlete to resume competition as quickly as possible. Obviously a conditioning program can make muscles stronger, but a certain amount of rehabilitation should be dedicated to the improvement of technique efficiency.

REFERENCES

1. Groppel, J.L.: Tennis for advanced players: and those who would like to be, Champaign, Ill., 1984, Human Kinetics Publishers.
2. Hay, J.G.: Biomechanics of sports techniques, Englewood Cliffs, N.J., 1982, Prentice-Hall.

5. The utilization of proper racket sport mechanics to avoid upper extremity injury

Jack L. Groppel

Because of the size of various sport implements, proper mechanics are essential to the athlete's longevity in his or her respective sport. The force loads and excessive torques created from improper movement mechanics are often severe and can cause an injury. The goal of any racket sport athlete is to be as efficient and effective as possible yet always minimize the potential for injury.[1] Efficiency of movement can be defined as the attempt at reaching an optimal outcome by use of a few moving parts in an economical fashion. This implies that the motion involved in performance should be efficient from two standpoints: (1) avoidance of excessive muscular stress and joint duress and (2) avoidance of excessive movements, which tend to drain one's energy level. Effectiveness of movement in racket sports implies that the athlete attempts to be as deliberate as possible in winning a point at hand, either by hitting with a greater velocity or with greater control to impede the opponent's performance.

The goal of sports biomechanics is to examine the technique of an athletic activity and assess the technique involved. This analysis must include the skilled, able-bodied athlete; the unskilled, able-bodied performer; the skilled, disabled athlete; and the unskilled, disabled competitor. Each of the aforementioned persons have, within their limitations, specific requirements unique to performance in any racket sport they might undertake. However, it is essential that the sport scientist realize that the same principles of human motion apply regardless of how those forces might be transferred through the body.

Most forces in racket sport movements are initiated from the ground in the form of a ground reaction force. In Fig. 5-1, one can see how this force is created by a push-off against the ground. Newton's third law states that for every action there is an equal and opposite reaction. Therefore, as the athlete pushes against the ground, the ground pushes back with an equal and opposite force. This force is then transferred through the body's linked system. Each body part then acts as a link in a series of chain links that transfers force from one segment to another. For example, in a tennis stroke the force begins with a ground reaction force. Once the ground reaction force is created, that force is transferred through the legs to the hips and then to the trunk on

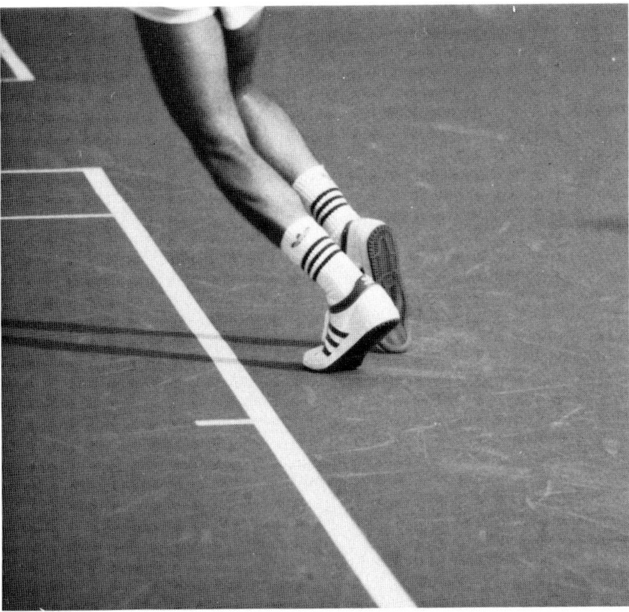

Fig. 5-1. During the serve in tennis, there is flexion of the knees followed by a forceful extension of the ground reaction force necessary for an effective serve.

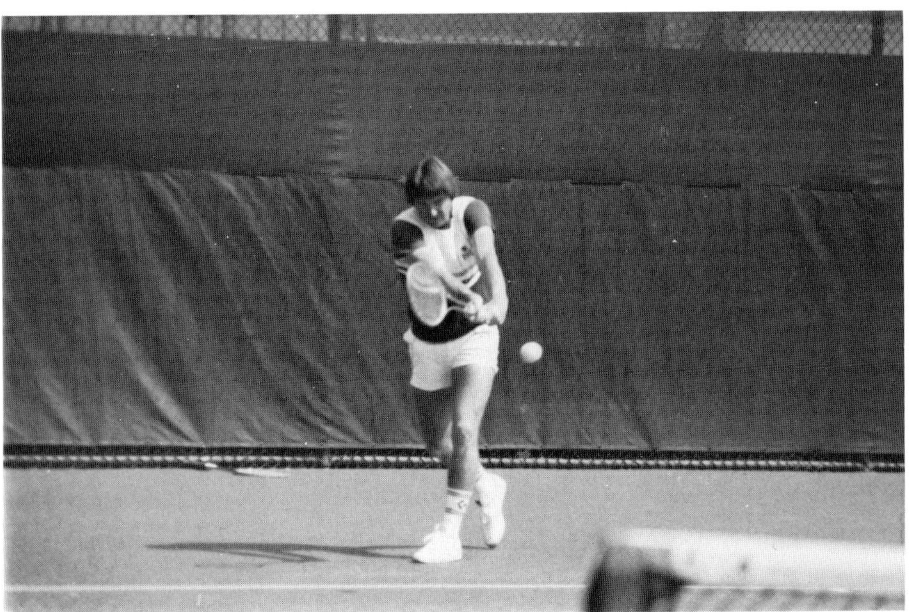

Fig. 5-2. This is an efficient stroking action that utilizes the ground reaction force and body momentum well.

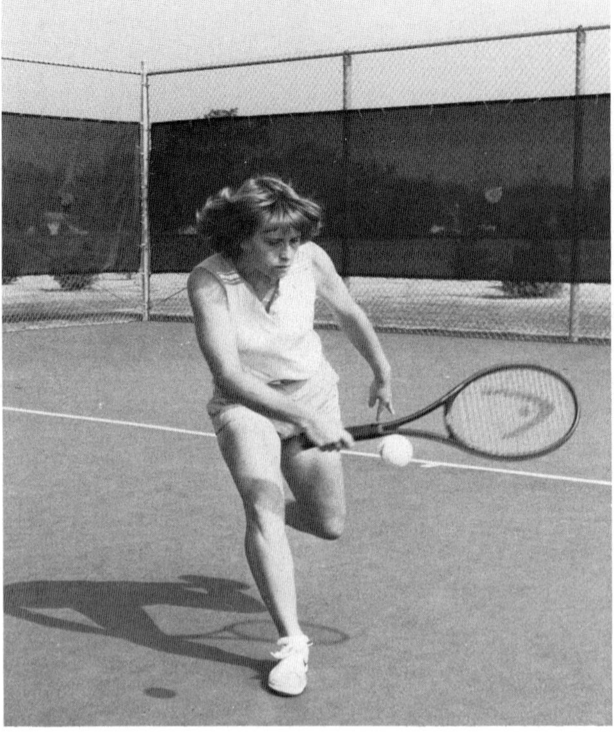

Fig. 5-3. Notice the difficulty this athlete has in manipulating the racket efficiently.

to the upper limb and racket. The point to bear in mind is that each segment not only transfers force from the previous segment to the next but also contributes to the force obtained from the previous body parts; that is, there is a summation of joint forces that occurs and not simply a transfer of force. It is the summation of joint forces that dictates the efficiency and effectiveness of performance.

Problems that occur in a stroke sequence may involve the summation of forces, the continuity of joint forces, and the timing of these forces. Problems in the summation of force occur when a body part does not contribute an adequate amount to the transmission of force out to the racket or when a body part is omitted from a movement. For example, in Fig. 5-2, you can see how this athlete properly utilizes all the body parts creating a ground reaction force and transferring that force efficiently to the racket. In Fig. 5-3 you can see how some difficulties may exist when an athlete does not perform in an efficient manner.

The continuity of joint forces is also extremely important in the final outcome of a movement. That is, forces may be created at a certain body part but not transmitted effectively. Without this continuity of forces there can be no total summation of the actions of the body parts.

The timing of the joint forces is also necessary for optimal performance. Each body

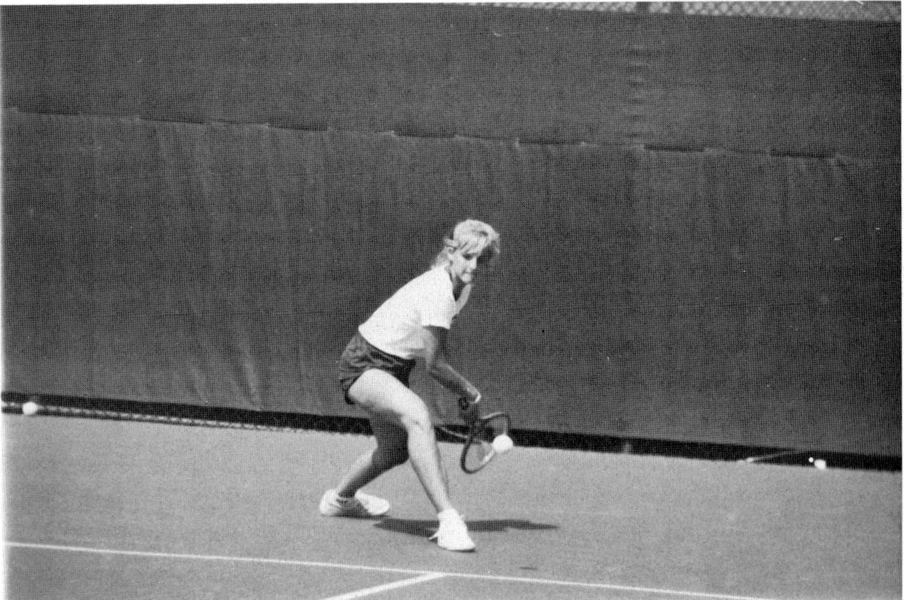

Fig. 5-4. The step toward the ball initiates the transfer of linear momentum.

part could create its optimal force production but if the transmission of force from one body part to another does not occur at the correct time, the summation of force will be poor. Each body part must accelerate within its limitations, and, once an optimal velocity is reached, that force must be transferred on to the next body part. It is this poorly timed transfer that can create problems in the summation of joint forces.

Two other concepts of mechanics come into play during a performance: linear momentum and angular momentum. These entities are essential to the optimal outcome of a racket sport stroke. For example, as the person in Fig. 5-4 transfers her body momentum forward (notice how she steps toward the direction of the shot), a certain amount of momentum is created in that direction. This linear momentum is equal to mass times velocity. As she steps toward the shot, transferring her body weight in that direction, her momentum is moving in a straight line. Once this is done effectively, angular momentum comes into play. Angular momentum is equal to a body's moment of inertia multiplied by its angular velocity. Although the moment of inertia will change very little during a stroke, the angular velocity plays a large role in how the racket will be brought into the proper impact zone (where the ball will be contacted). Notice in Fig. 5-5, *A*, how this athlete has transferred her body weight toward the shot and how the hips are rotated to the side. In Fig. 5-5, *B*, notice how there is no difference in the positioning of the legs, but observe how the hips and trunk have rotated vigorously to bring the racket into the proper hitting position. Problems in performance can occur when linear momentum and angular momentum are not combined properly. In fact, it has been said that if the lower body and the

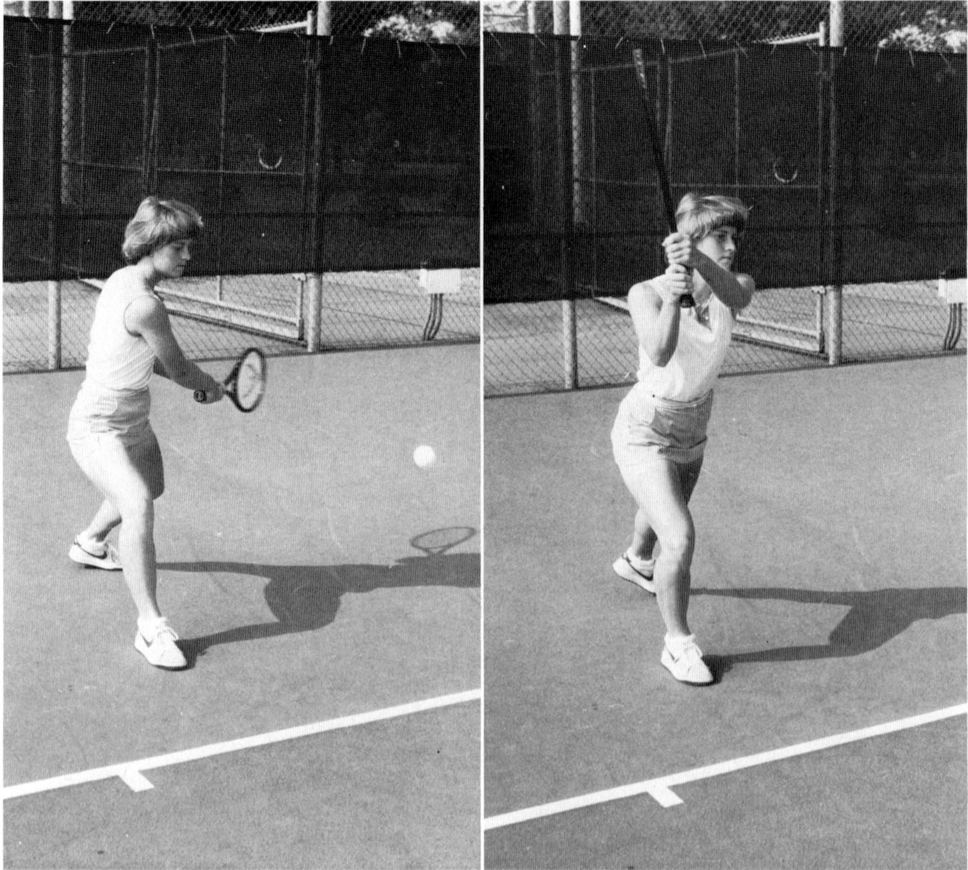

Fig. 5-5. Observe how the hips and trunk become involved following the step forward.

upper body are used properly in a racket sports stroke, the upper limb will not have to work as hard to produce force.

Examples of improper mechanics that may lead to upper extremity injuries include (1) timing the body to the ball instead of the stroke,[1] (2) exhibiting a "tray effect" when one is serving a ball,[2] (3) hitting off the back foot and so disallowing any use of linear momentum,[1] (4) hitting with a one-handed backhand stroke while leading with the elbow,[1] (5) deviating the wrist at the last second to supplement the racket velocity generated during a poor stroke,[1] and (6) attempting to do too much, too soon, too fast. This merely emphasizes the need for warm-up and conditioning when one is competing in the racket sports.[2]

The goal of any racket sport athlete is to hit with a sufficient amount of force and control to keep the opponent on the defensive. By performing each stroke in an efficient and effective manner, the athlete will hopefully be able to minimize the potential for upper extremity injury. Through an understanding of the body's linked system and how forces are transmitted from one body part to another, the sport scientist can be made aware of how problems in stroke production generating in legs, hips, or trunk can actually create physical trauma to the upper limb. Therefore it is essential that when prescribing a new technique within an activity the prescriber must be aware of how essential the lower body, hips, and trunk are to performance in the racket sports.

REFERENCES

1. Groppel, J.L.: Tennis for advance players: and those who would like to be, Champaign, Ill., 1984, Human Kinetics Publishers.
2. Nirschl, R.P.: Arm care, Arlington, Va., 1982, Medical Sports, Inc.,

6. The upper extremity in swimming

David C. Johnson

Swimming is the most popular participant sport in the United States. Last year over 200,000 swimmers under 25 years of age trained year around for serious competition. This included an estimated 15,000 20 years of age to well over 80 years who competed under the auspices of the master's swimming program. Add to this another 500,000 who swim only part of the year (high school or country club leagues and so on), and the number of competitors exceeds 700,000. How many swimmers who don't train for competition but who do swim as a form of exercise is not known, but a recent Neilson poll indicated that over 105 million Americans swim recreationally. This represents almost half of the United States population.

It is therefore appropriate that health care professionals interested in recognizing and treating the musculoskeletal problems of the active population be conversant with the mechanics and training methods of swimming because the training techniques employed and the motions required to swim various strokes have a direct relationship on the production of musculoskeletal problems in swimmers.

TRAINING CONSIDERATIONS

Johnny Weissmuller, perhaps the most celebrated swimmer of the past 5 decades, set records lasting 24 years with a training regimen consisting in swimming an easy 400 yards four times a week.[14]

Competitive swimming today would be unrecognizable in Weissmuller's era. Today serious competitive swimmers train between 14,000 and 24,000 meters a day (between 8 and 14 miles per day) 6 days a week. In addition, most competitive swimmers train with weights or weight machines. The equipment and accoutrements of swimming also have changed (Fig. 6-1). Now there are goggles, pull buoys, drag suits, hand paddles, and kickboards, all designed either to add resistance in the water or increase the work required to overcome the already long distances of a workout.

Because swimmers propel themselves primarily with their upper extremities, it is no wonder that shoulder problems predominate. It has been estimated that an average competitive swimmer subjects each of his or her shoulders to up to 16,000 revolutions per week or up to 660,000 strokes per season.[12] This competitive stress far

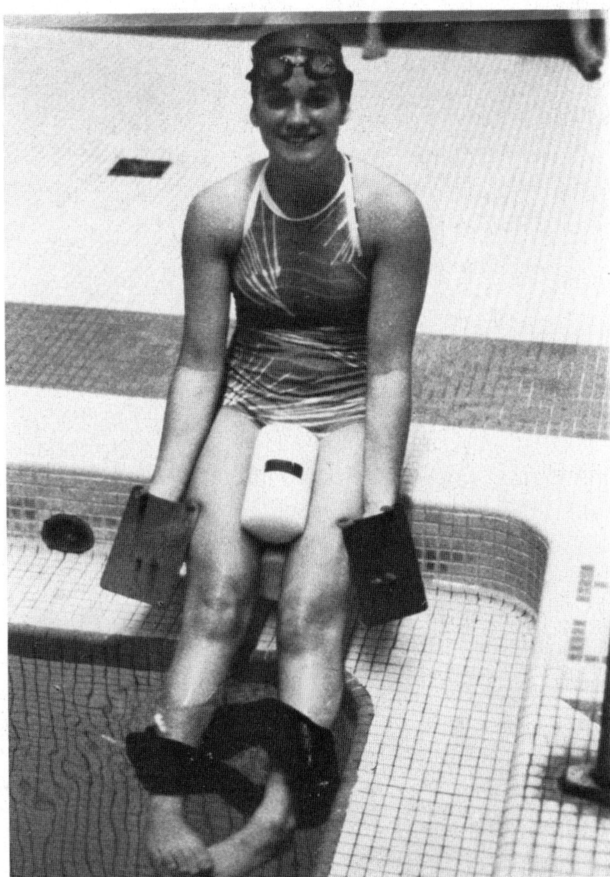

Fig. 6-1. Accoutrements of the modern swimmer include pull buoys, hand paddles, goggles, and kickboards (not shown). The pull buoys and hand paddles are designed to add resistance in the water or increase the work required to negotiate the already long distances of a practice session.

exceeds that encountered in any other sport (Table 6-1). Because of the distances swum and the training techniques employed, it is no wonder therefore that overuse syndromes develop.

CLINICAL CONSIDERATIONS

It is now recognized that the most common overuse syndrome in a competitive swimmer is that of impingement of the rotator cuff and biceps tendons beneath the coracoacromial arch.[2-5,9,11,12] Neer has described the stages of progression of the impingement syndrome, identifying edema and hemorrhage in stage 1, fibrosis and tendinitis in stage 2, and tendon degeneration, bony changes, and tendon ruptures in stage 3.[10]

It has been estimated that approximately a half to two thirds of élite swimmers of

Table 6-1. Shoulder stress (revolutions/week) in sports

golf	150
javelin	200
baseball	600
tennis	1,000
swimming	16,000

national or world-class calibre have or have had significant complaints referable to the shoulder.[12] It seems to be age related; those who have been swimming the longest seem to have the highest incidence. There does not appear to be any sexual predominance though some studies have shown girls to be more frequently affected than boys.[12] An impingement syndrome of the shoulder predominates in those swimmers who swim freestyle, butterfly, and backstroke, with breaststrokers (unless they train in freestyle) being relatively immune. Sprinters and middle-distance freestylers are the most commonly afflicted; distance swimmers surprisingly have a lower incidence.

Shoulder problems are correlated with the use of hand paddles,[12] probably because the pull phase of swimming is slowed and rotation of the body is prevented (thus producing more of an impingement at the shoulder during the recovery phase).

Symptoms usually present in the early and midportions of the competitive season. Initially the swimmer will have a dull ache after but not during the workout. It usually is of short duration and is completely reversible with rest. However, these symptoms can become progressively more severe after each workout until pain occurs during and after workout. Discomfort has been described as occurring in the recovery and early pull phases and at first may be more annoying than disabling. Finally, a full impingement syndrome becomes established, and the swimmer is unable to continue swimming. Clinically the pain may be very ill defined, but on examination there may be point tenderness anterolaterally over the rotator cuff and over the biceps tendon anteriorly just below the coracoacromial ligament. This tenderness does not seem to shift with rotation of the shoulder.

Full forward flexion of the shoulders (bringing the rotator cuff and biceps tendon against the sharp leading edge of the coracoacromial ligament) if painful constitutes what Neer has described as an "impingement sign."[10] This position is duplicated at the start of every stroke in butterfly, backstroke, breaststroke, and freestyle (Figs. 6-3, *a*, 6-4, *a*, and 6-5, *a*).

Another impingement sign, described by Hawkins and Kennedy,[5] is internal rotation of the forward flexed shoulder, again with the rotator cuff and biceps groove area being brought beneath the coracoacromial ligament. This "impingement sign" is also reproduced in the "catch position" of the beginning of the pull-through in freestyle, butterfly, and breaststroke (Fig. 6-2).

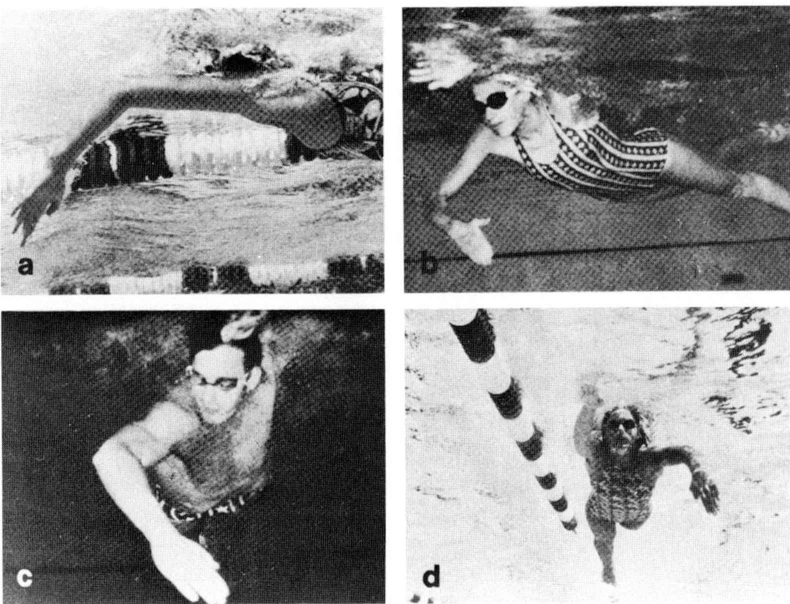

Fig. 6-2. The high elbow position of the "catch" phase of the beginning of the freestyle pull involves abduction and internal rotation of the shoulder. This position can bring the rotator cuff and biceps tendon against the sharp leading edge of the coracoacromial ligament and anterior acromion if the shoulder is in too much flexion. (From Counsilman, J.: Complete book of swimming, New York, 1977, Atheneum Publishers.)

STROKE MECHANICS

In studying the mechanics of the shoulder in swimming, Richardson observed remarkable similarities of shoulder motion in freestyle, butterfly, and backstroke.[12] All three involve internal rotation and adduction during the pull-through and external rotation and abduction during recovery. In freestyle, the beginning of the pull-through involves adduction and internal rotation as is illustrated in Fig. 6-3, *a* to *c*. This motion, as mentioned previously, brings the rotator cuff and biceps tendon against the sharp leading edge of the coracoacromial ligament. At the midpoint of the pull (Fig. 6-3, *d* to *e*) the elbow is flexed to 90 degrees, and the humerus begins its adduction against the chest. Although Schleihauf[13] computed a theoretical hand propulsive force of 4 kg at this phase of the stroke, Counsilman[1] measured the actual amount of thrust generated with each arm to be between 25 and 30 pounds. If the fingertips cross the midline in the midportion of the stroke, impingement beneath the coracoacromial arch is maximized. The body roll throughout the pull is important in decompressing the coracoacromial arch and in maximizing the efficiency of the pull as well. In the butterfly (Fig. 6-4) no such body roll exists, and the addition of the dolphin kick places a hyperflexion force on the shoulders as well (Fig. 6-4, *b* and *c*).

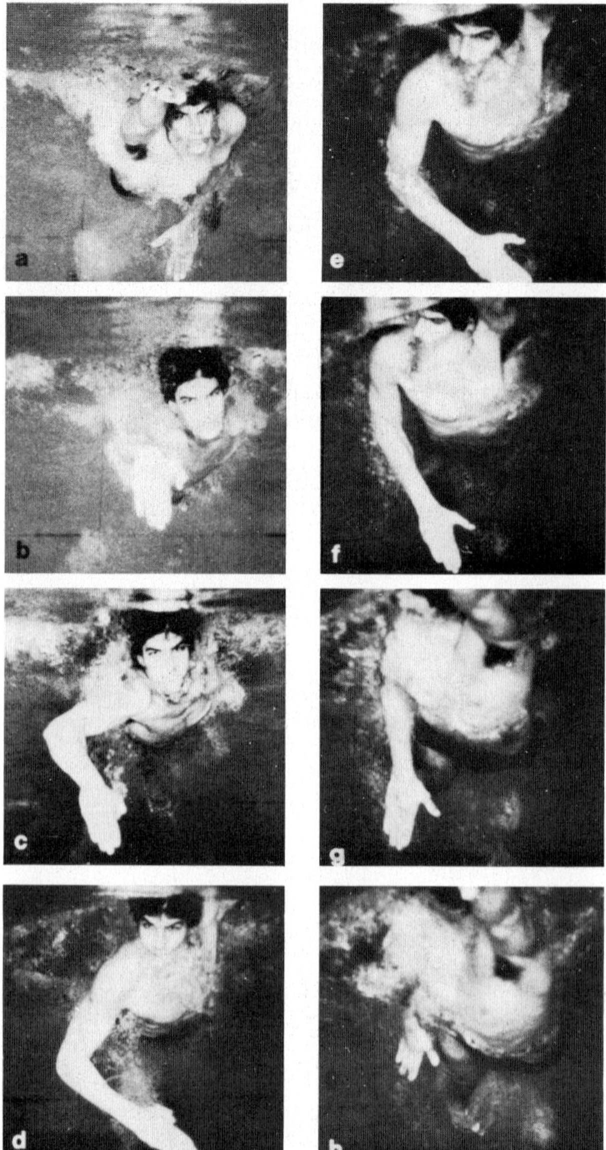

Fig.6-3. A head-on underwater view of the freestyle stroke. **a,** The right shoulder is in full flexion and does not cross in front of the face. **b,** The wrist is cocked forward to begin the catch phase of the start of the pull. **c,** The hand is anchored in the water, and the body is pulled over the hand by flexing of the elbow to 90 degrees and initiation of adduction of the humerus against the side of the body. **d** and **e,** The midportion of the pull is the most powerful part of the stroke, and the forces on the palm are maximized in this position. If the fingertips cross the midline of the body too far, coracoacromial arch impingement may be increased. The speed of pull-through in the water accelerates during this phase. **f** to **h,** Adduction of the humerus against the side of the body is completed, and the triceps muscle continues to provide forward propulsion. Body roll lengthens the effective stroke and readies the shoulder for the over-the-water recovery to initiate the next pull. (From Counsilman, J.: Complete book of swimming, New York, 1977, Atheneum Publishers.)

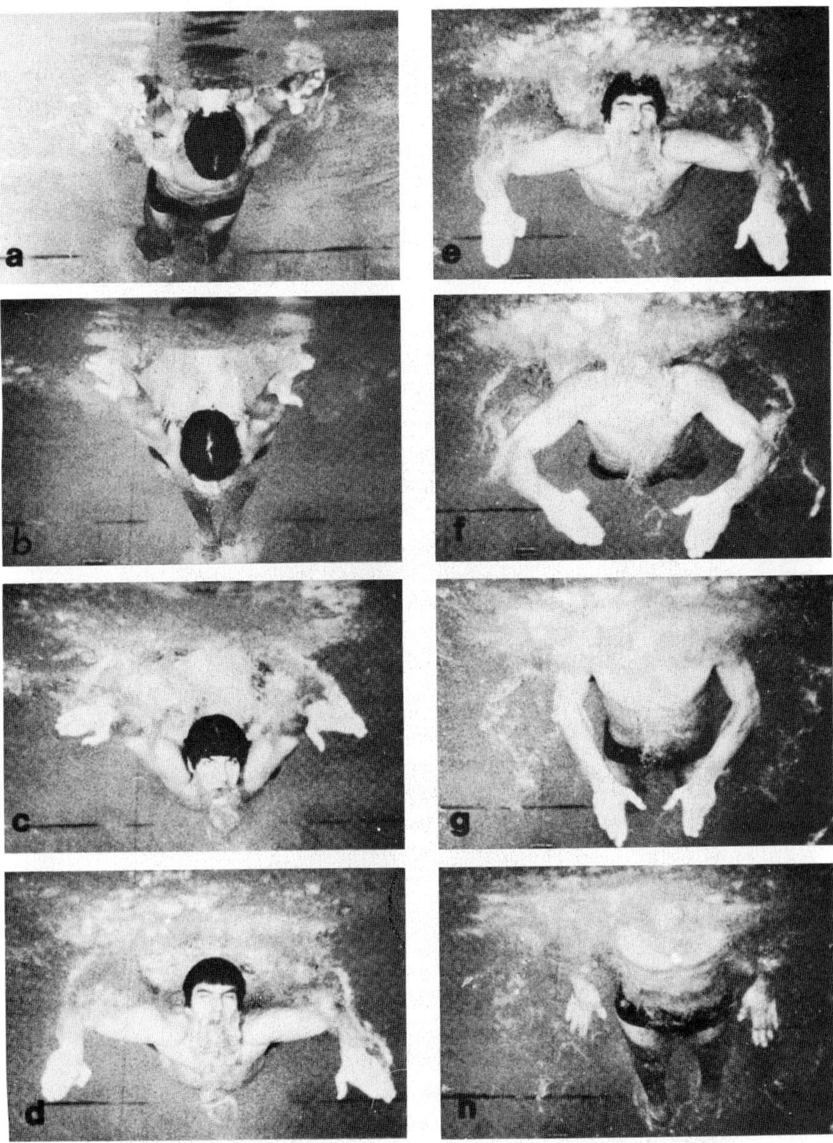

Fig. 6-4. Head-on underwater view of the butterfly stroke. Many of the same components in freestyle are identified here though both arms are working in tandum. **a** and **b,** Entry into the water in the "thumbs-down position." **c,** The catch phase is initiated with the elbows higher than the shoulders. **d,** The elbows remain in a high position as the elbows begin to flex at the start of the power portion of the stroke. **e** and **f,** The humeri are adducted toward the sides as the fingertips approach midline position and accelerate the body forward. **g** and **h,** The conclusion of the stroke involves extension of the elbows and adduction of the humerus. This provides clearance of the upper extremities from the water to allow for stroke recovery before the beginning of the next underwater pull. (From Counsilman, J.: Complete book of swimming, New York, 1977, Atheneum Publishers.)

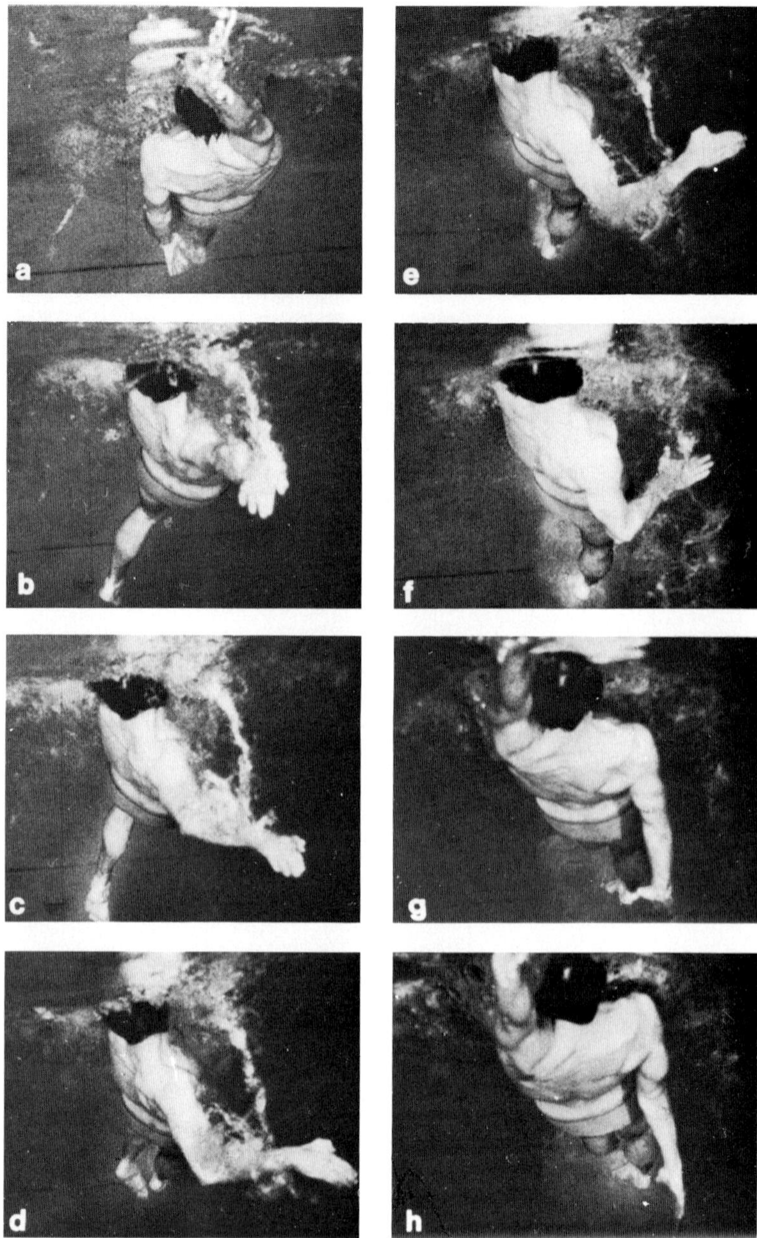

Fig. 6-5. Head-on underwater view of backstroke. **a,** Full abduction of the shoulder at the start of the stroke. **b,** Body roll aids in the initiation of the catch phase. **c,** The humerus begins adduction against the body when the elbow begins its flexion. **d** and **e,** At the midportion of the backstroke pull, the elbow approaches 90 degrees and the shoulder internally rotates. **f** to **h,** The completion of the stroke, in combination with the body roll, produces more of an internal rotation of the shoulder than in any other stroke. The elbow is fully extended at the completion of the stroke because of the strong action of the triceps and the hand finishes well below the buttocks with the shoulder in extension. (From Counsilman, J.: Complete book of swimming, New York, 1977, Atheneum Publishers.)

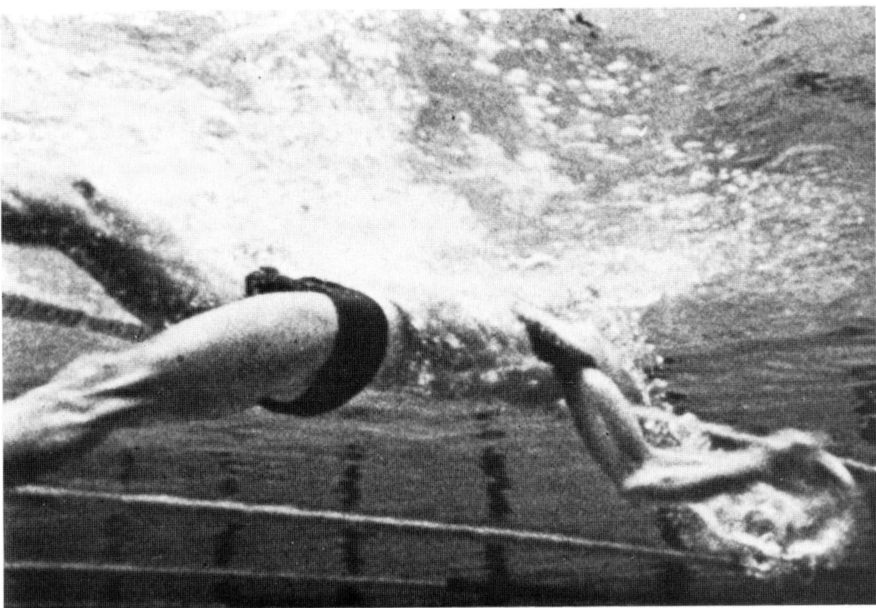

Fig. 6-6. Underwater view of the midportion of the backstroke pull as the elbow is flexing and the humerus is beginning its internal rotation. The brachioradialis, biceps, brachii, and forearm flexors are maximally active during this part of the stroke. Patients prone to posterior subluxation of the shoulder have symptoms at this portion of the stroke.

Again, the beginning of the pull is internal rotation and adduction done in tandem. At the terminal phase (Fig. 6-4, *g* to *h*) the pull must also provide body lift; poor timing here may strain the abductors of the shoulder.

In back stroke, the start of the pull is at maximum flexion and abduction of the shoulders, again duplicating the position of Neer's "impingement sign" maneuver (Fig. 6-5, *a*). The remainder of the pull involves adduction of the humerus and internal rotation. At the terminal phases of the pull, the internal rotation of the shoulders exceeds that of freestyle and butterfly (Fig. 6-5, *g*).

In discussing backstroke, it is of interest to note that many backstrokers complain of a dull ache in the anteromedial portion of the elbow, especially after sprinting. Fig. 6-6 illustrates that at the midportion of the backstroke pull-through the forces are maximized at the brachioradialis and biceps as well as at the medial ligaments of the elbow, leading to strain involving these structures. Many backstrokers also complain of pain in the posterior aspects of the elbow at the tip of the olecranon at the conclusion of their pull (Fig. 6-5, *g*) when the elbow is fully extended. This may represent strain of the triceps tendon as it attaches to the olecranon, or possibly pinching of the synovium in the olecranon fossa.

Not all shoulder pain in swimmers is secondary to impingement. Muscle strains can also be a cause of shoulder pain, especially in the young swimmer who injures himself in the exuberant (and frequently unsupervised) use of free weights and weight machines during training. Marathon swimmers are also at risk of abductor or external

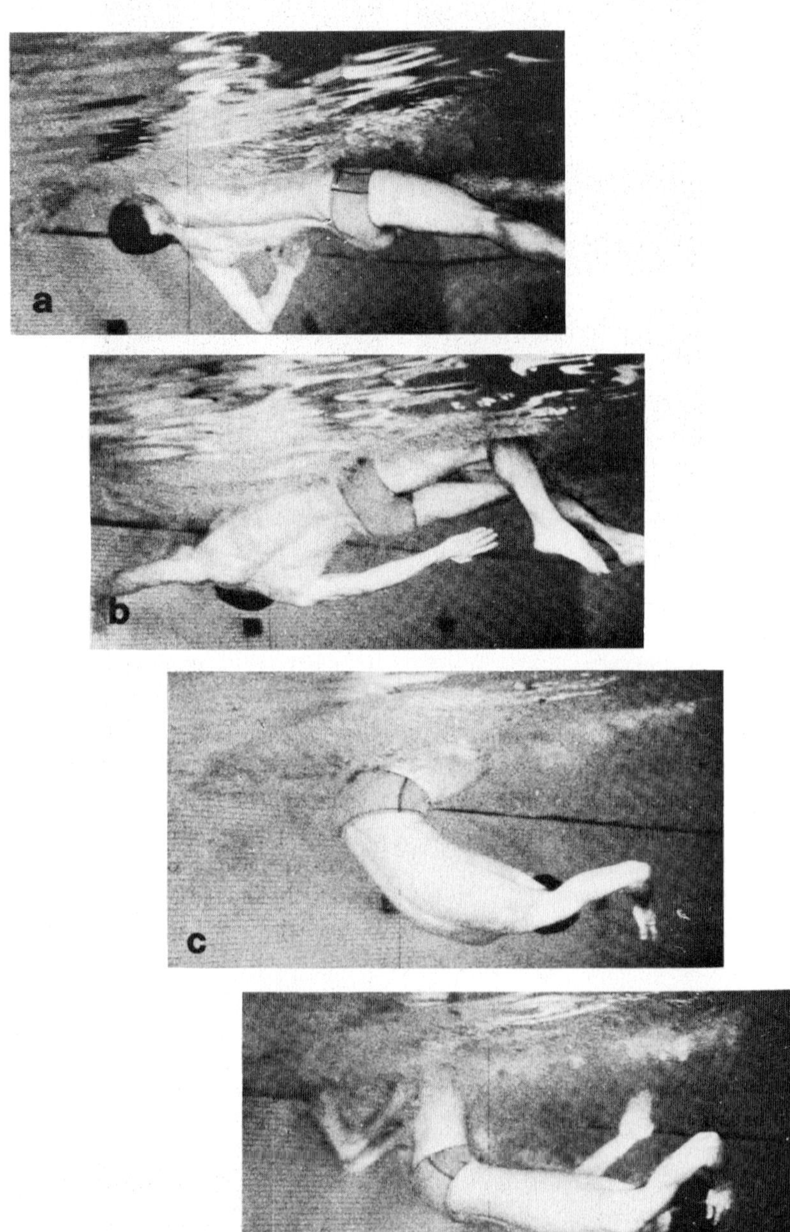

Fig. 6-7. Underwater view of backstroke flip turn. (From Counsilman, J.: Complete book of swimming, New York, 1977, Atheneum Publishers.)

rotator muscle pulls of the shoulder when their stroke recovery is abruptly halted by rough or choppy water.

Shoulder instability, with or without accompanying impingement tendinitis, can be a source of pain as well. In anterior instability of the shoulder, symptoms are brought on especially during the backstroke flip turn when, at wall strike, the body is levered about the shoulder (Fig. 6-7, *a* to *c*). In susceptible shoulders, this maneuver can lever the humeral head anteroinferiorly out of the glenoid. Posterior subluxation of the shoulder can be a source of pain and weakness at the midportion of the backstroke pull when the forces on internal rotation of the shoulder are maximized (Figs. 6-5, *e*, and 6-6).

TREATMENT

Treatment of overuse syndromes of the upper extremities in swimmers involves ice applications after training sessions followed by a 10- to 14-day course of anti-inflammatory medication. During this time it may be wise to diminish the distance swum and to avoid those strokes that are the most painful. Proper coaching is very important because even minor changes in technique may exert a profound difference in stress at the shoulder or elbow. Strengthening exercises with the use of rubber tubing is a safer alternative to free weights, but all weight training should probably be suspended during symptomatic periods. Richardson[12] and Hawkins,[5] however, have noted improvement in symptoms with strengthening and stretching exercises. In severe or recalcitrant cases of impingement tendinitis, ultrasound treatments have been useful. Local injections of steroid and Xylocaine (lidocaine) are rarely indicated and then only in a skeletally mature swimmer who also will take the time to rest the shoulder. Surgery, very helpful in impingement syndromes in throwing sports,[7] is generally disappointing in swimmers.[8] The operation usually consists in resection of the coracoacromial ligament with or without an anterior acromioplasty. Although there are reports of good results in the literature,[3] Kennedy recorded 16 operations involving the transsection of the coracoacromial ligament resulting in a return to the previous level of competition in only 50% of the swimmers so treated. Even so, all symptoms returned within 2 years in that series.[8]

Shoulder instability can be successfully treated with appropriate exercises. In anterior subluxation of the shoulder, internal rotation and strengthening exercises may be of significant help in relieving symptoms. In persistent cases, surgical stabilization of the anteriorly unstable shoulder can return the swimmer to a full competitive level. In posterior subluxation of the shoulder, external rotation strengthening exercises are very helpful, but surgery here may be less useful.[6]

A relatively uncommon affliction is thoracic outlet syndrome. It usually is precipitated by hypertrophy of the pectoralis minor muscle, though occasionally anterior scalene hypertrophy is implicated. It is generally symptomatic while one holds a kickboard with the shoulders fully forward flexed (particularly after a heavy period of sprinting), or during the early phases of butterfly pull when the shoulders are hyperflexed. Most of these symptoms abate as the season progresses, but in persistent cases resection of the first rib is generally curative.

SUMMARY

In summary, swimming has come a long way since the days of Johnny Weissmuller, not only in stroke mechanics and training techniques but also in popularity as a participant sport. Because of the long distances surmounted in training and the motions of the upper extremities required to execute the various strokes, the upper extremities in swimmers are exposed to more stress than that in any other sport. Good coaching is vital in preventing these overuse syndromes, but the expertise of the family physician, orthopedist, or pediatrician in diagnosing and treating these overuse syndromes will be critical in returning the injured swimmer to his or her chosen sport.

REFERENCES

1. Counsilman, J.E.: Personal communication, 1982, Indianapolis, Indiana.
2. Dominguez, R.H.: Shoulder pain in age group swimmers. In Eriksson, B., and Furberg, B., editors: Swimming medicine IV, Baltimore, 1978, University Park Press, vol. 6, p. 105.
3. Dominguez, R.H.: Coracoacromial ligament resection for severe swimmers' shoulder. In Eriksson, B., and Furberg, B., editors: Swimming medicine IV, Baltimore, 1978, University Park Press, vol. 6, p. 110.
4. Dominguez, R.H.: Shoulder pain in swimmers, Physician Sports Med. 8:37, 1980.
5. Hawkins, R.J., and Kennedy, J.C.: Impingement syndromes in athletes, Am. J. Sports Med. 8:151, 1980.
6. Hawkins, R.J., Koppert, G., and Johnston, G.: Recurrent posterior instability (subluxation) of the shoulder, J. Bone Joint Surg. 66A:169, 1984.
7. Jackson, D.W.: Chronic rotator cuff impingement in the throwing athlete, Orthop. Trans. 1:24, 1977.
8. Kennedy, J.C.: Personal communication, 1983.
9. Kennedy, J.C., Hawkins, R.J., and Krissoff, W.B.: Orthopedic manifestations of swimming, Am. J. Sports Med. 6:309, 1978.
10. Neer, C.S., and Welsh, R.P.: The shoulder in sports, Orthop. Clin. North Am. 8:583, 1977.
11. Penny, N.J., and Welsh, R.P.: Shoulder impingement syndromes in athletes and their surgical management, Am. J. Sports Med. 9:11, 1981.
12. Richardson, A.B., Jobe, F.W., and Collins, H.R.: The shoulder in competitive swimming, Am. J. Sports Med. 8:159, 1980.
13. Schleihauf, R.E.: A hydrodynamic analysis of swimming propulsion. In Terauds, J., and Bedingfield, E.W., editors: Swimming III, Proceedings of the Third International Symposium of Biomechanics in Swimming, Baltimore, 1978, University Park Press, p. 70.
14. Weissmüller, J.: Personal communication, 1969, New Haven, Conn.

7. Tennis strokes

Rod Dulany

When the tennis professional deals with upper extremity injuries, he must look at the player's stroke production, equipment, warm-up habits, and playing tendencies. These aspects must be examined all together, as a unit, in order to get an overall view of the athlete and the cause and effect of his playing characteristics.

STROKE PRODUCTION

In the area of stroke production, the professional's job is to analyze each stroke and ascertain whether the student is using his whole body or just the arm. Several key factors are involved in making the correct stroke. The first is that the player always must be in the proper ready position with weight on the balls of the feet, knees bent, and the racket in front of the body pointing to the other side of the court (Fig. 7-1). This is the same stance a basketball player would take when guarding his opponent. This is very important because a quick, first body movement will either make or break the ability to get into the proper hitting position.

Once the player knows where the opponent is going to hit the ball (remember that the first instinct is usually right), I like to tell the student to let his shoulders take the racket back (Fig. 7-2). This shoulder turn keeps the backswing in a smooth, controlled sequence with the whole body. Again, in this part of the stroke, the knees are bent, and the weight is on the balls of the feet for a smooth movement. Balance is very important during the whole stroke.

Now that the shoulder is turned and the side is to the net, the racket, both handle and head, should drop to the thigh level (Fig. 7-3). Since the first rule of tennis is to get the ball over the net, the player must therefore be *under* the ball before he starts his forward swing. The player now steps over and into the ball while he swings up and meets the ball off his left knee (Figs. 7-4 and 7-5). The head still remains at the contact point for as long as it is comfortable afterward to ensure that the racket's path remains consistent. The mind has already computed the flight of the ball to make that solid contact. If the player's head comes up at or before contact, it pulls the whole body and changes the flight of the racket. This action results in arm-jarring mis-hits.

Tennis players don't hit the ball—they hit *through* the ball. Think of it as hitting seven balls in a row. The wrist should be laid back so that the racket handle and racket

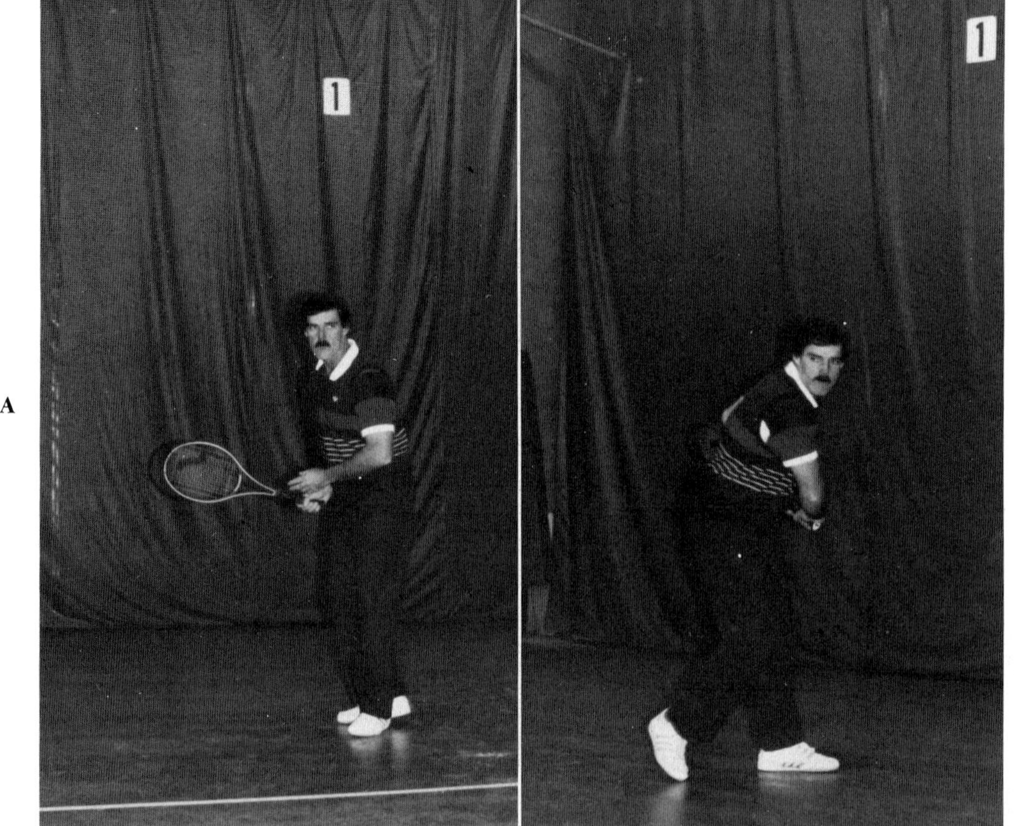

Fig. 7-1. Starting forehand, **A,** and backhand, **B,** shoulder turn to get the racket back early.

head are even through the contact area of all seven balls. With the wrist solid, the player hits out and through the ball. If the elbow flies away from the body through the motion, the player will lose an awareness of where the racket head is and will create a whip action in follow-through. The racket and shoulder should be solidly behind the ball with the thumb ending up at eye level as the stroke is completed. This ensures a complete follow-through, with the ball going over the net with top spin and good placement, all by hitting *through* the ball.

This all sounds relatively simple, until the ball actually comes over the net. Then everyone wants to "punish" the ball! Of course, when this happens, the body jumps, the head comes off the ball, and the ball is mis-hit, which causes torque in the racket. This is the reason why the professional must make the player understand that he should hit the ball *solidly*, not hard.

Placement is more important than power. It won't matter how hard the player can hit the ball if it doesn't go into the opponent's court. Hitting with a smooth, solid stroke, will give both power and placement in one.

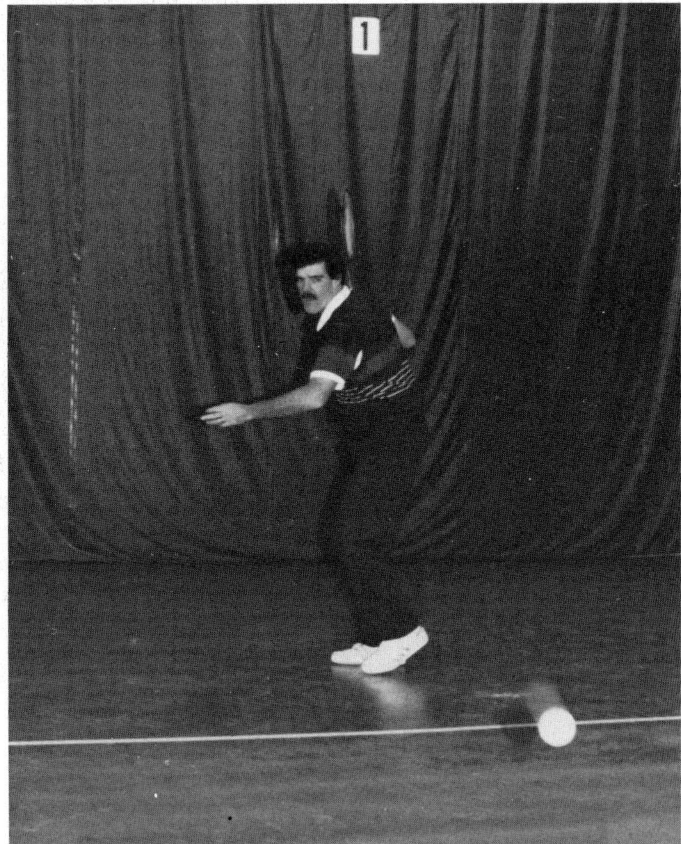

Fig. 7-2. Complete shoulder turn in backswing.

Timing is another problem for weekend players. The more exaggerated the motion, the more chance for error. Instruction therefore should be kept simple and uncomplicated.

THE SERVE

The two vital elements of the serve are toss and hitting *up* to the ball. The toss is a misnomer because the player is not actually tossing the ball but placing it up into the proper hitting area. When you hear the word "toss," it brings to mind the idea of flipping the ball up with the wrist. With a placement motion, the left arm reaches up and the natural arm speed will give the ball enough momentum to reach the proper placement (Figs. 7-6 to 7-8). To obtain controlled power, the ball should be in front and to the right of the body so that it is in front of the right shoulder as the player swings to strike the ball (Fig. 7-9). The height of the ball should be a little higher than the extended racket (Figs. 7-10 and 7-11). Only when the placement of the ball is correct is there a smooth, full body stroke.

One of the myths of tennis is that the service motion is like that of a pitcher

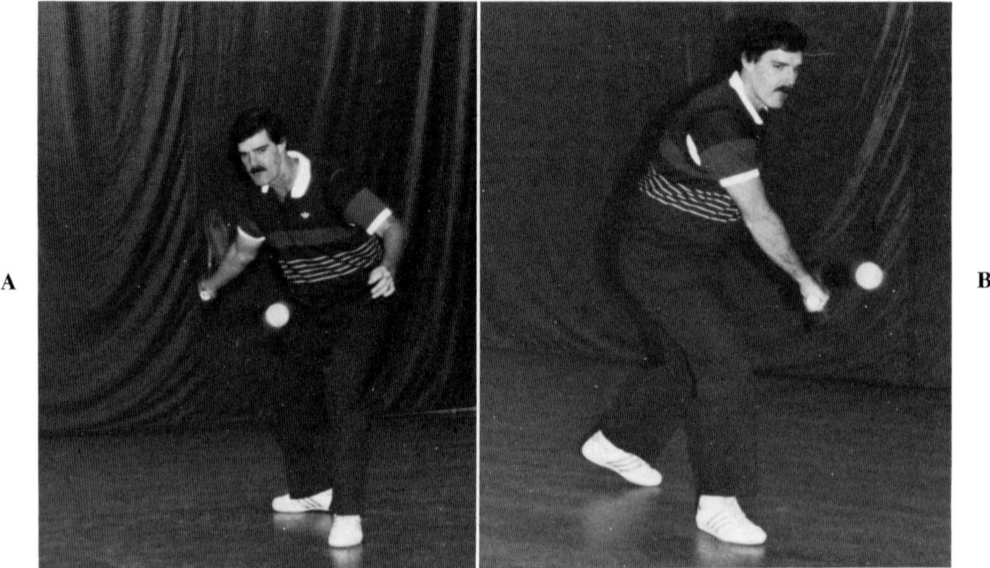

Fig. 7-3. The racket drops to thigh level as the player comes under the ball. **A,** Forehand. **B,** Backhand.

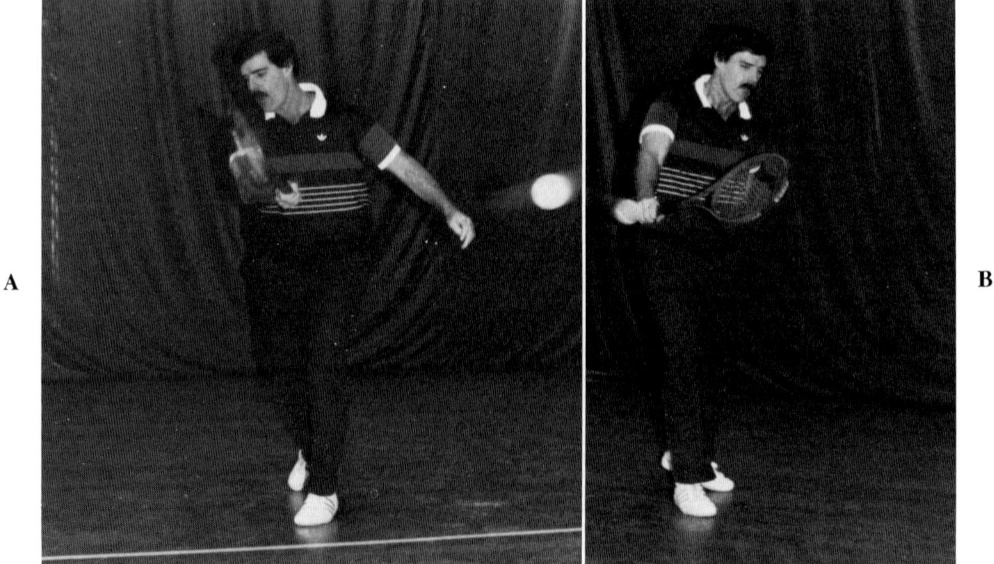

Fig. 7-4. The player swings up and into the ball. **A,** Forehand. **B,** Backhand.

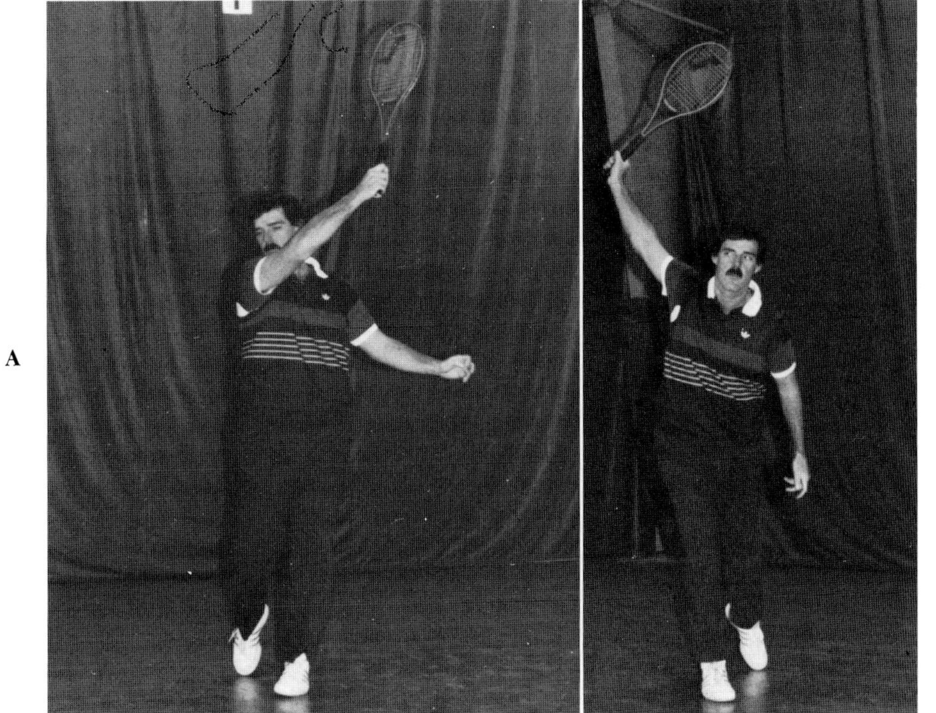

Fig. 7-5. Follow-through swing. **A,** Forehand. **B,** Backhand.

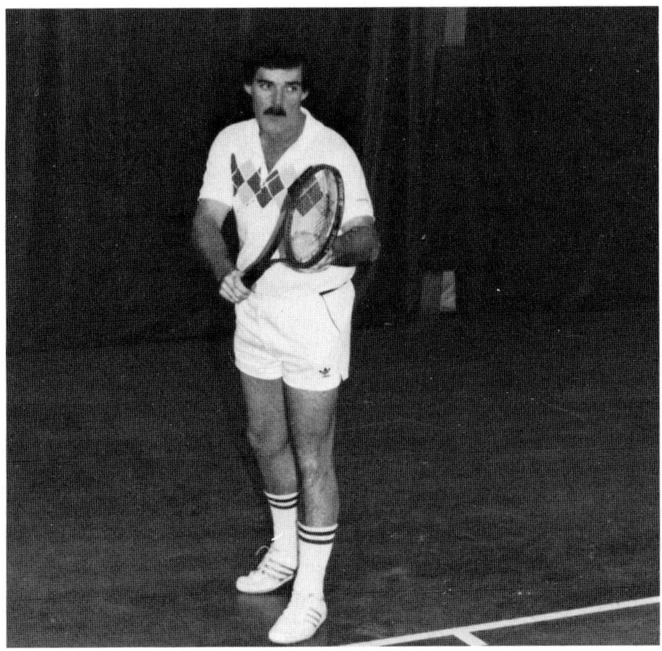

Fig. 7-6. Preparing for the serve.

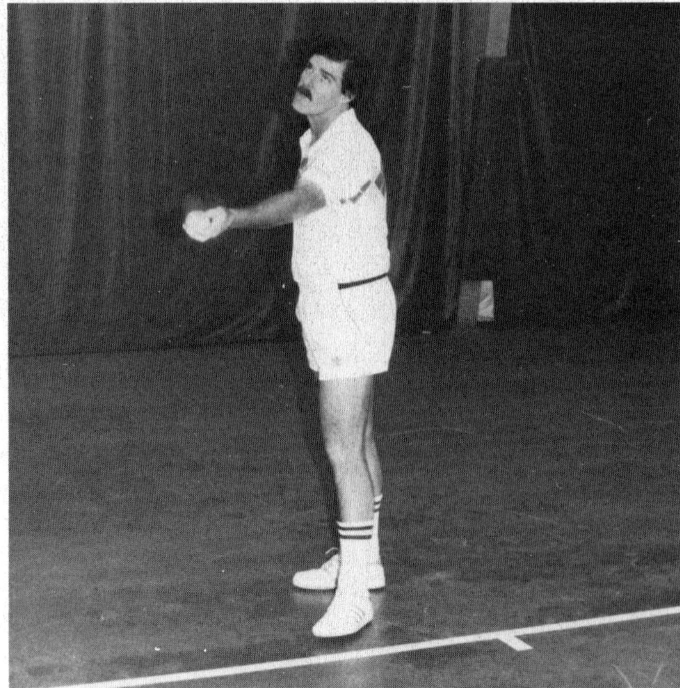

Fig. 7-7. The extended arm begins to raise the ball for proper placement.

throwing a baseball. A pitcher throws from a mound that is 4 to 6 inches high, and he throws downward at a gradual incline. If a tennis player served that way, he would be hitting his own service line with every serve. A correct service motion is like that of an outfielder throwing to home plate. The outfielder must throw with a slight upward motion in order to reach the plate. The server needs to do the same thing in order to get the ball over the net.

RACKETS

Another area in which a tennis professional can assist is in offering advice in choosing the proper racket. There is no single racket that is right for everyone. Therefore it is necessary for a prospective buyer to practice with various demonstration rackets. It is not wise to make a quick decision when buying a racket. Remember that when the player is considering a new racket, no one knows his game better than the professional coach. He should help with the playing characteristics of the various types of rackets available.

As the player begins looking for a racket, he should keep in mind five features that will affect his playing style: head size, material, grip size, weight, and string tension.

The trend in the last several years has been toward a midsize or oversize racket

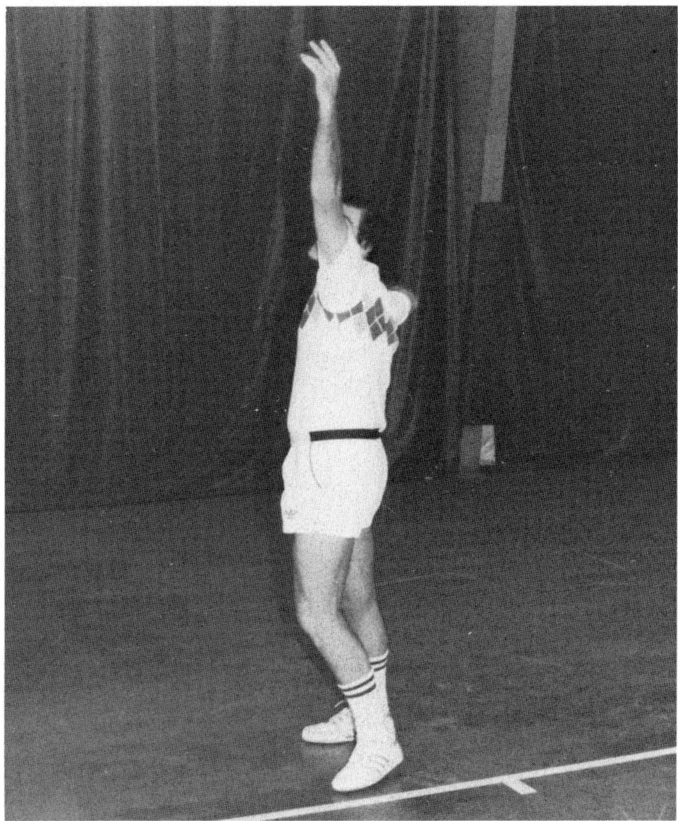

Fig. 7-8. Proper placement of the ball for service is in front and to the right of the body (in a right-handed player).

head and away from the traditional size. The midsize has a 20% larger racket head, and subsequently a larger sweet spot than the traditional racket. Most have open-throat construction, which cuts down on the twisting on off-center hits. This racket should be strung between 62 and 67 pounds. Nylon strings are recommended since the tighter the gut is strung, the less responsive it is. With the midsize and oversize rackets, the strings will not last as long because the higher tension causes greater stress on them. There is also a greater tendency for the strings to shift, causing friction and resulting in breakage. The midsize is a good racket for the all-around player because it is solid enough for the groundstroke and still maneuverable for volleys.

The biggest advantages of an oversize racket are the large sweet spot and the tremendous psychological boost. The larger sweet spot gives back to the recreational player the one thing he loses by getting to play only once or twice a week—timing! It makes it a little more forgiving and, at the net, gives him the feeling that he can't miss. As with the midsize, the oversize racket has an open throat to help prevent

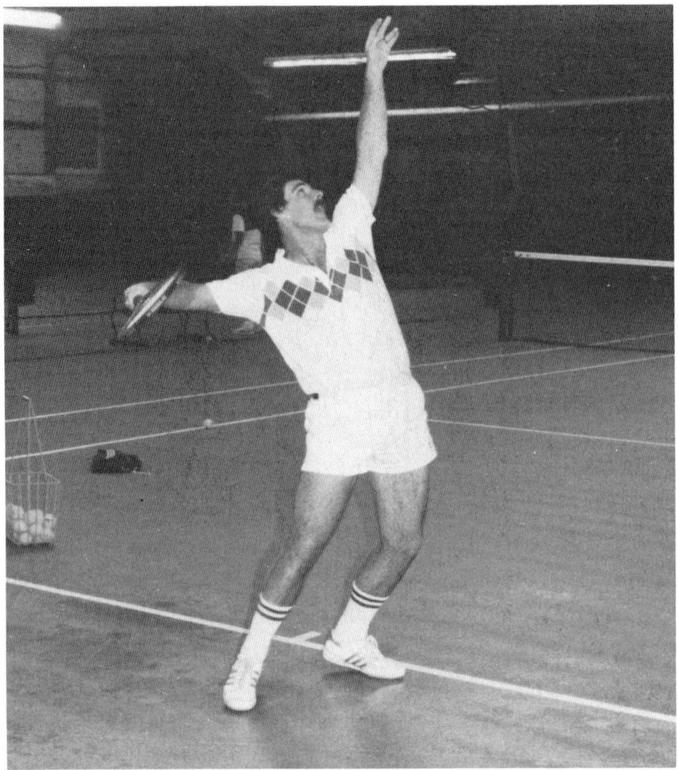

Fig. 7-9. The player stretches and begins the swing.

twisting in the hand. These rackets should be strung from 72 to 80 pounds with nylon, since, again, tightly strung gut will be less responsive. Stringing companies have had to keep pace with the market trend and are therefore coming out with strong strings and different techniques of making nylon for better playability.

The graphite racket is the most expensive racket on the market. Good graphite rackets will run between $150 and $200. Some are available for as little as $75, but as the price goes down, it usually means the quality and amount of graphite decrease. Graphite has the best vibration-dampening characteristics, and most graphite rackets have foam pallet handles. Both factors are good on the arm. Graphite is a strong material, making the racket solid without being bulky, and therefore even oversize graphite rackets will be maneuverable.

A good leather grip is important to cushion the shock. It should be long enough to accommodate a two-handed grip (Fig. 7-12). Grips should be replaced every 6 months, since a worn grip will become smooth and have the tendency to turn in the hand. Getting the proper size grip is an important factor and one of the most misunderstood. The simplest method for doing so is to take a ruler and measure the open palm from the top of the ring finger (on the side of the ring finger closest to the middle

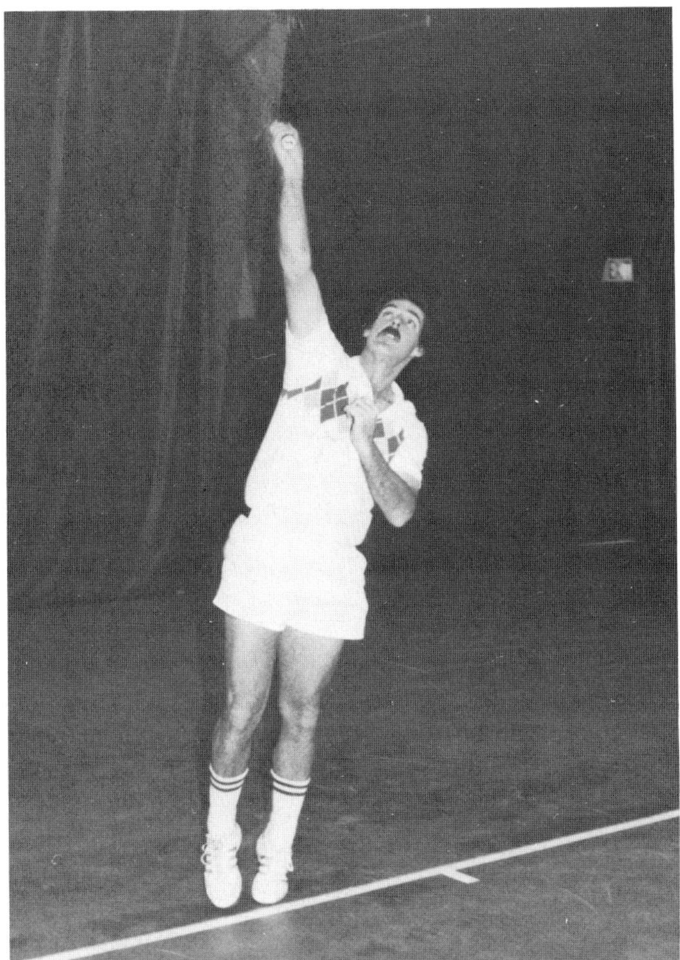

Fig. 7-10. The ball should be slightly higher than the extended racket.

finger) down to the second line running across the palm. That exact measurement will be the grip size.

The player should be more concerned with the balance of the racket than with the weight. A lighter head is recommended. Although it is true that a heavy-headed racket produces more power, this is all predicated on the player hitting the racket through the ball. Since many injuries are created by the player hitting the ball *late*, it follows that a lighter head will make the racket more mobile through three sets of play.

The largest influx into the current market is the junior player, 4 to 7 years of age. Smaller, lighter rackets as short as 16 inches are now available for tiny tots. No little one should be sent out with Dad's old racket!

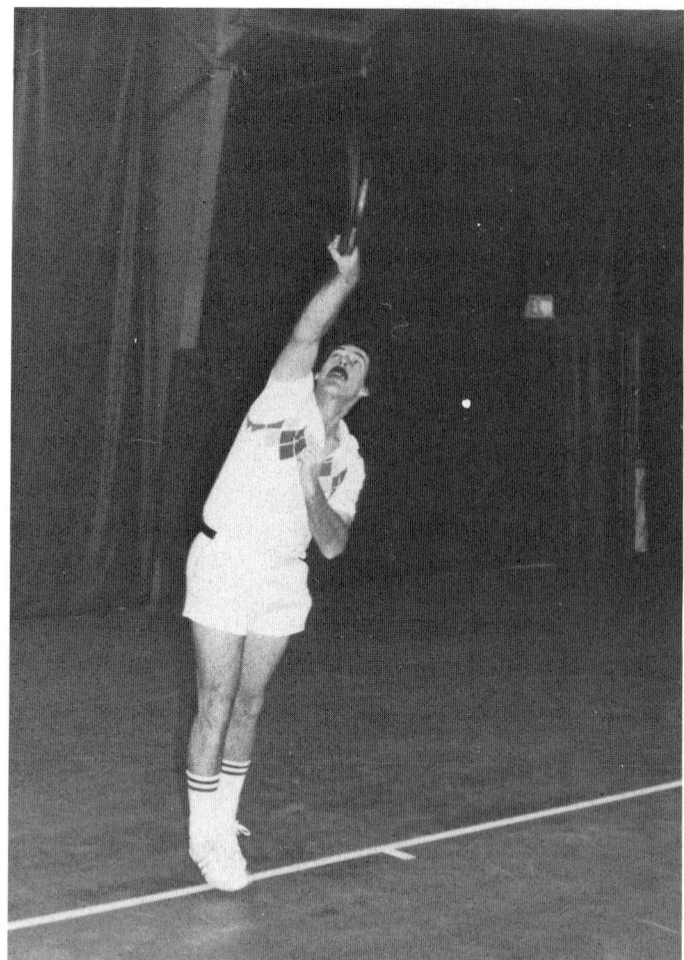

Fig. 7-11. The server hits up and through the ball.

WARM-UP

A player with good strokes and a good racket can still have injuries because of a poor warm-up or poor playing habits.

Picture the body as a can of lard that's been refrigerated. It is still and restricted in motion. One needs a 10 to 15-minute warm-up to loosen up before ever stepping foot onto the court. This warm-up should include a series of easy running in place, jumping jacks and steady stretches, starting out nice and smooth with no jerky motions. By the time the player is on the court, he will have already "broken a sweat." On-court warm-up should be a process of loosening up the arm and body by hitting all the strokes easy to begin with and then gradually working up to game speed. The body should be prepared *slowly* for the game so as not to pull any muscles.

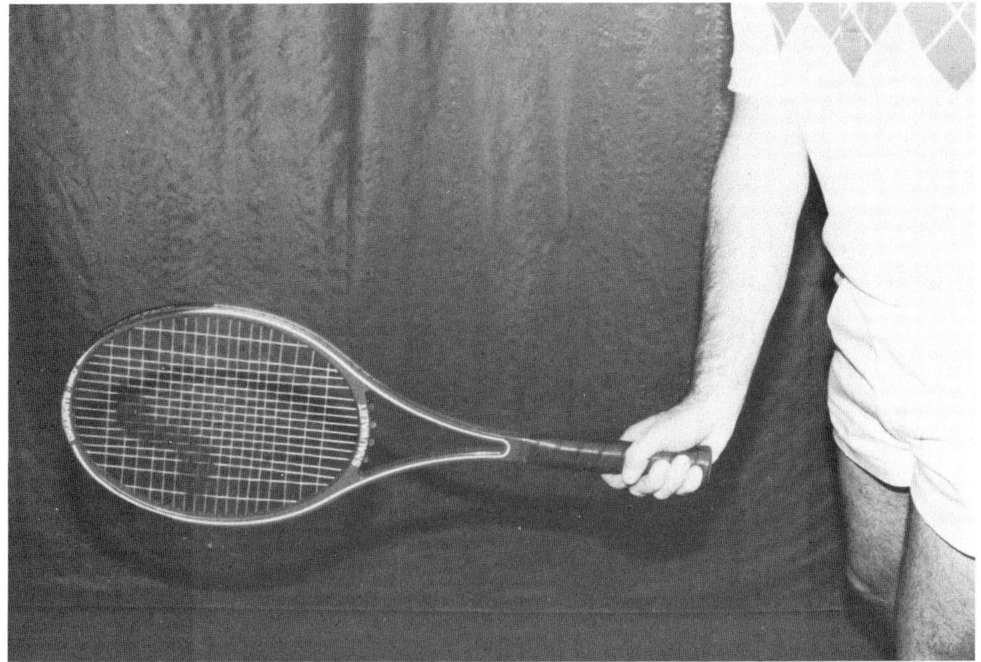

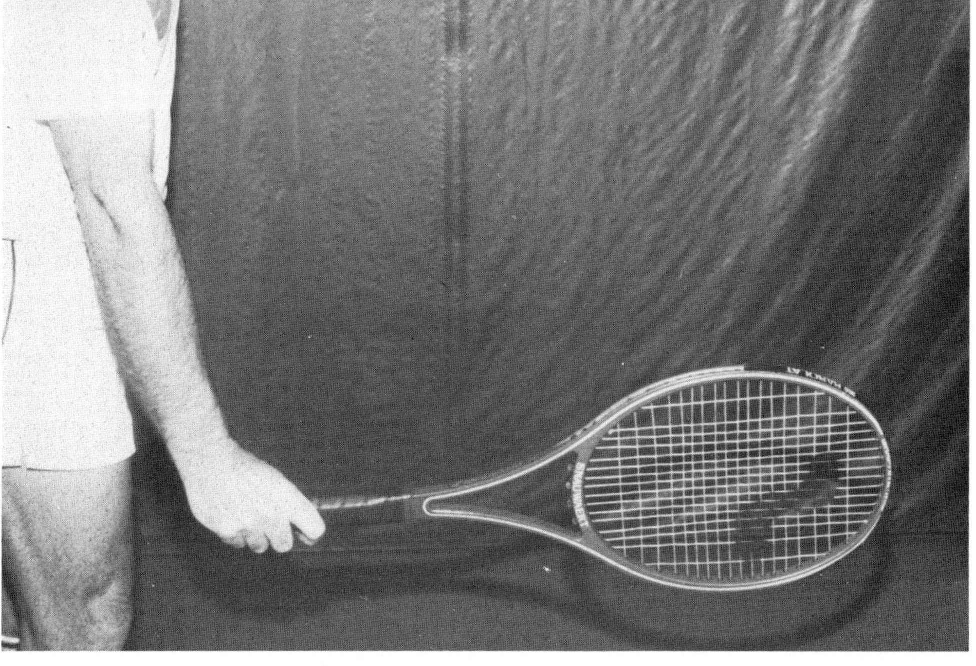

OVEREXERTION

It happens every weekend. A player goes out to play after having no exercise all week. He plays three sets of tennis on Saturday and three more on Sunday. He goes back to work on Monday, and his arm is killing him. "Discretion is the better part of valor!" The occasional player should approach his athletic activities with moderation. It is wise to space tennis outings evenly throughout the week. Timing will be better because of it too. It will help to eliminate those off-center hits that are so prevalent in causing arm injury.

SUMMARY

Tennis is a fast game with quick starts and stops, played mostly by weekend athletes for recreation and not necessarily to improve their game. That aspect alone is responsible for many arm and shoulder injuries, since the arm and shoulder always do most of the work.

All we can do as professionals is instill the correct methods into the minds of our players and hope they cultivate them for their own good.

8. The pitching motion

Frank A. Pettrone

The throwing motion achieves tremendous levels of angular velocity and kinetic energy. The pitcher can develop an acceleration of 90 mph in $1/10$ second. The repetitive action with these significant forces predisposes the shoulder girdle to injuries from abuse or overuse.

The throwing motion may be divided into four phases: windup, cocking, acceleration, and follow-through. (1) The windup commences the motion. This phase ends with the removal of the ball from the glove (Fig. 8-1). (2) The cocking phase brings the shoulder into extreme abduction and external rotation, ending at its maximum point (Fig. 8-2). (3) The acceleration phase begins from this extreme position and continues as the ball is brought forward by the upper extremity and released (Fig. 8-3). (4) The follow-through phase completes the throwing motion (Fig. 8-4).

WINDUP

Windups are for initiation of the momentum of the throwing motion. From a beginning position of equal weight on both lower extremities, weight is transferred to the ipsilateral side and trunk motion is initiated. The shoulder is relatively unstressed with little muscular activity.

COCKING PHASE

As the windup progresses, the shoulder is brought backward as it is maximally externally rotated and abducted. The shoulder also moves backward from flexion into full extension, and trunk rotation continues. During this phase, first the deltoid and then the rotator cuff (supraspinatus, infraspinatus, teres minor) fire and become active. Last, the subscapularis fires to end this external rotation motion.

During this phase of the throwing motion, arch impingement of the rotator cuff can occur. At the extremes of external rotation and abduction the greater tuberosity of the humerus compresses the cuff under the coracoacromial ligament or acromion, or both. With this movement to an extreme position, biceps and triceps tendinitis can be identified. Frequently restriction of internal rotation of the throwing arm is seen in professional pitchers.

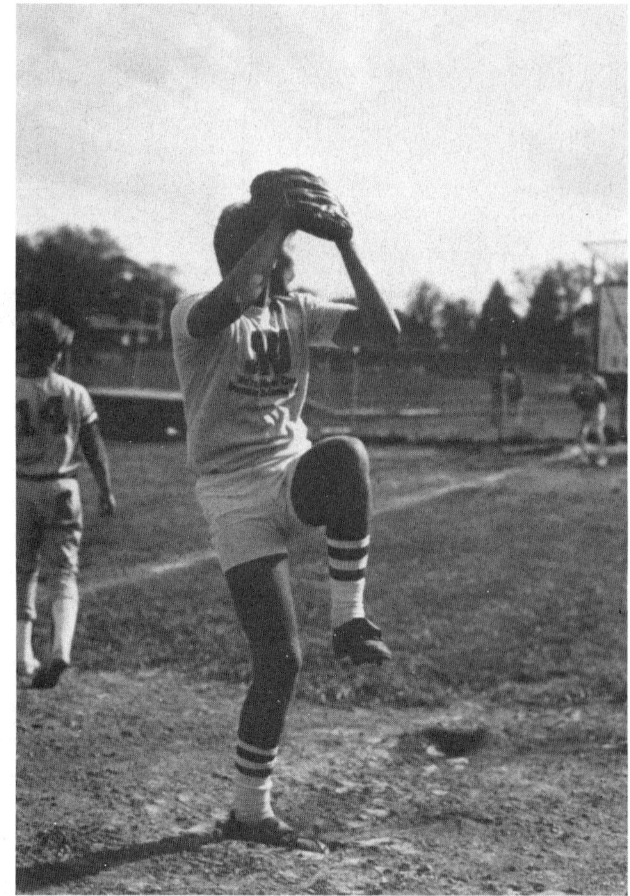

Fig. 8-1. Wind-up.

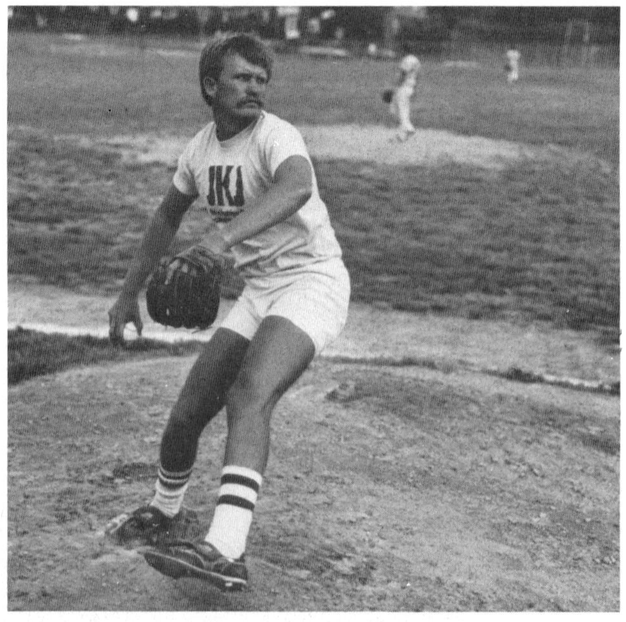

Fig. 8-2. Cocking.

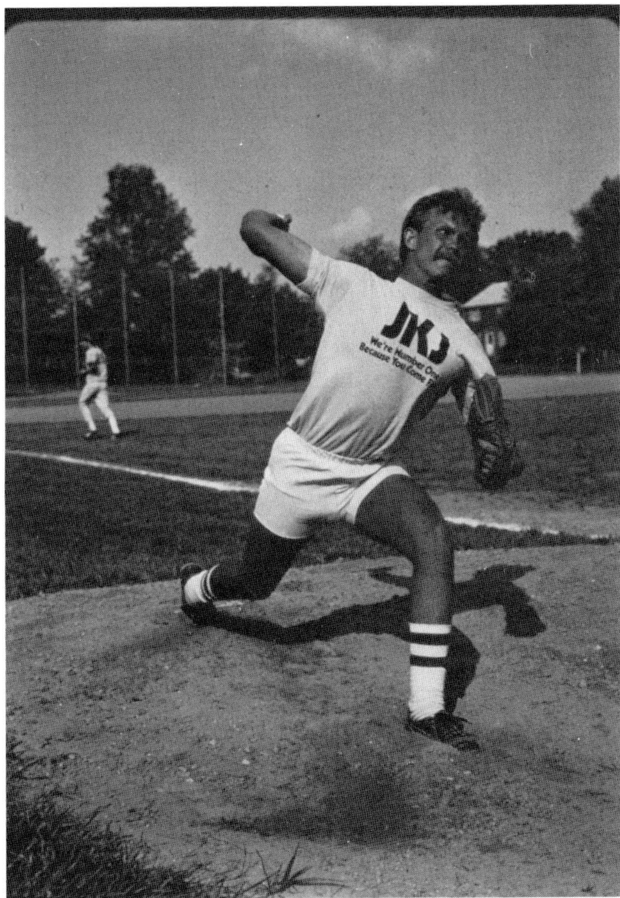

Fig. 8-3. Acceleration.

Further trunk rotation occurs also. The elbow is flexed approximately 90 degrees. As the cocking phase ends, the forward foot contacts the ground again.

ACCELERATION

The shoulder capsule after it has been wound up tight in external rotation during the cocking phase is violently released like a coiled spring. This is a short phase of less than 1/10 second. However, in this short period the shoulder forces (primarily extrinsic) generate a ball velocity of 90 mph. The forward motion of the trunk fixed by the forward foot initiates the phase, and the shoulder then goes into internal rotation and longitudinal flexion. As has been pointed out by Jobe with electromyogram studies,[1,2] this phase is characterized by a noticeable lack of muscle activity in the rotator cuff even though this arm is accelerating forward. It is thus suggested that the rotator cuff serves to stabilize or fine tune the shoulder at this phase. This phase ends with ball

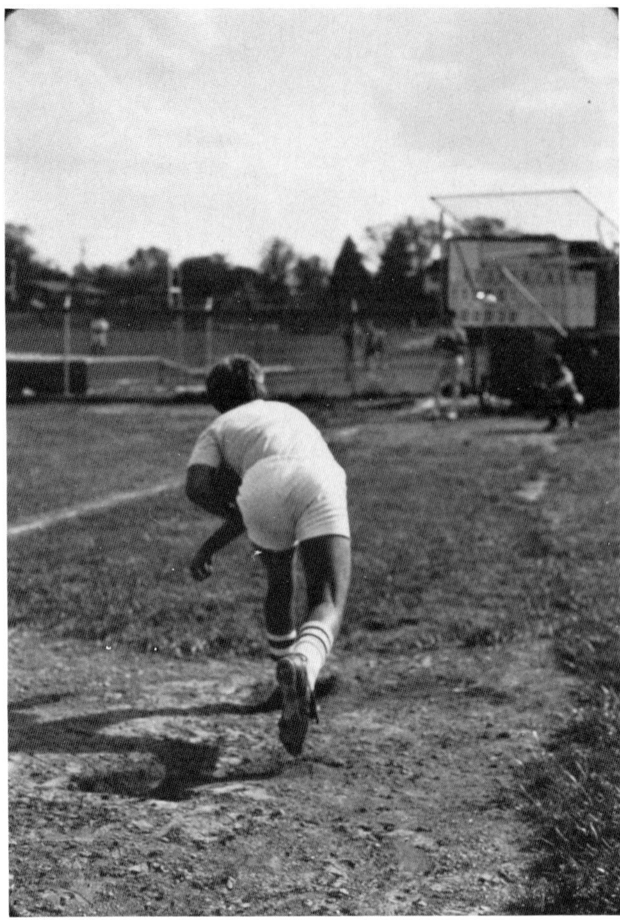

Fig. 8-4. Follow-through.

release, which occurs at about head level. However, the ball and hand move simultaneously farther forward together though apart briefly.

During this phase of the throwing motion, tendinitis of the extrinsic muscles (pectoralis major, latissimus dorsi, serratus anterior), which are active, can occur. Also spontaneous spiral fractures of the humerus in adults may occur because of this tremendous rotatory violence.

Severe valgus strain is imparted to the elbow. This yields significant medial tensile forces and lateral elbow compressive forces. Medial (flexor) tendinitis and osteochondral problems at the capitellum may then occur.

FOLLOW-THROUGH PHASE

After the ball release the shoulder continues to rotate internally and flex horizontally. This is the most active phase with all muscle groups firing intensely. The forces are arm deceleration and forearm rotation. This yields traction injuries to the posterior capsule (traction spurs). The rotator cuff and deltoid firing to decelerate the arm contributes to their involvement in overuse syndrome. Similarly, forces at the elbow are significant and continue tensile strain.

The follow-through phase is primarily concerned with ball rotation (curve, slider, fast ball). Finger position on the ball and wristsnap on motion impart this subtle though significant alteration of ball release. Proper completion of follow-through should allow the pitcher to end with weight balanced on both feet, head up facing the plate, and ready to field a ball hit to him.

REFERENCES

1. Jobe, F., et al.: An EMG analysis of the shoulder in throwing and pitching, Am. J. Sports Med. **11**(1):3-5, 1983.
2. Jobe, F., et al.: An EMG analysis of the shoulder in pitching, a second report, Am. J. Sports Med. **12**(3):218-220, 1984.
3. Tullos, H., and Bennett, J.: The shoulder in sports. In Scott, N., Nisonson, B., and Nicholas, J., editors: Principles of sports medicine, Baltimore, 1984, Williams & Wilkins.

PART TWO

Hand, forearm, and wrist

9. Functional anatomy of the forearm and hand

George P. Bogumill

DORSAL SKIN AND COMPARTMENTS

The skin of the hand is frequently injured because of its exposed position. It is the most frequent point of contact of the body with the environment. Dorsally the skin is loose and extensible to allow for the increased length needed for simultaneous flexion of wrist and digits. It is separated from the extensor tendon plane by a subcutaneous space in which blood and lymphatic vessels are situated (Figs. 9-1, *B*, and 9-4, *A*). The tendons are also separated from the dorsum of the metacarpals by a potential subaponeurotic space (Fig. 9-4, *B*). When this latter space is obliterated by adhesions after fracture, infection, or hematoma, the tendons are unable to glide, and so an extension contracture of the metacarpophalangeal joint results. The skin on the dorsum of the hand tears easily especially over the metacarpophalangeal joint because of its absence of stable attachments to deeper structures. On the fingers, the dorsal skin is attached to this skeleton along the sides of the fingers by Cleland's and Greyson's ligaments. More distally, the nail bed is thin and adherent to the terminal phalanx; it is easily disrupted with any fracture, and so open fractures are particularly common.

EXTENSOR RETINACULUM

The extensor retinaculum consists of transversely placed reinforcing fibers in the deep fascia at the distal forearm level (Fig. 9-1, *A*). These fibers attach strongly to the distal end of the radius but pass obliquely and distally to bypass the distal ulna, attaching instead to the ulnar collateral ligament and pisohamate capsule. This pattern permits travel of the radius about the ulna during pronation and supination without need for change in length of retinacular fibers. Extending anteriorly from the extensor retinaculum are a number of strong short fibrous septa, which attach firmly to the radius, creating five dorsal compartments (Fig. 9-1, *B* and *C*). A sixth compartment is attached to the dorsum of the distal ulna.

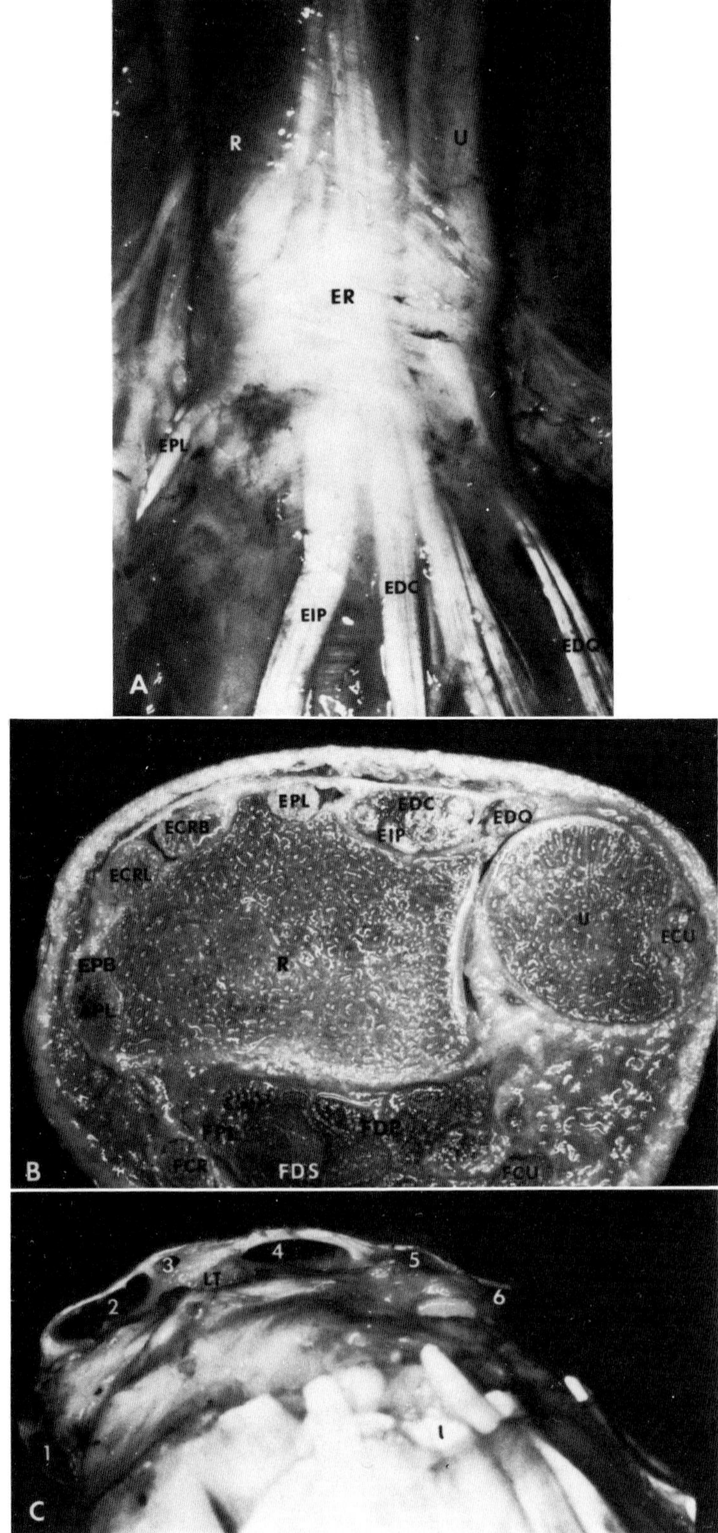

Fig. 9-1. For legend see top of opposite page.

Fig. 9-1. Extensor retinaculum. **A,** Dorsal view of oblique course of reinforcing fibers of forearm fascia that form extensor retinaculum. It is attached to the distal radius and to the ulnar collateral ligament of the wrist. **B,** Cross section through distal radioulnar joint. **C,** End view of six dorsal compartments of extensor retinaculum with tendons removed. *APL,* Abductor pollicis longus; *ECRB,* extensor carpi radialis brevis; *ECRL,* extensor carpi radialis longus; *ECU,* extensor carpi ulnaris; *EDC,* extensor digitorum communis; *EDQ,* extensor digiti quinti; *EIP,* extensor indicis proprius; *EPB,* extensor pollicis brevis; *EPL,* extensor pollicis longus; *ER,* extensor retinaculum; *FCR,* flexor carpi radialis; *FCU,* flexor carpi ulnaris; *FDP,* flexor digitorum profundus; *FDS,* flexor digitorum superficialis; *FPL,* flexor pollicis longus; *LT,* Lister's tubercle; *R,* radius; *U,* ulna.

EXTENSOR TENDONS

The extensor tendons are quite variable in pattern. Four or five to the fingers is the usual number, but there may be as many as nine or ten. The tendons traverse the six compartments in the extensor retinaculum and diverge to reach their final insertions. As they pass beneath the retinaculum, they are surrounded by synovial sheaths, which extend a short distance proximally and distally to the retinaculum. Across the dorsum of the hand, they are loosely surrounded by paratenon, which forms a mesotenon conveying blood vessels to the tendon for its nutrition. The common digital extensors are attached to each other over the metacarpal region by juncturae tendinum. These can be utilized after tendon injury by appropriate splinting of adjacent fingers to stabilize a lacerated tendon through its juncturae.

As the digital extensor tendons approach the metacarpophalangeal joint, each is reinforced by transverse fibers that pass from the common extensor tendon around the sides of the head of the metacarpal to attach to the volar plate and transverse metacarpal ligament (Fig. 9-2, A). These transverse fibers extend the proximal phalanx by lifting it around the curve of the metacarpal head. Slightly more distal in the extensor hood are transverse fibers from the interosseous muscles, which function as the primary flexor of the metacarpophalangeal joint. In addition, there are oblique fibers from the interossei and the lumbrical to each finger (Fig. 9-2). These pass more distally, blending with fibers from the central slip to act as extensors of the proximal interphalangeal (PIP) and distal interphalangeal (DIP) joints. Over the proximal phalanx, the hood mechanism becomes fairly complex in that the central slip divides into three portions, the central part inserting into the base of the middle phalanx and the other two bypassing it on either side. These lateral slips blend with the fibers from the lumbrical and interossei to bypass the PIP joint and insert into the distal phalanx.

The interossei are short bulky muscles with limited excursion but significant power. They are the powerful primary flexors of the metacarpophalangeal joints. On the radial side of the index and middle fingers, the major portion of the first and second dorsal interosseous tendons insert directly into the proximal phalanx where they act as flexors but also strong abductors of these two digits to resist forces exerted by the thumb during pinch.

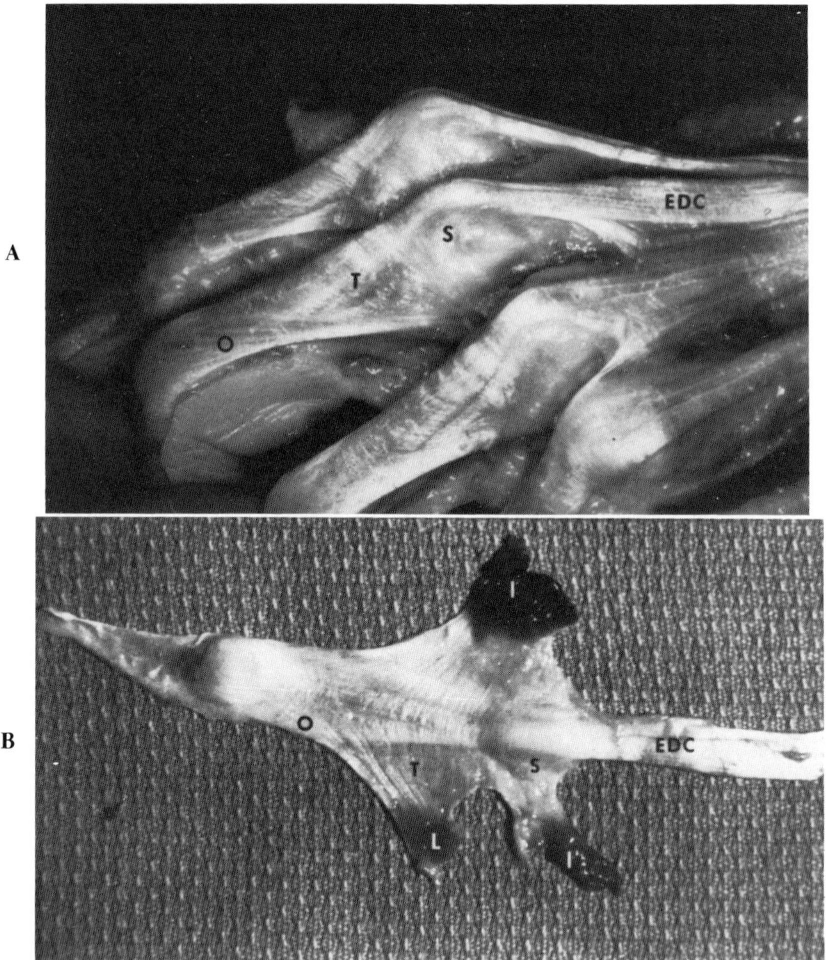

Fig. 9-2. Extensor hood mechanism of the fingers. **A,** Long extensor tendon blends with fibers from interossei and lumbricals to provide flexion *and* extension at metacarpophalangeal joint, as well as extension at interphalangeal joints. **B,** Hood mechanism for one finger. *EDC,* Extensor digitorum communis; *O,* oblique fibers from interossei and lumbrical that extend interphalangeal joints; *S,* sagittal fibers from extensor that extend proximal phalanx; *T,* transverse fibers from interossei that flex proximal phalanx.

The lumbrical muscles are also flexors of the metacarpophalangeal joints and extensors of the interphalangeal joints. They pass volarly to the transverse metacarpal ligament in the lumbrical canals formed by dorsal septa from the palmar aponeurosis. The lumbrical acts as an extensor of the terminal joint in part by drawing the long flexor distally during extension of the finger.

At the PIP joint level, the extensor mechanism becomes rather complex and interesting. The lateral bands lie dorsally to the axis of PIP joint flexion/extension and thus are extensors of that joint. For economy of movement, the lateral bands slide volarly slightly during flexion of both interphalangeal joints; this sliding allows both to flex simultaneously. When the central slip is ruptured, the lateral bands slide below the axis of flexion/extension of the PIP joint and thus lose their extensor capability at the PIP joint. In fact, they become flexors. The harder one tries to overcome the loss of central slip by pull on the interossei, the more extension one gets of the terminal joint but the greater the flexion forces at the proximal interphalangeal joint; thus a boutonnière deformity is created. The lateral bands are normally retained in position by the transverse retinacula, which become shortened in the boutonnière deformity. Extension of the interphalangeal joints can be accomplished by either the long extensor tendons or the interossei, depending on the position of the metacarpophalangeal joint. The long extensors will accomplish PIP extension when the metacarpophalangeal joint is flexed, and the interossei will accomplish PIP extension when the metacarpophalangeal joint is extended. The interossei and long extensors have opposite effects at the metacarpophalangeal joint, with the interossei being the primary flexors of that joint.

The oblique retinacular ligament is said to be a passive extensor of the DIP joint; however, this is true only if there is a contracture of this oblique retinacular ligament. Normally we can extend our PIP joint fully and still flex the DIP joint 60 to 70 degrees.

PALMAR SKIN AND COMPARTMENTS

The skin is bound to the palmar aponeurosis by numerous short vertical septa. Since the aponeurosis is fixed to the skeleton by various attachments, the skin also is relatively fixed and does not glide with grasping activities. The blood supply to the palmar skin comes with the fibrous septa, which makes skin loss more likely if there is extensive tearing or elevation of the palmer skin surgically. The septa attaching the skin to the distal phalanx also carry numerous blood vessels to the bone. The spaces between these septa are filled with fat, which provides for padding the pulp of the finger while still holding the skin relatively secure during grasping activities.

CARPAL TUNNEL

The carpal tunnel is made up of bone on three sides, and the fourth is bridged by a firm unyielding ligament extending from the hamate to the trapezium and scaphoid (Fig. 9-3). Through this rigid-walled tunnel pass nine flexor tendons plus the median nerve in a synovium-lined compartment. Also passing through this tunnel is the flexor carpi radialis in its own separate synovium-lined tunnel. The flexor retinaculum, like the extensor retinaculum, is designed to prevent bowstringing of the tendons that cross the wrist during flexion and extension activities.

The flexor carpi ulnaris and palmaris longus pass superficially to the transverse retinaculum. The flexor carpi radialis passes in a tunnel through the trapezium but outside the carpal tunnel (Fig. 9-3, *B*). The flexor carpi ulnaris attaches to the pisiform and then through the pisometacarpal and pisohamate ligaments gains insertion dis-

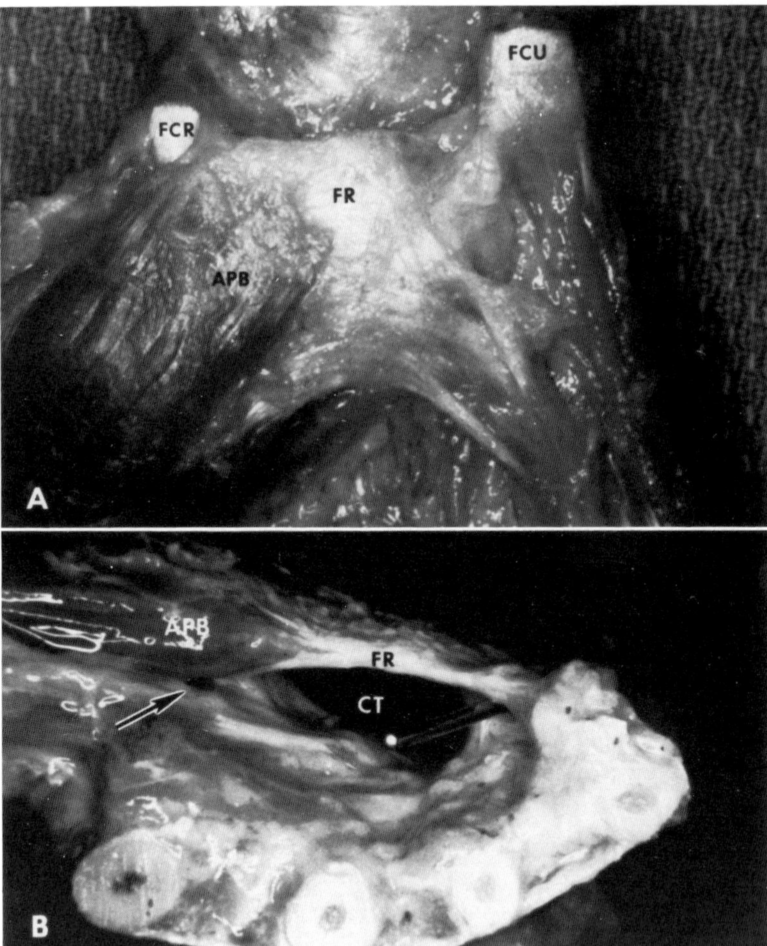

Fig. 9-3. Carpal tunnel. **A,** Palmar view of extent and location of flexor retinaculum. **B,** End-on view of carpal tunnel. Probe in canal in origin of flexor digiti minimi brevis through which passes the deep motor branch of ulnar nerve. *APB,* Abductor pollicis brevis; *FCR,* flexor carpi radialis; *FCU,* flexor carpi ulnaris; *FR,* flexor retinaculum; *arrow,* separate tunnel for FCR across carpus.

tally. This is the only muscle that is attached directly to a carpal bone; the rest of the muscles all bypass the carpus. Basically, all the long powerful wrist flexors and extensors bypass the carpus, with the result that the carpus functions as an intercalated segment acted upon by muscles not attached to it. The carpal bones assume positions depending on the relative stresses that are applied around them.

Wrist and finger motions are synergistic; in order to obtain maximum wrist extension, one must relax the long finger flexors. In making a fist, greater wrist extension is possible as the fingers flex, and more power can be exerted by the fingers as the wrist extends. Oppositely, maximum wrist flexion requires finger extension. Thus movements of the wrist are used to augment the power and excursion of the finger flexors and extensors and must be considered when doing tendon transfers. These wrist and finger motions are synergistic and automatic.

FLEXOR PULLEYS AND SHEATH

Five annular pulleys are described, but only three are important. These are the A2 pulley at the proximal phalanx level, and A4 pulley at the middle phalanx level, and the A1 pulley at the metacarpophalangeal joint. The synovial flexor sheaths end proximally to the A1 pulley in the palm by reflecting from the tendon surface to the pulley surface. Infections tend to collect in this cul-de-sac, and failure to drain this area may result in chronic and persisting infection. The A1 pulley is attached firmly to the volar plate of the metacarpophalangeal joint (Fig. 9-4). At the same level are attached the collateral ligaments, the transverse fibers of the extensor hood, and the transverse metacarpal ligaments. The posterior surface of the flexor tendon sheath is also the periosteum of the phalanges. Fractures of the phalanges can cause flexor tendon adherence by disrupting this tendon sheath.

The tendons themselves have an arrangement whereby the flexor digitorum superficialis splits to enclose the flexor digitorum profundus. This is done in a manner that does not occlude the space of the decussation during longitudinal tension on the flexor superficialis. The flexor superficialis attaches to the midshaft of the middle phalanx rather than to its base (Fig. 9-5); thus fractures of the volar lip of the middle phalanx do not become displaced by muscle pull. This is not true at the terminal phalanx where the flexor digitorum profundus attaches nearer the base of the distal phalanx and fractures are frequently displaced by muscle pull, particularly avulsions of the ring finger profundus during strong grasping activities. The vincula act as intermittent mesotenons in the flexor sheath and provide blood supply, which enters the dorsal aspect of the tendons.

HAND SKELETON

The hand skeleton is constructed of carpals, metacarpals, and phalanges connected and separated by appropriate joints. The second and third metacarpals are rigidly fixed to the trapezoid and capitate at their base, providing a stable central point of the hand. The arches of the hand are based on these two metacarpals and are both transverse and longitudinal. The fourth, fifth, and first metacarpals are quite mobile at their base of attachment and move a fair distance with power grip. The fingertips point to the scaphoid tuberosity when the fingers are flexed individually, but the distal metacarpal arch flattens when all fingers are brought down together, and thus the tips cannot all point to the same area simultaneously.

DIGITAL JOINTS

Metacarpophalangeal joints. The metacarpal head is rounded and the origin of the collateral ligament is eccentric and dorsally placed. This position makes the ligament looser in extension than in flexion and allows side-to-side motion or distraction

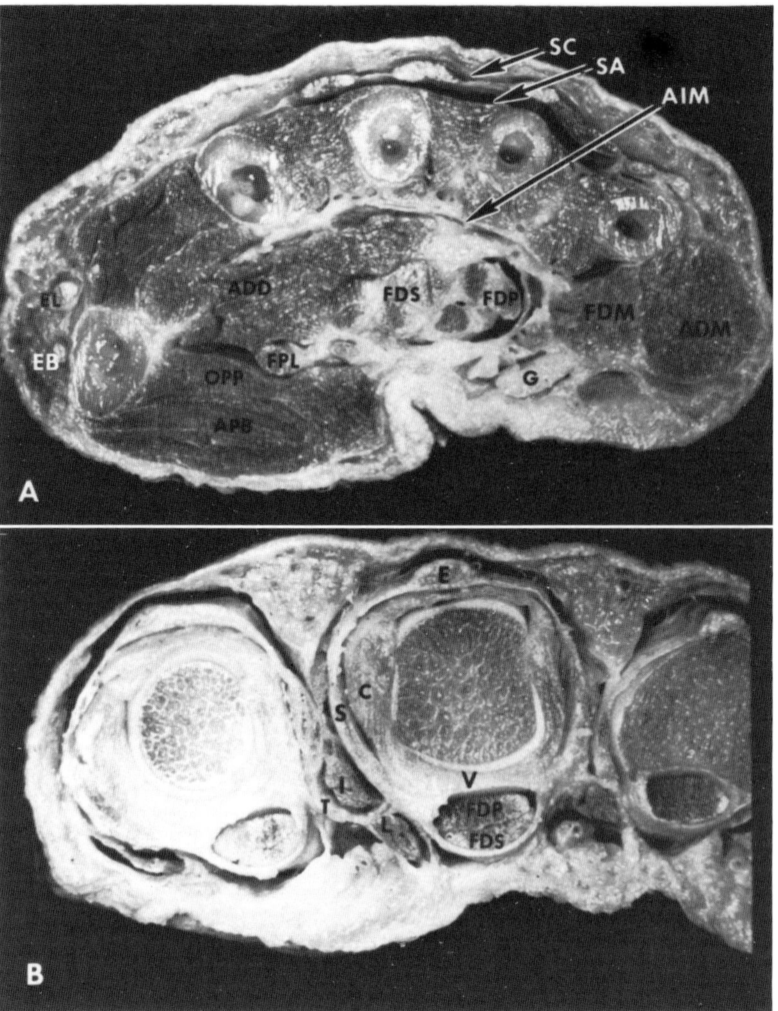

Fig. 9-4. Cross sections through the hand. **A,** Proximal part of palm. **B,** Distal part of palm. *ADD,* Adductor pollicis; *ADM,* abductor digiti minimi; *AIM,* anterior interosseous membrane; *APB,* abductor pollicis brevis; *C,* collateral ligament; *E,* extensor digitorum communis; *EB,* extensor pollicis brevis; *EL,* extensor pollicis longus; *FDM,* flexor digiti minimi brevis; *FDP,* flexor digitorum profundus; *FDS,* flexor digitorum superficialis; *FPL,* flexor pollicis longus; *G,* Guyon's canal with ulnar artery and nerve; *I,* interosseous tendon; *L,* lumbrical tendon; *OPP,* opponens pollicis; *S,* sagittal fibers of extensor hood; *SA,* subaponeurotic space; *SC,* subcutaneous space; *T,* transverse metacarpal ligament; *V,* volar plate.

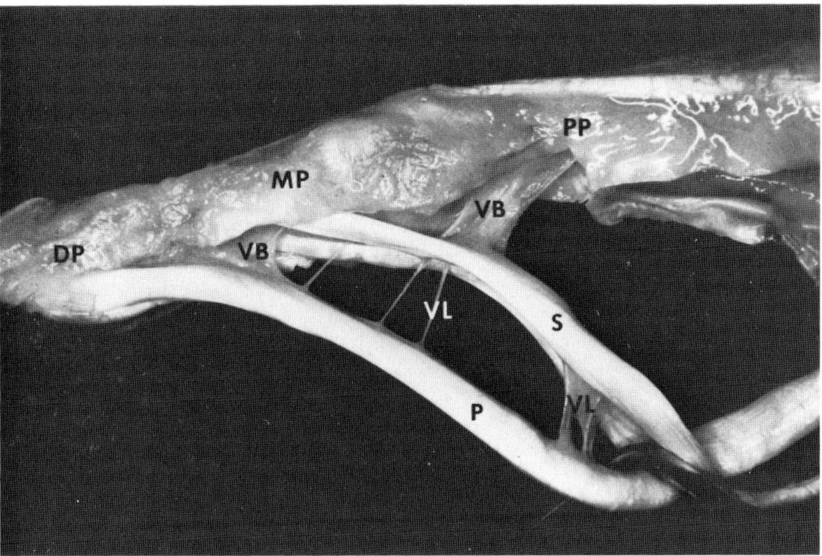

Fig. 9-5. Flexor tendon mechanism in the finger. The margins of the opened A2 and A4 pulleys are evident at proximal and middle phalangeal levels. *DP*, Distal phalanx; *P*, flexor digitorum profundus; *PP*, proximal phalanx; *S*, flexor digitorum superficialis; *VB*, vinculum breve; *VL*, vinculum longum.

of the phalanx on the metacarpal head when the joint is extended (Fig. 9-6, *A* and *B*) but not when the joint is flexed. The metacarpophalangeal joint must be splinted in flexion to prevent an extension contracture after treatment is finished.

Interphalangeal joints. The head of the phalanx is broader transversely than in the anteroposterior direction. The ligaments are taut in flexion and extension and allow no distraction of the joint in either position (Fig. 9-6, *C* and *D*). Collateral ligaments develop in situ.

PRECISION AND POWER GRIP

Position of function of the hand is actually a position of preparation for function. Precision grip is usually done between the thumb and the radial two fingers. This is median nerve territory. Power grip is usually done primarily with the ulnar digits though it can be with all digits. Precision grip and power grip can be combined or alternated between the hands or even portions of the hand.

WRIST JOINTS

The wrist is made up of multiple joints, separated into distal radioulnar, radiocarpal, intercarpal, carpometacarpal, and pisotriquetral. This is a complex arrangement of bones and ligaments that provides for stability and mobility. The joints are acted upon by muscles that cross the carpus but do not attach to it. Therefore positioning of the carpal bones is passive in response to muscles forces applied to the

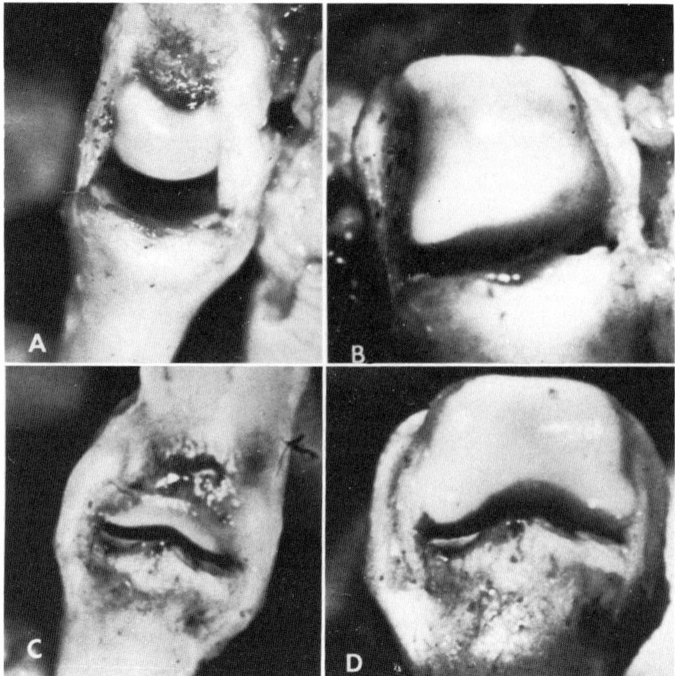

Fig. 9-6. Collateral ligaments at metacarpophalangeal and interphalangeal joints with longitudinal traction applied. **A** and **B,** Metacarpophalangeal joint in extension and flexion. Eccentric attachment of ligament and shape of metacarpal head allow distraction of joint in extension. **B** and **C,** Proximal interphalangeal joint in extension and flexion. Collateral ligaments allow no distraction in either position.

metacarpals. The distal radioulnar joint is separated from the proximal carpal row by the triangular fibrocartilage complex (TFCC) (Fig. 9-7). The radial and ulnar collateral ligaments are relatively lax in neutral position of the wrist and tighten at extremes of radial and ulnar deviation. The dorsal capsule is looser than the volar and has fewer ligaments (Fig. 9-7, *B*), which extend from the radius to the proximal carpal row. The dorsal ligaments between the two carpal rows are quite small and irregular. Interosseous ligaments attach proximally on the scaphoid, lunate, and triquetrum and help the proximal row act as a unit with the scaphoid connecting between proximal and distal rows. These interosseous ligaments separate the radiocarpal joint from the midcarpal joint. The triangular fibrocartilage complex separates the radiocarpal joint from the distal radioulnar joint. An arthrogram of radiocarpal joint will not have dye extending into the distal radioulnar joint unless there is a tear in the TFCC. However, radiopaque medium will extend from the radiocarpal joint into the pisotriquetral joint in approximately one third of normal wrists.

The volar capsule has numerous strong ligaments extending from the radius and TFCC to the capitate, hamate, lunate, and triquetrum (Fig. 9-7, *A*). These volar

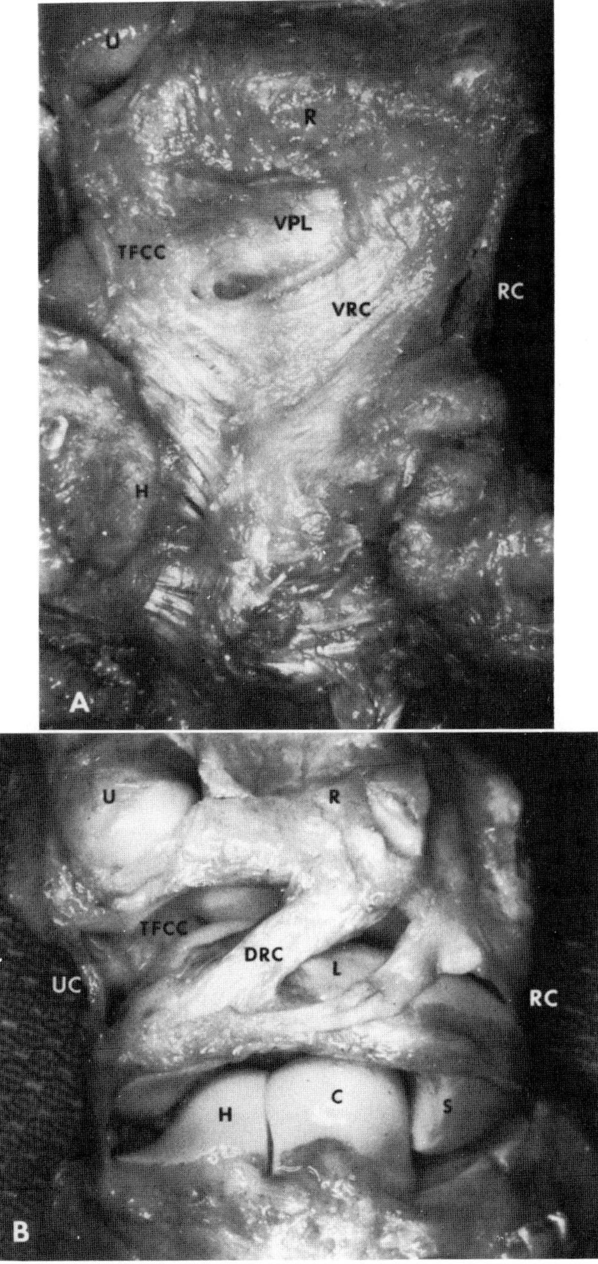

Fig. 9-7. Ligaments of wrist. **A,** Volar. **B,** Dorsal. *C,* Capitate; *DRC,* dorsal radiocarpal; *H,* hamate; *L,* lunate; *R,* radius; *RC,* radial collateral; *S,* scaphoid; *TFCC,* triangular fibrocartilage complex with its volar extension to triquetrum, hamate, and capitate; *U,* ulna; *UC,* ulnar collateral; *VPL,* volar radiolunate; *VRC,* volar radiocapitate.

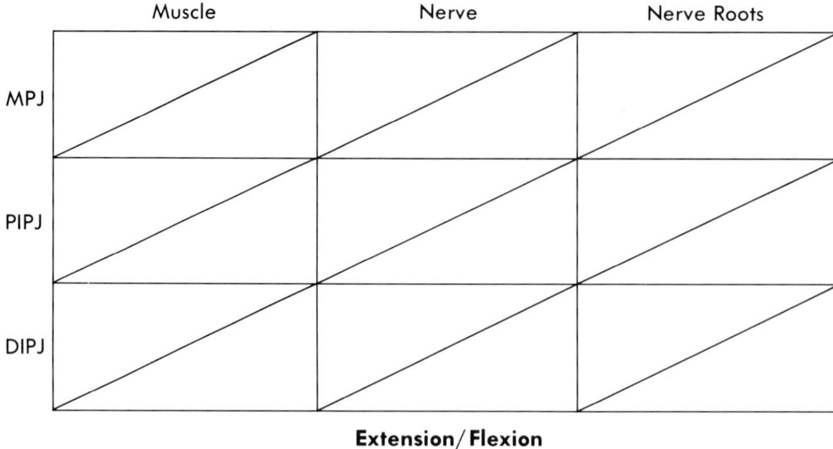

Fig. 9-8. Exercise in analysis of motor function of a digit. Filling in the blanks and utilizing the long finger as an example aid in understanding the complexity of flexor and extensor function. (Concept by Dr. Monroe Levine, Augusta, Ga., 1980.)

ligaments are very strong and heavy and provide most of the stability of the wrist. Since both the dorsal and volar ligaments originate from the radius and attach to the carpus, the hand must passively follow the radius as it rotates around the ulna in pronation and supination. Wrist movements are centered about axes through the head of the capitate in both flexion and extension and radioulnar deviation.

NERVES

The superficial nerves are primarily sensory, and the patterns are somewhat variable. The deeper nerves are both motor and sensory. The pattern is more constant, but there is some variability and communication between nerves, such as the Martin Gruber anastomosis in the forearm between median and ulnar nerve. The median, ulnar, and radial nerves each enter the forearm between two heads of a muscle and are subject to compression at that point. Other areas of compression are Guyon's canal, the carpal tunnel, the area beneath the flexor digitorum superficialis origin, the area beneath the lacertus fibrosus, and the ligament of Struthers.

An excellent method for study and for testing our understanding of the flexion and extension mechanisms of the digits was proposed by Dr. Monroe Levine. Filling in the blank spaces of Fig. 9-8 requires a knowledge of muscle and nerve anatomy and is useful clinically for locating a source of dysfunction.

ARTERIES

Arteries are more constant in pattern and location than veins. The interosseous arteries supply the muscles of the forearm, both dorsal and volar as they pass down the interosseous membrane. The radial and ulnar ateries make up the superficial and deep arches of the hand from which originate the metacarpal and digital arteries.

10. Soft-tissue injuries to the hand

Frank C. McCue III
Gary A. Miller

Hand injuries are common in athletes because the hand typically precedes the athlete in most sports and frequently absorbs initial contact. Any injury may occur in any sport, but certain injuries are prone to occur in specific sports because of the nature of the activity, the regulations, protective devices, equipment, and equipment failure (Fig. 10-1). Even in noncontact sports the digits are often in a vulnerable position.

There is a tendency to minimize the severity and significance of some hand injuries because they only rarely disable the athlete. Unfortunately this is often the case with young, poorly supervised athletes who may return to forceful, unprotected use of the extremity long before adequate healing has occurred. Proper care of hand injuries hinges upon precise diagnosis and treatment, followed by appropriate rehabilitation. This chapter is a summary of the recognition and treatment of soft-tissue injuries of the hand in athletes and a consideration of the protective measures, devices, and splints, which are of value in their prevention.

PERIPHERAL NERVE PROBLEMS

Entrapment syndromes in the general population most often occur at the carpal or cubital tunnels. The carpal tunnel is by far the most common location of median nerve entrapment. Carpal tunnel syndrome is more common in women than in men and usually occurs in the dominant hand. Ulnar nerve compression at the wrist is not so common as carpal tunnel syndrome. A common type of entrapment within Guyon's canal is median nerve entrapment in the carpal tunnel among patients with inflammatory synovitis such as rheumatoid arthritis. The nerve may also be compressed by a lipoma, ganglion, ulnar artery thrombosis, or aneurysm. Other entrapment syndromes are found below the brachial plexus, but they are relatively rare.

The relative incidences and causes of peripheral nerve involvement among athletes differ greatly from those among the population at large. These differences are pointed out in the discussion that follows. Peripheral nerve involvement among ath-

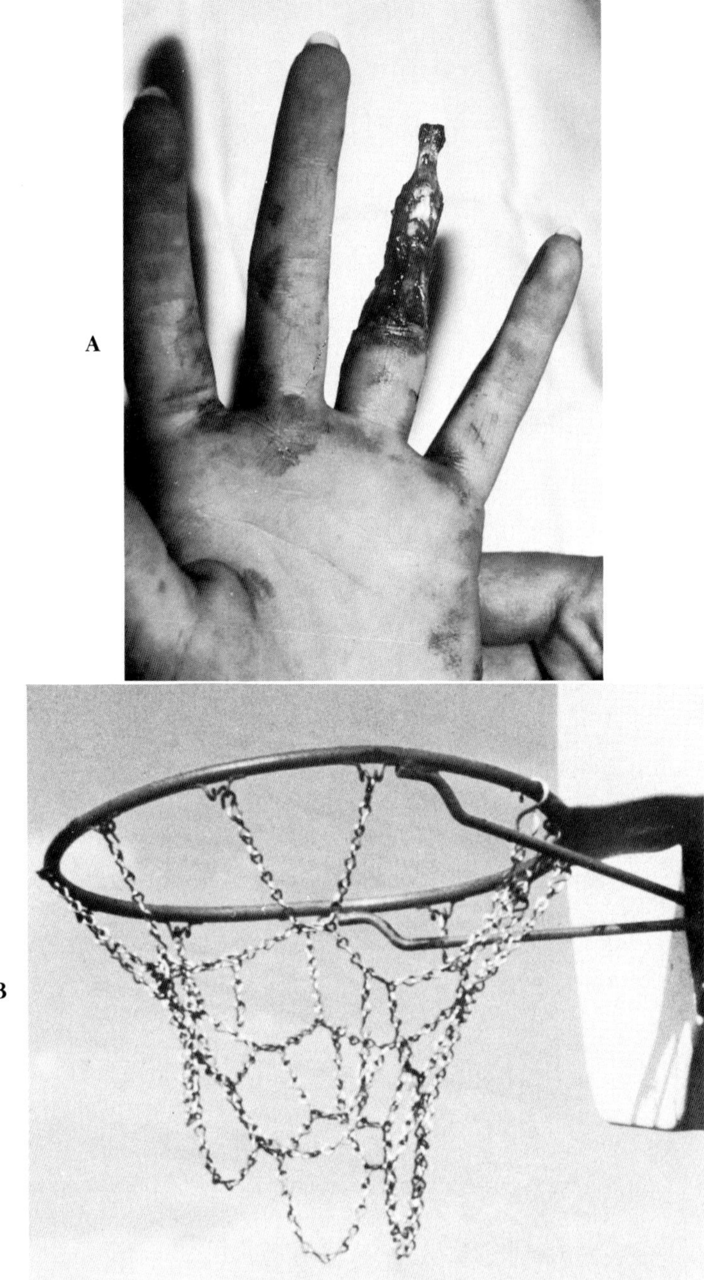

Fig. 10-1. A, Ring avulsion of the finger, the result of attempting to dunk a basketball through a chain net, **B.**

letes usually results from continuous compression and repeated trauma to the involved nerve. It typically presents as an entrapment neuropathy.[10]

The ulnar nerve is the one most frequently injured in athletic activities involving the upper extremity. The nerve may be affected at the elbow or wrist, as well as at the hand. The ulnar nerve is most vulnerable at the elbow, and injury may result from direct trauma as well as from repetitive motion and swelling within the confined canal. The latter situation is most frequently encountered in the throwing athlete in baseball but is also observed in skiing, weightlifting, and stick-handling sports. The nerve may be compressed within the cubital tunnel, particularly if there is a tight groove. The nerve may be naturally hypermobile or may become so by stretching of the ulnar groove ligament. The hypermobile nerve becomes subject to repetitive trauma in the groove and over the bony prominence of the medial epicondyle. The ulnar nerve is not frequently involved in the forearm, though direct blows, lacerations, and occasionally muscle hypertrophy or edema may compromise the nerve in this region.

The nerve may be compressed in the canal of Guyon at the wrist. The canal is bordered distally and laterally by the hook of the hamate and medially and proximally by the pisiform and is covered by the volar carpal ligament. The superficial branch of the nerve provides sensation to the ulnar half of the ring and little fingers, whereas the deep branch supplies the hypothenar muscles, all the interossei, the lumbricals of the ring and little fingers, the deep head of the flexor pollicis brevis, and the adductor pollicis. Compromise of the nerve most commonly results from chronic overuse. Symptoms include pain along the hypothenar eminence and in the ring and little fingers, along with ulnar intrinsic muscle weakness. The syndrome is distinguished from more proximal involvement by sparing of the flexor carpi ulnaris and flexor digitorum profundus to the ring and little fingers. Touring cyclists often develop this syndrome because of sustained pressure of the handlebars on the ulnar nerve[8,14] (Fig. 10-2). The numbness and weakness may be relieved by wearing of cycling gloves, padding of the handlegrips, alteration of the handle angle, and adjustment of the seat height. This treatment in association with rest will relieve symptoms in most cases without need for surgical decompression of the canal. However, not all cases respond to conservative therapy. The authors have seen persistent ulnar nerve palsy some 12 months after onset during a transcontinental bicycle ride.

The ulnar nerve may be compressed after a fracture of the pisiform or the hamate. The hook of the hamate may be fractured in a fall but breaks more typically during a tennis, baseball, or golf swing.[32] A carpal tunnel view with the wrist in maximum dorsiflexion will demonstrate the fracture (Fig. 10-3). It is imperative to visualize the base of the hamate because most fractures occur at this site. Blunt, repetitive compression to the heel of the palm may also result in scarring and compression within the canal of Guyon.

Acute trauma may produce false aneurysm, arteriovenous fistula, or thrombosis of the ulnar artery, any of which can compress the ulnar nerve[11] (Fig. 10-4). Treatment includes decompression of the canal with vascular repair as indicated.

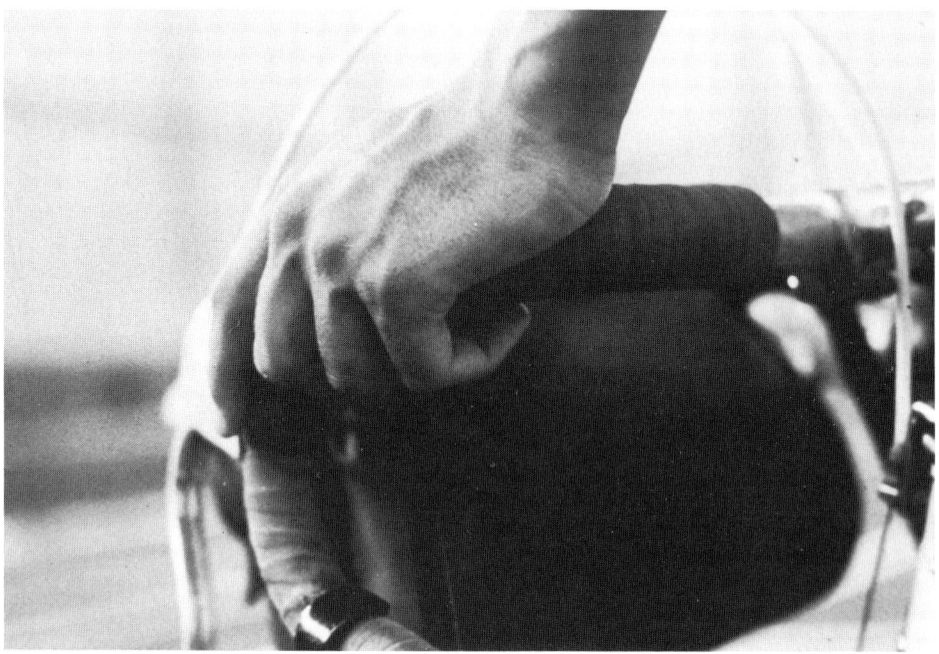

Fig. 10-2. Sustained pressure of the handlebars may result in compromise of the ulnar nerve in Guyon's canal.

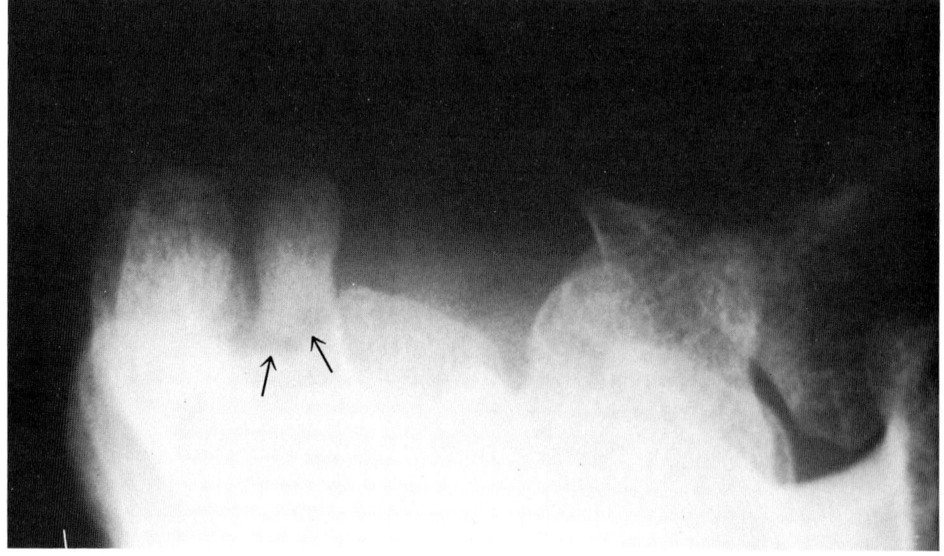

Fig. 10-3. Carpal tunnel view demonstrating fracture of the hook of the hamate.

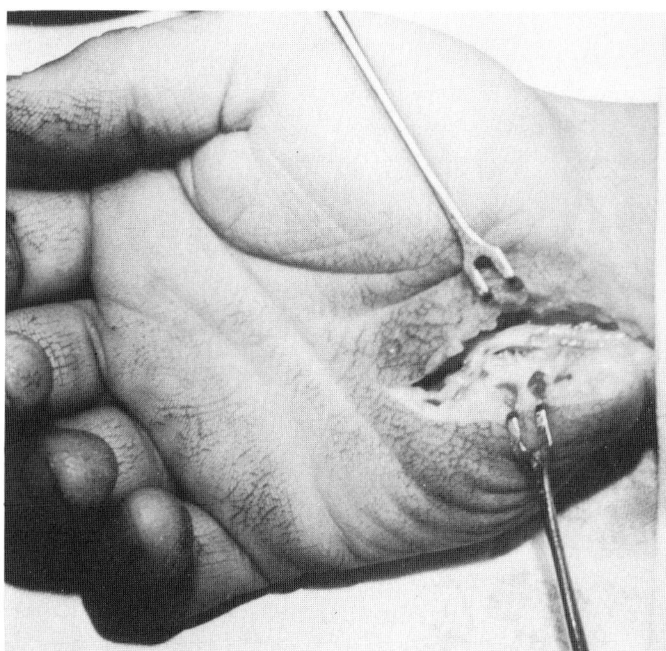

Fig. 10-4. Thrombosis of the ulnar artery.

The median nerve is not so commonly involved as the ulnar during athletic activities though injury from direct and repetitive trauma does occur. The median nerve may be compressed in a tight carpal canal, particularly with repetitive activities such as gripping, cycling, throwing, and repetitive wrist flexion and extension in weight lifting and fly casting.[21] The nerve may also be compromised by direct trauma and secondary swelling or hypertrophy of the flexor synovium. Women or girls engaged in repetitious activities such as fishing and cycling are particularly predisposed. Most cases respond to rest, anti-inflammatory medication, and other symptomatic measures.

The median nerve enters the forearm medially to the lacertus fibrosus in proximity to the brachial artery and biceps tendon. Entrapment of the nerve at this site is termed the "pronator syndrome" and may result from repetitive exercise and resultant hypertrophy of the flexor-pronator group. Patients complain of pain and tenderness over the area of compression as well as paresthesias in the median distribution of the hand. Motor involvement is generally mild with sporadic sparing of individual muscles.

The pronator syndrome is often a difficult diagnosis and must be distinguished from carpal tunnel syndrome. Tinel's sign will be positive over the area of compression. There is variable intrinsic involvement and usually sparing of muscles innervated by the anterior interosseous nerve. There will be pain in the proximal volar forearm increased by pronation and wrist flexion against resistance. Electromyography is often useful in the determination of the level of involvement. Compression most often occurs at the level of the pronator teres but may develop at the lacertus fibrosus and the origin of the flexor digitorum sublimus arch. Diagnostic features helpful in localization are reproduction of pain with resisted elbow flexion and forearm supination, an indication of compression at the level of the lacertus. Pain reproduced by resistance to flexion of the long finger flexor sublimus is suggestive of involvement at the sublimus arch.

The anterior interosseous nerve innervates the flexor pollicis longus, the flexor profundus of the index and long fingers, and the pronator quadratus. The nerve may be compressed at its origin some 5 to 8 cm distal to the lateral epicondyle or farther distally. The anterior interosseous nerve is most commonly injured in repetitive activities such as throwing, racket sports, or weight lifting. There may be characteristic weakness of flexion of the distal phalanx of the thumb and index and long fingers and of the pronator quadratus. The clinical picture may be variable because of the presence of interneural communications in the forearm such as the Martin-Gruber anastomosis between the median and ulnar nerves.

As with other neural compression syndromes, rest, anti-inflammatory medications, and other symptomatic treatment will usually relieve median nerve compression, but surgical decompression and neurolysis will be required in some cases.

The radial nerve may be contused, compressed, or severed in athletic injuries. The nerve may be damaged in the spiral groove as it courses around the humerus. The nerve is also vulnerable where it passes under the lateral head of the triceps bordered by the fibrous arcade. Compression can occur in this region with exercise, particularly throwing motions.

The nerve passes through the lateral septum over the epicondyle and divides into the superficial sensory branch, which travels distally over the extensor carpi radialis brevis, and the posterior interosseous branch, which passes through the supinator. Before entering the supinator, a sensory branch (the recurrent radial nerve) emerges. Irritation of this nerve is believed to be a cause of lateral epicondylitis. The posterior interosseous nerve innervates the wrist extensors, finger and thumb extensors, abductor pollicis longus, and supinator. It is most commonly injured in throwing sports, skiing, and those activities that demand repetitive, tight gripping, such as golf, tennis, and weight lifting.

As for the aforementioned neuropathies, radial nerve compression syndromes usually respond to conservative measures. However, full muscle power may not return after surgical decompression for chronic radial palsy allowed to persist for prolonged periods of time.[21]

"Bowler's thumb" refers to neuropathy of the ulnar digital nerve of the thumb.[6,7,13,18,28,31] Repetitive pressure against the base of the bowler's thumb produces perineural fibrosis of this relatively subcutaneous nerve and the resulting neuropathy. The bowler will complain of pain, paresthesias on digital pressure, numbness of the ulnovolar aspect of the thumb and a tender, firm fusiform mass.[6] If

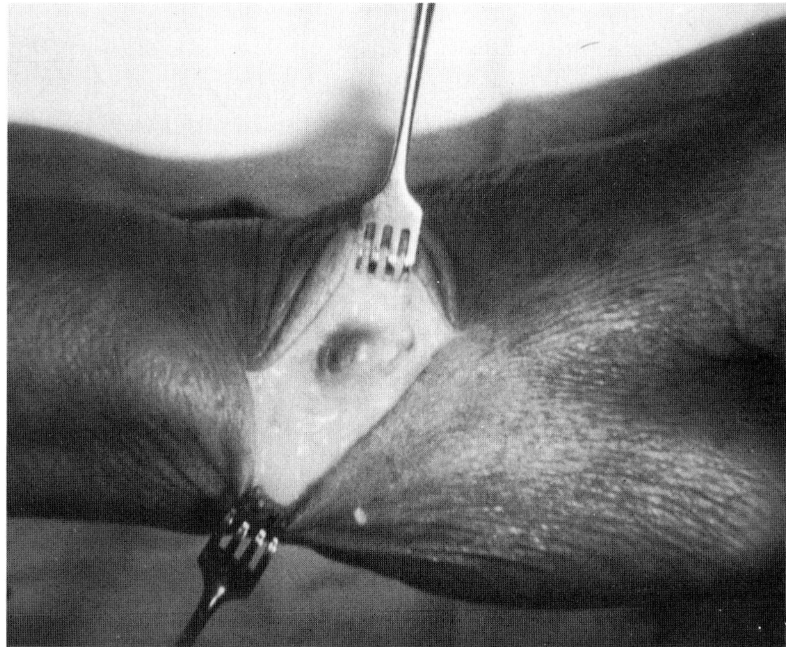

Fig. 10-5. Arteriovenous fistula of the superficial radial artery.

detected early, the condition usually responds to modification of the bowler's grip and use of a larger bored or padded thumb hole. If a mass has developed, surgical neurolysis under magnification is often required.[6] Transposition of the nerve to a more dorsoulnar aspect of the thumb is performed.[7] Awareness of this condition may prevent unnecessary removal of the neuroma. Symptoms may be relieved without excision of the neuroma, thereby maintaining sensation along the ulnar aspect of the thumb.

VASCULAR PROBLEMS

Vascular injuries may result from repeated trauma to any region yet are more prevalent in certain areas such as the canal of Guyon. Aneurysm and thrombosis of the ulnar artery have been reported by Millender and others.[27] Arteriovenous fistulas may also be encountered (Fig. 10-5).

The so-called hypothenar hammer syndrome is characterized by scarring, aneurysm, or thrombosis of the ulnar artery as the result of repeated trauma. It has been observed in industrial workers and particularly in handball players and baseball catchers. Symptoms develop from the thrombosis as well as the decrease in vascular flow and the secondary compression of the ulnar nerve.

Repeated compression injuries will sometimes cause perivascular fibrosis and decreased vascularity of the digits. Lowrey has reported decreased digital perfusion to the index finger of the glove hand of 13 of 22 baseball catchers examined by

Doppler flow and Allen's test.[17] Buckhout studied digital perfusion of handball players and observed that decreased perfusion may result from acute injury or repeated trauma but that players with more than 200 hours of accumulated playing time were at greater risk of developing symptomatic alteration in perfusion.[4] Symptoms may be improved by use of protective gloves. In baseball, modification of the glove lessens the force of impact. Additional padding and alterations in the webbing can be helpful.

The index fingers of baseball pitchers have been involved from stimulation of the local sympathetic nervous system with secondary diminished perfusion of the index finger. Symptoms of a cold, pale digit have been seen after a period of gripping the baseball. This can often be relieved by rest and vasodilators though sympathetic block has been indicated in certain cases. The ulcer that rarely develops on the fingertip should be protected from secondary infection. In one instance, chronic involvement in a catcher resulted in secondary osteomyelitis of the distal phalanx requiring excision of the sequestrum.

Vascular compromise stemming from acute compartment syndrome occurring after fracture is well recognized but must be remembered by physicians treating sports-related injuries. For example, a recent report documented volar compartment syndrome after Salter II distal radius fracture in an adolescent.[20]

TENDON

Tendinitis or tenosynovitis of the extensor tendons in the wrist and hand frequently occurs in the throwing and lifting sports. This is especially the case early in the season or after a particularly prolonged workout requiring a great number of repetitions. Most cases of extensor involvement clear with rest and other conservative measures. De Quervain's tenosynovitis is relatively uncommon in the young athlete. The flexor tendons are more often involved in the carpal tunnel, with secondary median nerve compression a possibility.

Trigger digits may result from chronic repetitive flexion of the fingers or trauma to the base of the fingers and the distal area of the palm. This is particularly common among handball players who frequently decline to use protective gloves. They develop thickening of the subcutaneous tissue with secondary triggering of digits. Most cases respond to conservative management, but those with chronic symptoms and pronounced soft-tissue thickening may require surgical release.

Recurrent subluxation of the extensor carpi ulnaris tendon may result from forearm hypersupination injuries sustained during athletics. Trauma is a relatively uncommon cause of this phenomenon. If the subluxation is chronic and sufficiently symptomatic, surgical reconstruction of the sixth dorsal compartment is indicated.[5]

KARATE

Karate means 'empty hand', originally 'Chinese boxing,' in Japanese. Karate veterans toughen their limbs, converting them into weapons for striking. One achieves this by hitting objects causing a progressive increase in the thickness of the scar tissue.[16] A correctly executed thrust and hand strike uses the index and long finger metacarpal heads. Axial compression forces are transmitted from the metacarpal to the distal carpal row, which is splinted by the taut tendons spanning the wrist. To minimize the risk of injury, the thumb is tucked out of the way and striking is done only with the index and long finger knuckles while the interphalangeal joints are maximally flexed and the fist maximally tightened.[21] At impact, the wrist is pronated.

Tenosynovitis may develop in areas of chronic use. The mass of scar tissue in some cases may entrap extensor tendons, so that surgical removal is necessary.[9]

Intra-articular fractures may occur.[15] Improper technique during thrusts, blows, and the blocking of kicks may produce angular torsional forces sufficient to produce fractures and joint injuries.[12,22-26] Management of such injuries is considered in other chapters of this symposium.

SKIN

A blister is a collection of fluid between separated epidermal layers. Callus refers to a protective accumulation of epidermis at sites of friction.

The hands of gymnasts require protection but also must be sufficiently unencumbered to retain a feel for the bar. Elastic tape or leather hand protection may be worn. Holes are cut through the tape for the index and middle fingers, and the tape is placed over the benzoin-coated palm. The tape is held at the wrist with adhesive tape. Calluses typically build up on the hands of the gymnast as the season progresses. Gymnasts follow a daily routine of cleansing and moisterizing their hands to control calluses. The callus should be trimmed by shaving with a razor or smoothed with sandpaper or file. The callus should be trimmed to the level of surrounding skin. If not trimmed, the callus may catch on equipment and tear. If it is completely removed, the underlying skin will be left tender and at risk of tearing. Gymnasts are advised to switch from one apparatus to another exercise when they notice hot spots developing on the hand.[3] After the workout, the hands are cleansed to remove gym chalk, which might otherwise dry the skin, increasing the likelihood of blisters and rips. Hand cream or glycerine-based lotion is also applied several times daily.

The possibility of infection beneath the callus must not be forgotten. If the skin rips, it should be cleansed and an antiseptic applied. The skin should be kept clean and lubricated with lotion to prevent cracking and breaking down.

Weight lifters are particularly prone to develop blisters across the palm at the base of the digits, especially when using a bar with deep knurling[21] (Fig. 10-6). Baseball pitchers are also frequently troubled by blister formation.[33] Blisters may develop on the thumb from repetitive throwing of the curve ball and on the fingertips from the fast ball. Blisters on the fingertips may indicate that the ball is being thrown correctly, but they can still interfere with throwing. Benzoin may be applied in order to toughen the fingers, particularly during the preseason and during prolonged layoffs from pitching. The early application of ice to hot spots or blisters may diminish the accumulation of fluid. Blisters may also be aspirated using sterile technique, and the outer

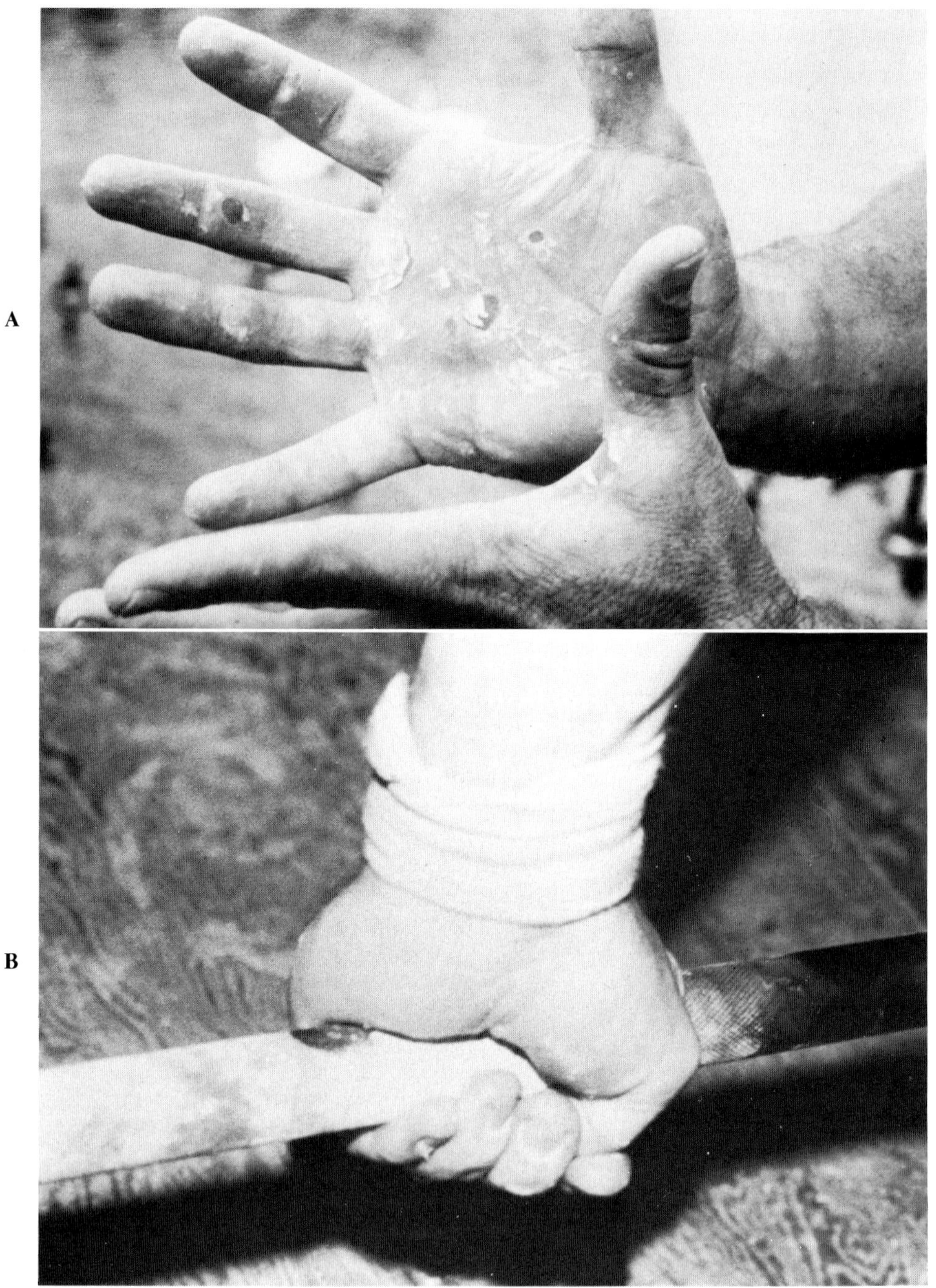

Fig. 10-6. This weightlifter developed extensive blister and callus formation, **A**, from repeated lifting of the deeply knurled bar, **B**.

layer held in place with moleskin attached with benzoin. Should a blister tear, it is cleansed and the shreds are removed. The main cover is then replaced with benzoin.[30]

Special mention must be made of the risk of infection when abrasions or other wounds occur on artificial turf. The small fibers in Astroturf may enter the wound and produce irritation. It is imperative that these wounds be thoroughly debrided and treated to prevent secondary infection.

GLOVES AND PROTECTIVE DEVICES

Gloves and other protective devices are used to protect the athlete's upper extremity, with the demands of the particular sport determining the nature of the protective device. For example, the glove used in lacrosse has a flexible thumb with extra padding over the carpal scaphoid. It is essential that the player have a feel for the stick, and accordingly the palm is left open. Some players gain an even better tactile control by excising the finger portion of the gloves out to the tips. This subjects the player to risk of injury to a finger and to risk of incurring a penalty because this practice is illegal.

There are gloves specific to the needs of a wide variety of sports (Fig. 10-7). Goalies, the sole member of the soccer team who are permitted to use their hands, have a specific type of glove. Cyclists use cycling gloves or alternatively pad the handlebars to prevent pressure on the ulnar nerve in the canal of Guyon. Fencers wear a gauntlet to protect their wrists from thrusts. Handball gloves are designed to prevent the repetitive direct trauma to the hand with secondary soft-tissue thickening, bone damage, soft-tissue injury, and decreased digital perfusion. Yet many players elect to compete without this protection because of their desire to achieve a greater feel for the ball. Wheelchair racers wear gloves to prevent damage to hands with impaired sensation. Participants in racket sports may wear light cotton gloves inside outer gloves to prevent skin irritation from excessive sweating and may go through several pairs of these during one match. Baseball players wear protective gloves to prevent blister and callus formation while batting. Some players rely on other gloves to protect the hands while sliding. Football receivers use a glove designed to permit surehandedness in cold weather (Fig. 10-8).

Long ski gloves protect not only from the cold and snow in freezing weather, but also protect the wrist from laceration, particularly from a sharp ski edge[19] (Fig. 10-9). Skiers should not wear short gloves. The young skier's gloves should be checked to be certain that he has not outgrown them, leaving his wrists susceptible to laceration from a ski edge. In skiing it is particularly important to protect the thumb because injuries there are very common.[29]

The boxing glove is actually a mitten because the thumb is separated from the other fingers. An extra pad guards the thumb, and a firm leather pad in the palm supports the finger metacarpals.

Platform tennis enthusiasts, who play in cold weather, frequently wear a mitten or

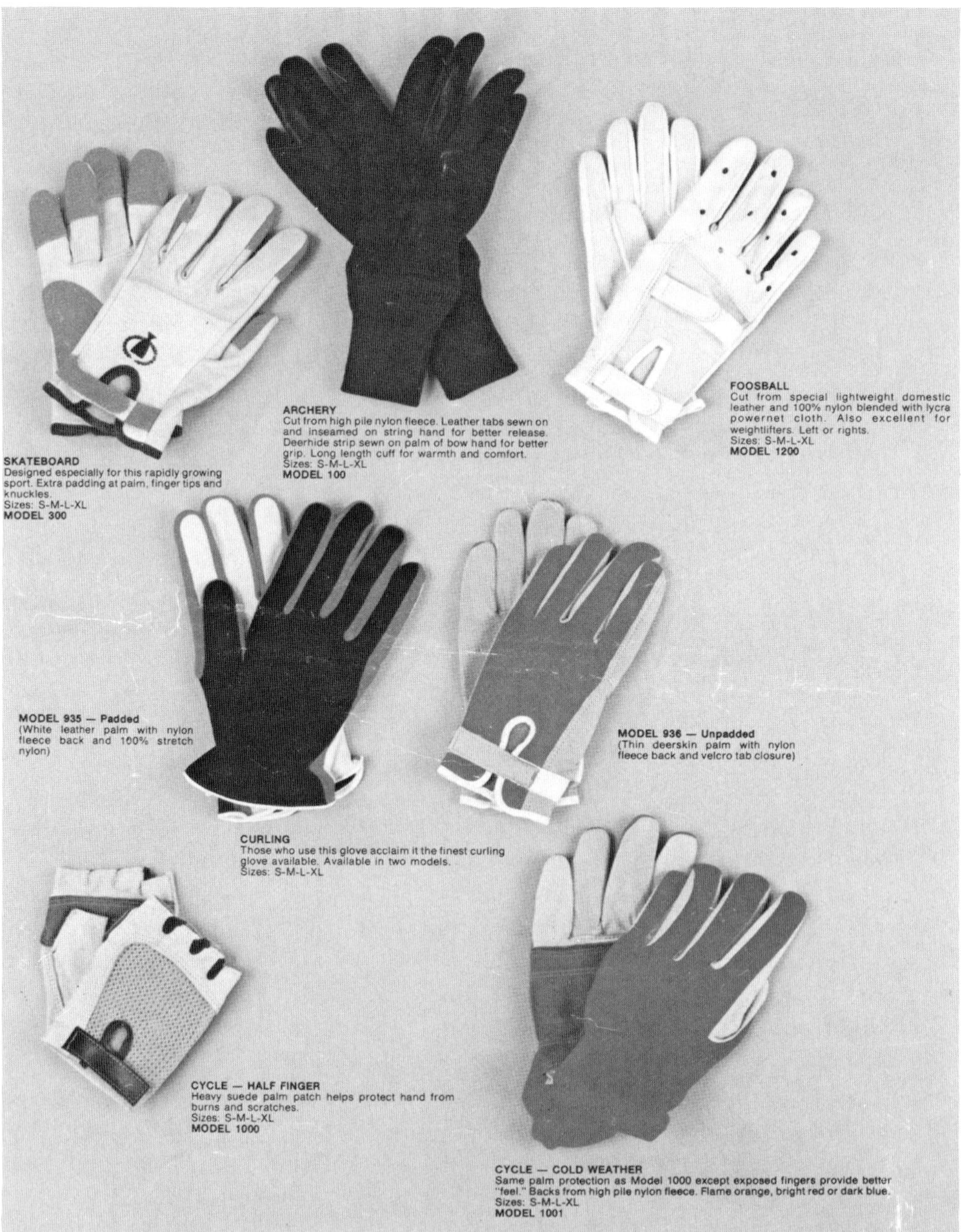

Fig. 10-7. Specialty gloves specific for various sports. (Courtesy The Trophy Glove Company, Albia, Iowa.)

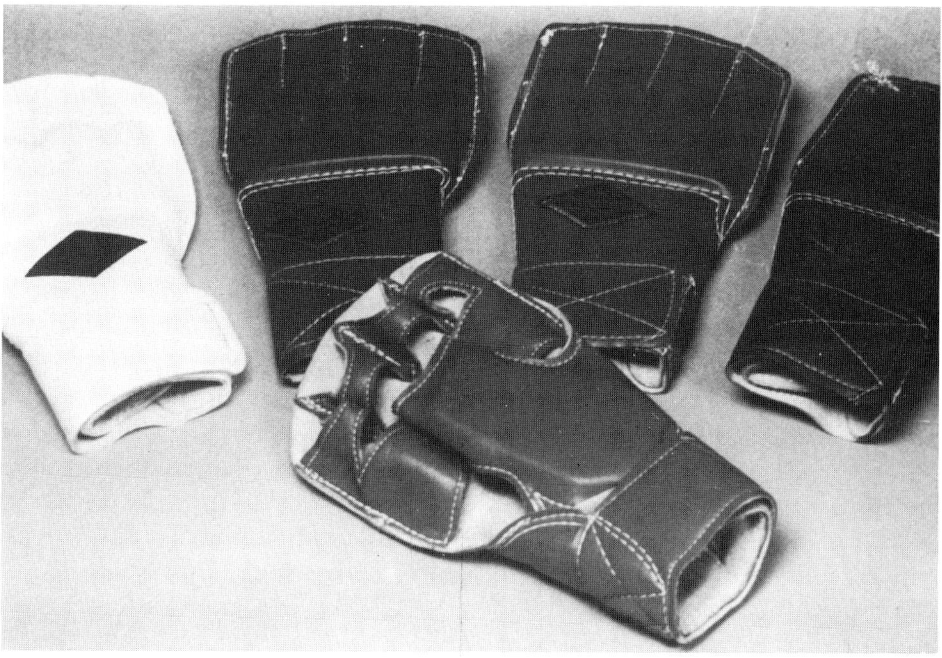

Fig. 10-8. Glove typically worn by football linemen.

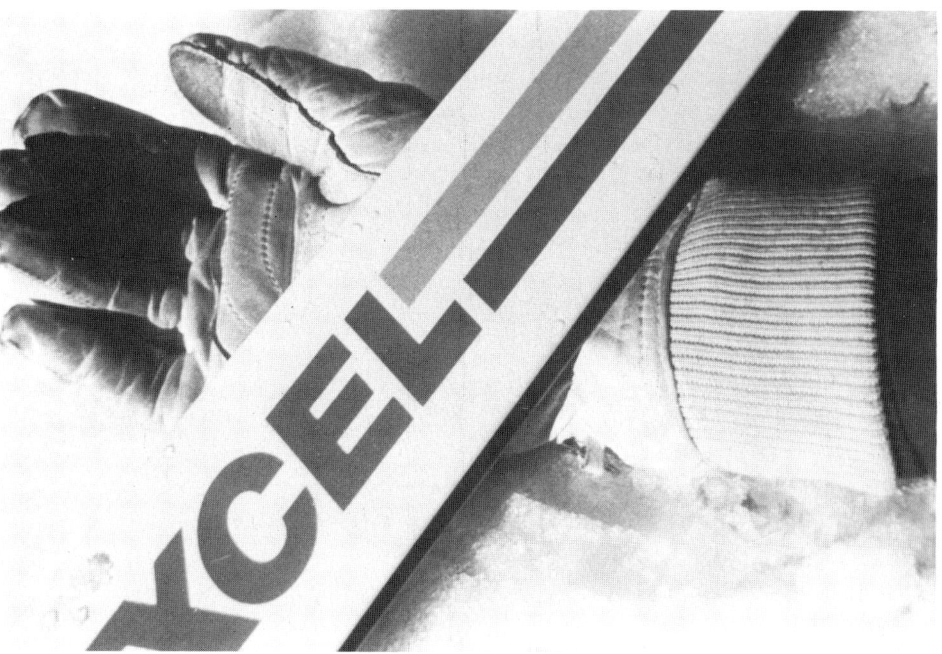

Fig. 10-9. Long gloves protect the skier's wrist against injury from a sharp ski edge.

wool sock with a hole in it to receive the handle of the paddle. This ingenious glove permits the player's hand to remain warm while retaining a feel for the paddle.[21]

There are specific gloves for sports such as curling and archery. There are many gloves designed for hunting, with the fingers in various parts of the hand left bare or rapidly accessible to permit firing of the gun when the occasion demands.

The baseball glove is specifically designed for the particular position. The catcher's mitt is flexible so that the player may catch one handed, thereby protecting his ungloved hand from injury. Gloves with specific padding are manufactured according to the requirements of the catcher.

Most catchers wear a pad inside the mitt to absorb shocks and to prevent thrombosis or aneurysm of the ulnar artery. The aneurysm is most likely to occur at the hook of the hamate where the vessel is least protected.

Protective devices are lighter and more durable than ever before. They have been of great help in preventing injury and protecting existing injuries sufficiently to allow the athlete to play. The nature and rules of the various sports determine the type of protective devices that may be employed. In professional football, a light or plaster cast is permissible provided that it is protected with an adequate thickness of a soft material, such as foam rubber. Under the rules of intercollegiate and interscholastic football, however, sole leather or other unyielding substances are prohibited on the hand, wrist or forearm, despite the extent to which they are insulated. This is ironic insofar as it is permissible to wrap the hand with multiple layers of iced tape producing the virtual equivalent of a maul and yet wearing even the most modest metal splint is a violation of the rules. Fortunately, a protective silicone rubber splint has been devised.[1,2,21] This permits the safe return to competition of athletes who have sustained injuries such as wrist sprains and healing fractures, or who have undergone recent surgical repair or reconstruction of soft tissue, bone, or joints.

The protective splint is constructed from gauze impregnated with a commercially available silicone rubber, RTV 11(GE) (Fig. 10-10). The splint conforms to the injured part and can be thickened as much as necessary to provide protection. The injured part may be further protected with underlying felt or foam rubber pads. The splint is extremely durable yet is not porous and has a tendency to produce maceration beneath the cast. It is therefore not used as a permanent cast but is worn only during practice and competition.[1,21]

The splint is easy to apply.[1] A thin coat of lubricant is first spread on the skin and gauze wrapped smoothly on the body part. A catalyst is mixed with the silicone, and a generous layer of silicone is applied. Generally, three or four thicknesses of gauze with the silicone worked into each layer with a spatula are used. The silicone requires about 3 hours in which to cure or harden at room temperature. Once cured, the splint is cut along the ulnar side to permit removal. It is secured for competition purposes with adhesive tape. Then a covering of soft materials, such as foam rubber, of at least one-half inch thickness is used to protect the cast. A bivalved hard cast is worn at all other times. The light plastic cast is customarily used because of its resistance to water.

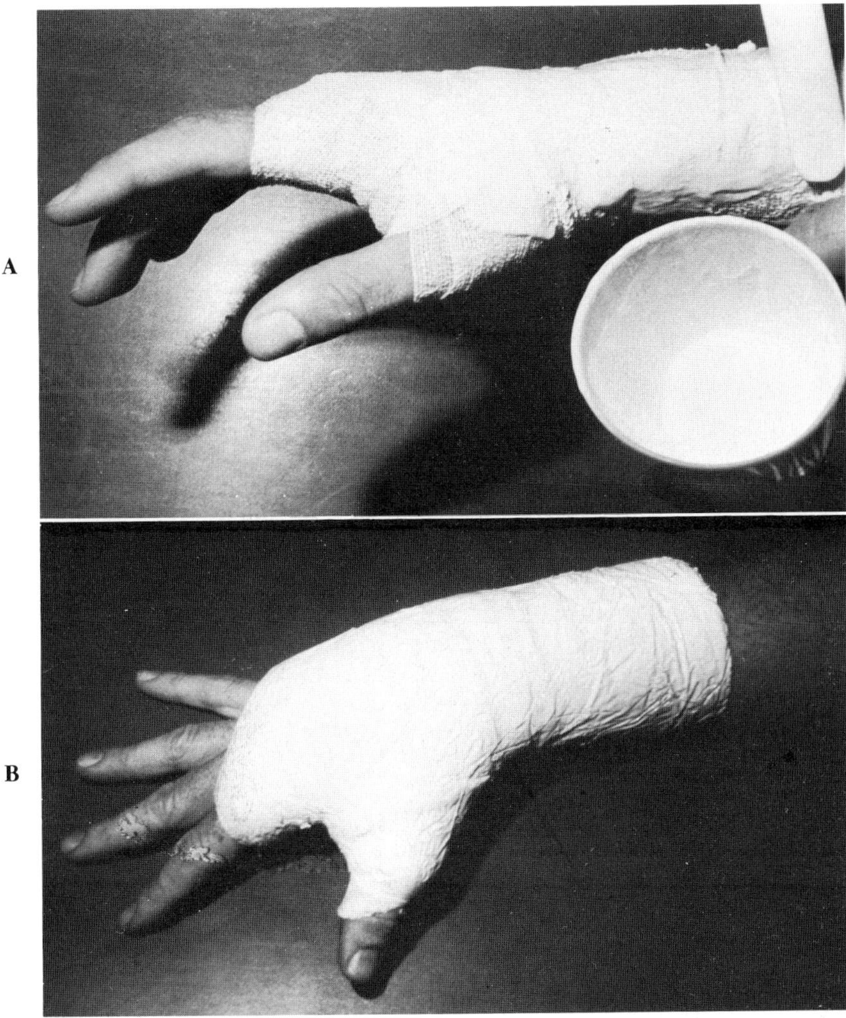

Fig. 10-10 Application of the silicone cast.

Other soft, slow-recoil, unicellular materials such as heat-moldable plastizote are useful in specific cases. The direct protection from blows afforded by these materials exceeds that of silicone, yet these materials have the disadvantage of not conforming to the extremity as readily.

REFERENCES

1. Bassett, F.H., et al.: A protective splint of silicone rubber, Am. J. Sports Med. 7:358-360, 1979.
2. Bergfeld, J.A., et al.: Soft playing splint for protection of significant hand and wrist injuries in sports, Am. J. Sports Med. 10:293-295, 1982.
3. Black, S.A.: Blistered and torn hands disrupt gymnast's training, First Aider, Cramer 48(6):10-11, 1979.
4. Buckhout, B.C., and Warner, M.A.: Digital perfusion of handball players: effects of repeated ball impact on structures of the hand, Am. J. Sports Med. 8:206-207, 1980.

5. Burkhart, S.S., et al.: Post-traumatic recurrent subluxation of the extensor carpi ulnaris tendon, J. Hand Surg. 7:1-3, 1982.

6. Dobyns, J.H., et al.: Bowler's thumb: diagnosis and treatment: a review of seventeen cases, J. Bone Joint Surg. (Am.) 54:751-755, 1972.

7. Dunham, W., et al.: Bowler's thumb, Clin. Orthop. (83):99-101, 1972.

8. Eckman, P.B., et al.: Ulnar neuropathy in bicycle riders, Arch. Neurol. 32:130-132, 1975.

9. Gardner, R.C.: Hypertrophic infiltrative tendinitis (HIT syndrome) of the long extensor: the abused karate hand, J.A.M.A. 211:1009-1010, 1970.

10. Hirasawa, Y., and Sakakeda, M.: Sports and peripheral nerve injury, Am. J. Sports Med. 11:420-426, 1983.

11. Kaplan, E.B., and Ziede, M.S.: Aneurysm of the ulnar artery: a case report, Bull. Hosp. Joint Dis. 33:197-199, 1972.

12. Kelly, D.W., et al.: Index metacarpal fractures in karate, Phys. Sportsmed. 8(3):103-106, 1980.

13. Kisner, W.H.: Thumb neuroma: a hazard of ten pin bowling, Br. J. Plast. Surg. 29:225-226, 1976.

14. Kulund, D.N., and Brubaker, C.E.: Injuries in the Bikecentennial Tour, Phys. Sportsmed 6(6):74-78, 1978.

15. LaRose, J.H., and Sik, K.D.: Knuckle fracture: a mechanism of injury, J.A.M.A. 296:893-894, 1968.

16. LaRose, J.H., and Sik, K.D.: Karate hand-conditioning, Med. Sci. Sports 1(2):95-98, 1969.

17. Lowery, C.W., et al.: Digital vessel trauma from repetitive impacts in baseball catchers, J. Hand Surg. 1:236-238, 1976.

18. Marmor, L.L.: Bowler's thumb, J. Bone Joint Surg. (Am.) 52:379-381, 1970.

19. Match, R.M.: Laceration of the median nerve from skiing, Am. J. Sports Med. 6:22-25, 1978.

20. Matthews, L.S.: Acute volar compartment syndrome secondary to distal radius fracture in an athlete, Am. J. Sports Med. 11:6-7, 1983.

21. McCue, F.C., III: The elbow, wrist and hand. In Kulund, D.: The injured athlete, Philadelphia, 1982, J.B. Lippincott Co.

22. McCue, F.C., III, and Abbott, J.L.: The treatment of mallet finger and boutonnière deformities, Va. Med. Monthly 94:623, 1967.

23. McCue, F.C., III, et al.: Athletic injuries of the proximal interphalangeal joint requiring surgical treatment, J. Bone Joint Surg. (Am.) 52:937-956, 1970.

24. McCue, F.C., III, et al.: The coach's finger, Am. J. Sports Med. 2:270-275, 1974.

25. McCue, F.C., III, et al.: Hand injuries in athletes, Surg. Rounds 2:24-30, Jan. 1979.

26. McCue, F.C., III, et al.: Hand injuries in athletics, Am. J. Sports Med. 7:275-286, 1979.

27. Millender, L.H., et al.: Aneurysms in thrombosis of the ulnar artery on the hand, Arch. Surg. 105:686-690, 1972.

28. Minkow, F.V., and Bassett, F.H., III: Bowler's thumb, Clin. Orthop. (83):115-117, 1972.

29. Mogan, J.V., and Davis, P.H.: Upper extremity injuries in skiing, Clin. Sports Med. 1:295-307, 1982.

30. Raymond, P.: Care of the hands, Oarsman 9(2):40-41, 1977.

31. Siegel, I.M.: Bowling thumb neuroma, J.A.M.A. 192:163, 1965.

32. Torisu, T.: Fracture of the hook of the hamate by a golfswing, Clin. Orthop. (83:)91-94, 1972.

33. Vere-Hodge, N.: Injuries in cricket. In Armstrong, J.R., and Tuckers, W.E., editors: Injury in sport, Springfield, Ill., 1964, Charles C Thomas, Publisher.

11. Fractures of the distal ends of radius and ulna

Charles P. Melone, Jr.
Joel B. Grad

Proficiency in athletics is frequently compromised by injury to the radius and ulna. These parallel bones with hinge and rotation joints at both ends constitute a unique anatomic unit that is essential to the mobility and stability of the elbow, wrist, and hand. Disruption of this unit at its distal end is prevalent in athletes because of the continual exposure to severe angular, rotatory, or compressive forces resulting from falls or direct blows.

In contrast to midforearm fractures, which typically involve both bones, those of the distal radius and ulna usually demonstrate obvious breakage of only one bone. Nonetheless, these seemingly isolated fractures seldom occur without injury to the soft-tissue attachments or articulations of the adjacent bone. The classic example of this distinctive pattern of injury is the Galeazzi fracture of the distal third of the radius that occurs with dislocation of the distal radioulnar joint, and a far more common occurrence is the articular fracture of the distal radius, which usually disrupts both the radioulnar and radiocarpal joints. Even the solitary nightstick fracture of the distal end of the ulna is prone to encroach on the interosseous membrane with consequential limitation of radial rotation. Optimal management of these fractures requires prompt recognition of the multiple components of injury and an accurate restoration of the skeletal architecture.

ROENTGENOGRAPHIC ANALYSIS

Despite similar mechanisms of injury that in many instances produce identical physical findings, fractures of the distal ends of the radius and ulna compose a diverse spectrum of severity. The key to an accurate diagnosis is a careful roentgenographic analysis of each injury. Also, since the functional result after fracture so closely parallels the accuracy of reduction, the roentgenograms provide a reliable guide for successful treatment.

It is axiomatic that the fracture and the joints above and below the obvious site of injury must be carefully scrutinized. High-quality anteroposterior (AP), posteroanterior (PA), lateral, oblique, and, in many instances, comparable contralateral views afford a thorough roentgenographic profile of the injured parts. The roentgenograms are inspected for displacement, angulation, comminution, and malrotation of the fracture as well as concomitant narrowing of the interosseous space, radioulnar subluxation, and in the younger patient epiphyseal separation.

Displaced diaphyseal and metaphyseal fractures invariably cause encroachment on the interosseous space, which is best detected on the AP roentgenogram taken with the forearm in full supination. In this projection the radius and ulna are in a position of maximum divergence, and the width of the interosseous space can be accurately assessed. Although some narrowing of the space is consistent with satisfactory function, obliteration of this interval causes a serious loss of forearm rotation. A prerequisite for maximum recovery is restoration of the interosseous space, which can only be accomplished by an accurate reduction.

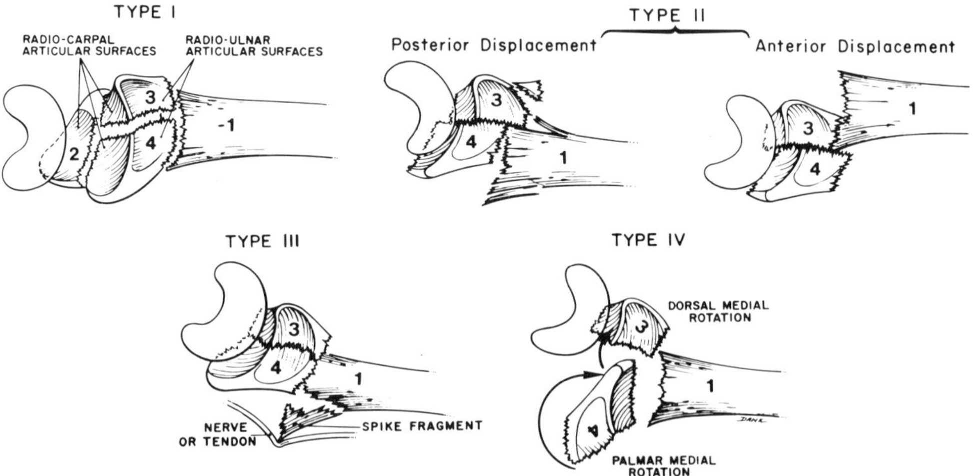

Fig. 11-1. Articular fractures of the distal radius consist of four basic components: the radial shaft, *1*; the radial styloid, *2*; the dorsal medial fragment, *3*; and the palmar medial fragment, *4*. Displacement of the key medial fragments causes a serious disruption of the distal radial articulations and is the basis for classification into four fracture types. Type II fractures are prevalent among adult athletes.

Fig. 11-2. Type II articular fracture demonstrating excessive shortening (9 mm) of the medial corner of the radius, **A,** and anterior displacement of the palmar medial fragment, **B.** Continuous skeletal traction employing pins and plaster, **C,** results in a stable reduction of the medial complex and excellent restoration of the radiocarpal and radioulnar joints, **D** and **E.** For numbers see Fig. 11-1.

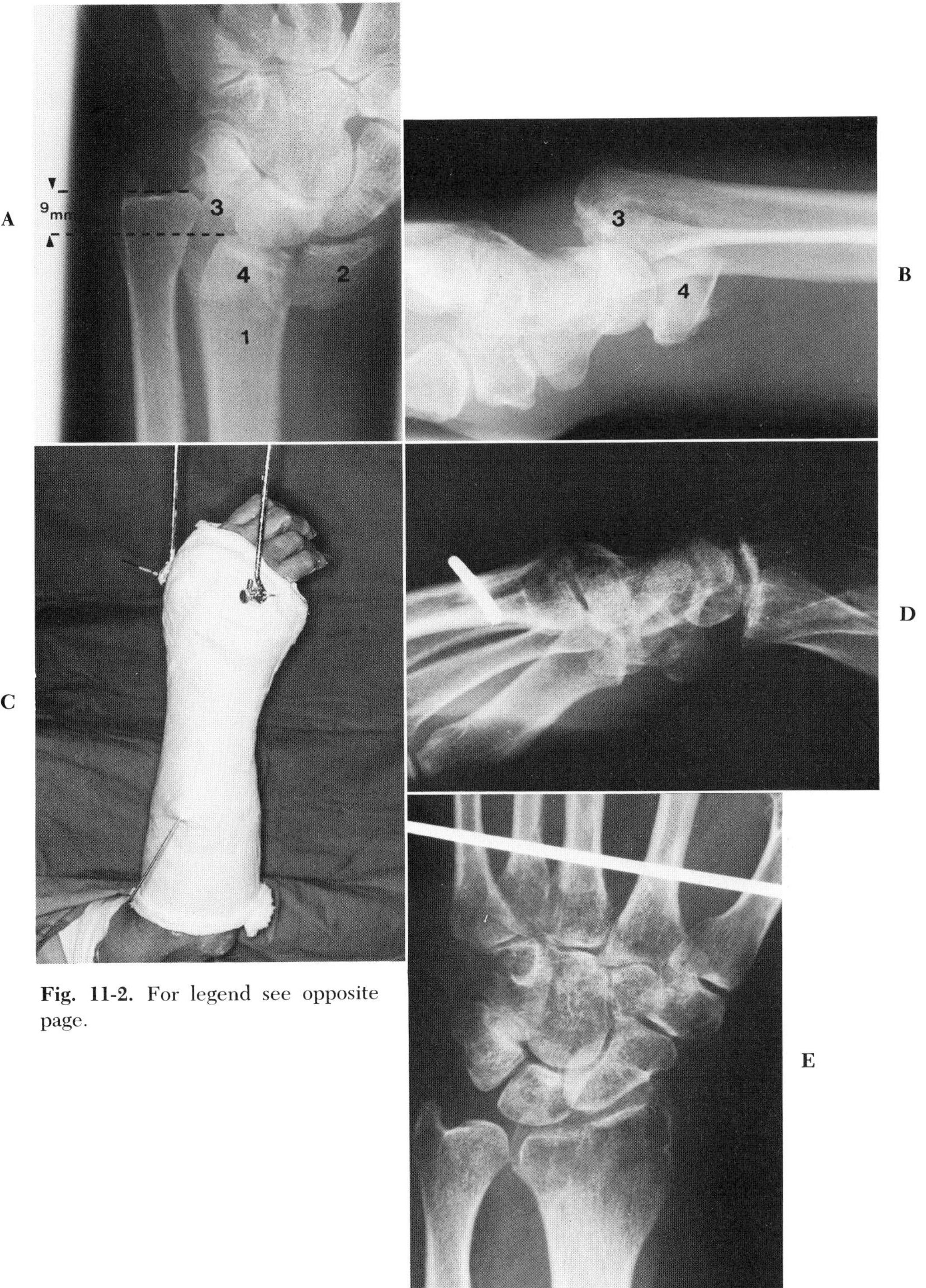

Fig. 11-2. For legend see opposite page.

Another fundamental goal of treatment is preservation of a stable distal radioulnar joint. Distal radial fractures at all levels—diaphyseal, metaphyseal, and articular—typically demonstrate proximal displacement, which is likely to cause subluxation of the radioulnar joint. Lidström,[17] in a roentgenographic review of distal radial fractures, determined that only a 6 mm collapse of the radius significantly disturbed function of the radioulnar articulation, and the studies of Palmer and Werner[22] indicate that even lesser discrepancies in radial and ulnar length may cause major alterations in load bearing and serious derangements of the wrist.

Radioulnar congruity is assessed by measurement of the ulnar length: the vertical distance between the distal ends of the medial corner of the radius and the ulnar head (Fig. 11-2, A). Since supination creates an illusory shortening of the ulna and pronation projects an image of increased ulnar length, this measurement, traditionally termed "ulnar variance," should be calculated on a PA roentgenogram with the wrist in neutral position.[21] Inspection of comparable views of the uninjured wrist is also necessary to determine normal ulnar length and avoid misinterpretations attributable to variations in anatomy or differences in roentgenographic techniques. Before injury the distal ulna and medial corner of the radius are usually at the same level (neutral variance), and after fracture one should strive to restore this relationship.

For many injuries, consistent roentgenographic observations have led to the formulation of classifications that serve to guide optimal treatment. For example, articular fractures of the distal end of the radius characteristically demonstrate four major components,[18] as follows: (1) the radial shaft, (2) the radial styloid, (3) a dorsal medial fragment, and (4) a palmar medial fragment (Figs. 11-1 to 11-3). The key medial fragments with their strong ligamentous attachments to the proximal carpals and ulnar styloid are in a pivotal position as the cornerstone of both the radiocarpal and radioulnar joints and have been designated as the medial complex. Displacement of this complex causes a serious biarticular disruption and is the basis for classification of articular fractures into four types (Fig. 11-1). Anatomic restitution of the medial complex is essential for preservation of the distal radial articulations and must be confirmed with postreduction roentgenograms.

Epiphyseal injuries are also categorized according to basic patterns of displacement (Table 11-1).[25] In most cases, classified as type II injuries, the distal radial epiphysis along with an attached metaphyseal fracture fragment is separated from the radial shaft and the extent of displacement is apparent on the roentgenograms (Fig. 11-4). However, when separation is minimal or spontaneous reduction occurs, the presence of the small metaphyseal fragment, termed the "Thurston Holland sign," may be the only obvious evidence of an injury that requires immobilization. Also the more severe epiphyseal injuries (types III, IV, and V) are often associated with subtle roentgenographic findings: minor displacement of the epiphysis or metaphysis, slight disruption of articular congruity, or inconspicuous narrowing of the epiphyseal plate. In these situations, comparison views of the contralateral normal epiphysis facilitate an accurate assessment of the complex chondrosseous anatomy of the injured side.

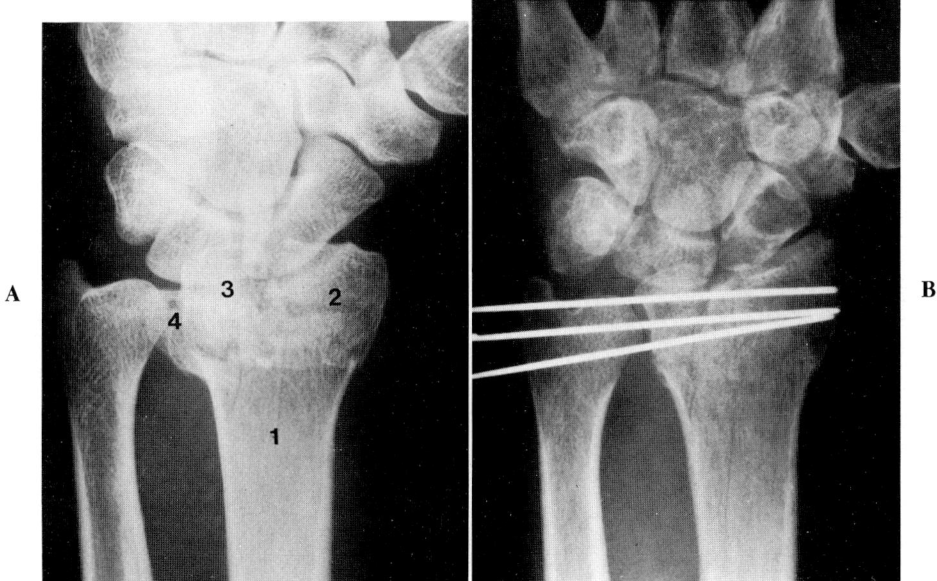

Fig. 11-3. A, Type IV articular fracture causing displacement of the medial fragments irreducible by closed techniques. **B,** Open treatment is necessary for restoration of the articular surfaces and decompression of a severely contused median nerve. Stabilization of the comminuted fragments is achieved with multiple Kirschner wires.

Table 11-1. Epiphyseal plate injuries (Salter-Harris classification)

Type	Description
I	Epiphyseal separation through the zone of provisional calcification.
II	Epiphyseal separation with a small metaphyseal fracture
III	Articular, epiphyseal, and epiphyseal plate separation
IV	Articular, epiphyseal, epiphyseal plate and metaphyseal separation
V	Epiphyseal plate crush injury

Preservation of a normal epiphyseal configuration on the PA roentgenogram is a critical objective of treatment.

SPECIFIC INJURIES
Articular fractures of distal end of radius

The type II fracture is the most frequent articular injury encountered among athletes (Fig. 11-2). A violent compression force transmitted primarily by the lunate accounts for pronounced displacement of the medial complex. In most instances the

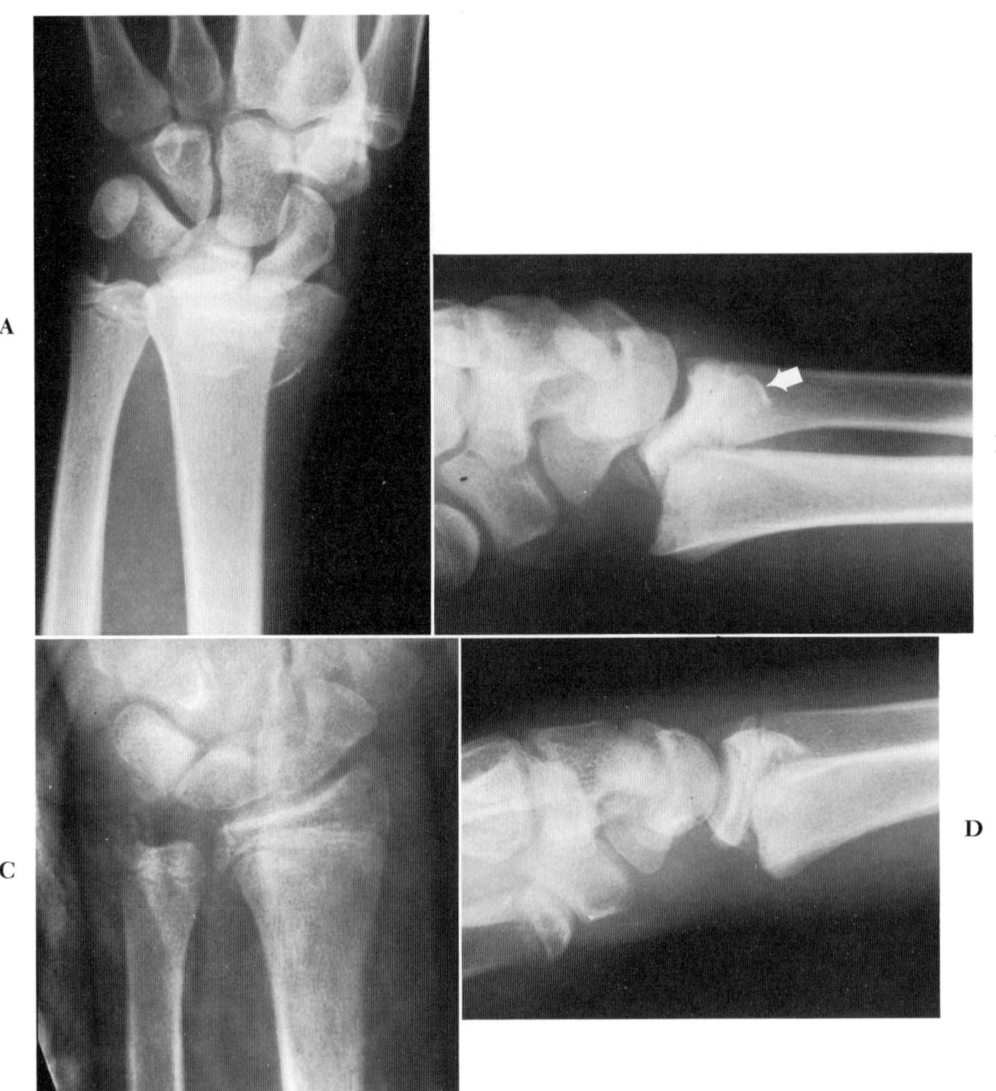

Fig. 11-4. Type II epiphyseal fracture of a 16-year-old football player. **A** and **B,** The roentgenograms demonstrate pronounced displacement of the distal radial epiphysis together with the typical metaphyseal fragment, *arrow.* **C,** After closed reduction the posteroanterior roentgenogram illustrates a normal epiphyseal configuration and normal radial length. **D,** Despite residual displacement on the lateral view, the reduction is satisfactory and repeated manipulations are unnecessary.

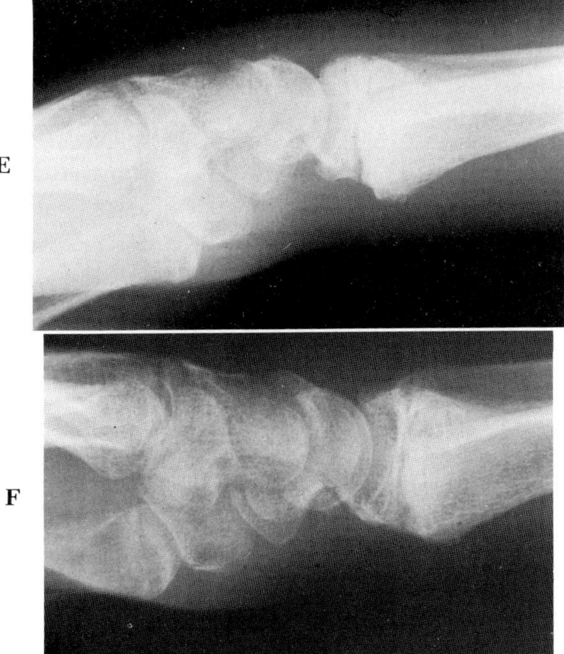

Fig. 11-4, cont'd. E and **F,** Progressive remodeling in the sagittal plane is observed over a period of 13 weeks.

dorsal medial fragment is impacted more than the palmar fragment and the roentgenograms demonstrate posterior displacement. Less often, the reverse mechanism causes greater compression of the palmar fragment resulting in anterior displacement of the complex. In either case the radioulnar articulations are severely disrupted and the magnitude of trauma results in considerable periarticular soft-tissue damage. Particularly prevalent are contusions of the median or ulnar nerves, which, in our experience, have occurred with nearly 20% of type II fractures.

In contrast to stable type I injuries, type II fractures are characteristically comminuted and unsuitable for closed reduction and cast immobilization. Without supplementary fixation of these unstable fractures, redisplacement—frequently to the prereduction position[12]—is a common occurrence. A stable reduction is best maintained by continuous skeletal traction using either pins and plaster or external fixators.[6-8,13,18] Successful traction is contingent on the strength of the ligament component of the medial complex, which remains essentially intact regardless of the severity of fracture.[8] Maintenance of these soft tissues under constant tension affords stability to the attached articular fragments.

Successful traction also depends on the skillful placement of transfixion pins, and one should not be misled by the apparent simplicity of pin fixation for articular fractures. In several large series, 15% to 33% of the cases have been complicated by pin loosening, pin-tract infection, osteomyelitis, or pin-site fracture.[6,7,13]

Our preferred method of traction employs two percutaneous ³⁄₃₂-inch smooth Steinman pins incorporated in a short arm cast.[18] Complications are avoided by observation of the following key technical points: always use a power drill to prevent excessive reaming, which is the major cause of pin loosening, infection, and fracture. Pass the distal pin transversely through the base of the index and middle finger metacarpals with the thumb and fingers held in maximum abduction. Careful positioning of the digits prevents the development of web-space contractures and subsequently facilitates digital motion. Pronate the forearm and place the second pin through the radius in the bare-bone interval just proximal to the abductor pollicis muscle. Be certain that this pin engages both radial cortices but does not pass more than several millimeters beyond the far cortex, so that the critical soft tissues of the forearm are avoided. Suspend the wrist in traction, gently manipulate the fracture, confirm the accuracy of reduction with roentgenograms and then incorporate the pins in a plaster cast leaving the fingers free for immediate active exercises. Do not disturb the pins for at least 6 weeks or until roentgenographic union is clearly demonstrated.

This technique of pins and plaster has proved successful for most type II articular fractures, including those with anterior displacement of the medial complex, which are commonly termed "Smith type II," or "Barton's, fractures."[11,27] Although the medial fragments may demonstrate considerable proximal displacement, they are not usually widely split or rotated and therefore can be accurately reduced by axial traction. In more than 80 cases, radial length and the distal radial articulations have been satisfactorily restored and pin-site infection or fracture has not been encountered. For those injuries with concomitant nerve contusions, a prompt and stable reduction of the medial complex has invariably been followed by complete recovery of nerve function over a period of several months.

Type III and IV articular fractures are relatively infrequent but reflect a greater magnitude of injury, which is likely to occur during sports activities. These injuries always result in serious soft-tissue damage and require open treatment for any nerve, tendon, or vascular repair as well as fracture reduction. Because of extensive comminution, the articular fragments are generally not suitable for rigid fixation, but successful stabilization can be achieved with multiple Kirschner wires (Fig. 11-3).

Metaphyseal fractures

Extra-articular fractures of the distal radius can usually be managed by closed manipulation, facilitated by a regional anesthetic and cast immobilization. Fractures demonstrating posterior displacement (Colles' fractures) are reduced by steady axial traction followed by palmar flexion, ulnar deviation, and pronation of the wrist; whereas those with anterior displacement (Smith's fractures) are reduced by traction and supination.[27] A stable reduction depends on restoration of a buttress provided by accurate apposition of at least one radial cortex. If both cortices are extensively comminuted, the injury must be recognized as inherently unstable and, despite an accurate reduction, redisplacement is inevitable. In such cases skeletal fixation, similar to that used for articular fractures, is necessary to maintain the reduction. After a successful reduction effective cast immobilization incorporates the base of the thumb and the humeral epicondyles so that the transmission of deforming forces is lessened across the fracture site.

Metaphyseal fractures of the preadolescent athlete usually involve both bones at a level several centimeters proximal to the wrist joint. These fractures invariably demonstrate posterior displacement, often with considerable shortening or anterior angulation. Facilitated by a general anesthetic for complete relaxation of the anxious child, steady traction followed by palmar flexion of the distal fragment usually achieves a satisfactory reduction. Remember that growth at the distal epiphyseal plates, coupled with motion in the flexion-extension arc of the intact wrist joint, induces remodeling of the injured bone that can ameliorate considerable displacement in the sagittal plane. Therefore a reduction that results in bayonnet apposition, or even slight overriding of the fragments, is acceptable and invariably leads to an excellent recovery. In contrast, angulation exceeding 25 degrees, axial rotation, and excessive narrowing of the interosseous space are not significantly influenced by the remodeling process and must be corrected by skillful manipulation and casting.

Epiphyseal injuries

Prevalent among adolescent athletes is the type II fracture-separation of the distal radial epiphysis (Fig. 11-4). The plane of this injury traverses the zone of provisional calcification, and an intact epiphysis displaces with the critical and basically undisturbed germinal layer of the epiphyseal plate. A successful closed reduction is usually accomplished by gentle manipulation, and the prognosis for normal growth is excellent.

In cases with minimal or moderate residual displacement, attempts to achieve a perfect reduction by repeated manipulations are liable to damage the growth plate and should be avoided. It is important to recognize that an epiphyseal injury can occur only in an immature skeleton that has the capacity for considerable remodeling of fractures. If normal configurations of the epiphysis and the radioulnar articulation are demonstrated on the PA roentgenogram, the reduction, regardless of persistent sagittal displacement, should be recognized as satisfactory. Epiphyseal fractures of girls as old at 14 years and boys as old as 16 years, demonstrating as much as 50% displacement on the lateral roentgenogram, consistently remodel to a normal-appearing epiphysis (Fig. 11-4, *E* and *F*).

The distal ulnar epiphysis is particularly vulnerable to type III (Fig. 11-5) and type IV (Fig. 11-6) injuries. These serious growth plate disruptions invariably occur with displaced distal third fractures of the radius and have been termed "Galeazzi equivalent lesions."[19,24] Since the plane of these fractures interrupts the growth zone of the epiphyseal plate, an anatomic reduction is essential to prevent a disabling deformity of the ulna. If closed reduction is unsuccessful, a prompt open reduction and internal fixation with fine Kirschner wires must correct residual articular, epiphyseal, or metaphyseal separation.

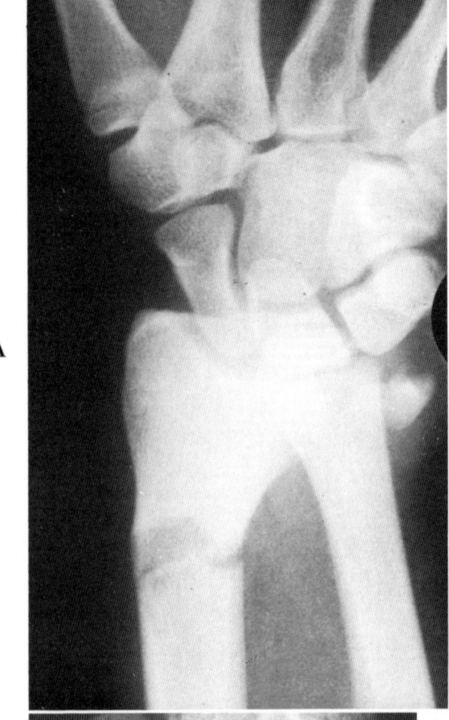

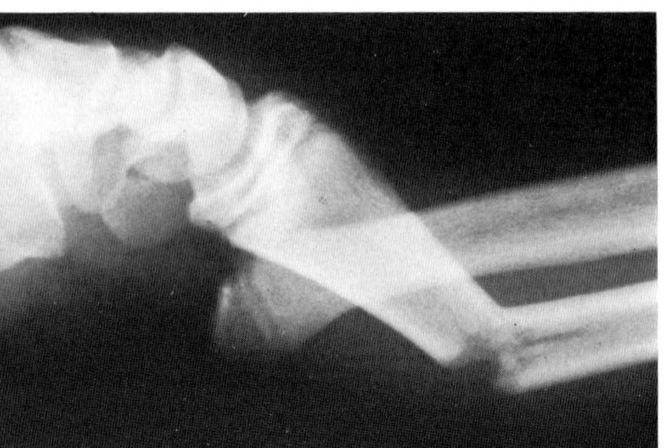

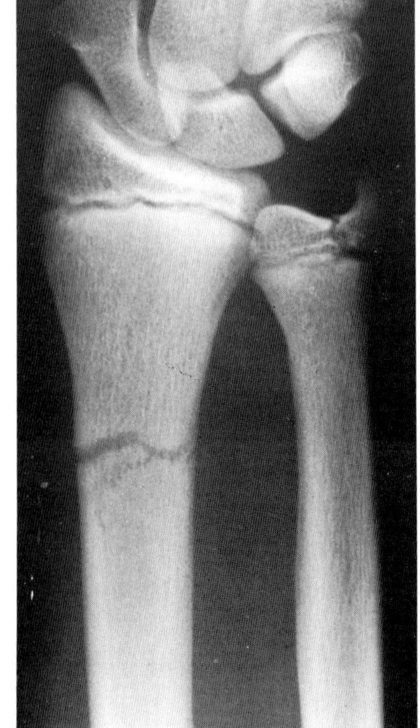

Fig. 11-5. **A** and **B**, A Galeazzi-equivalent lesion comprising a fracture of the distal third of the radius and a type III epiphyseal injury of the distal section of the ulna. **C**, Closed reduction successfully corrected the epiphyseal separation and led to an excellent recovery.

A

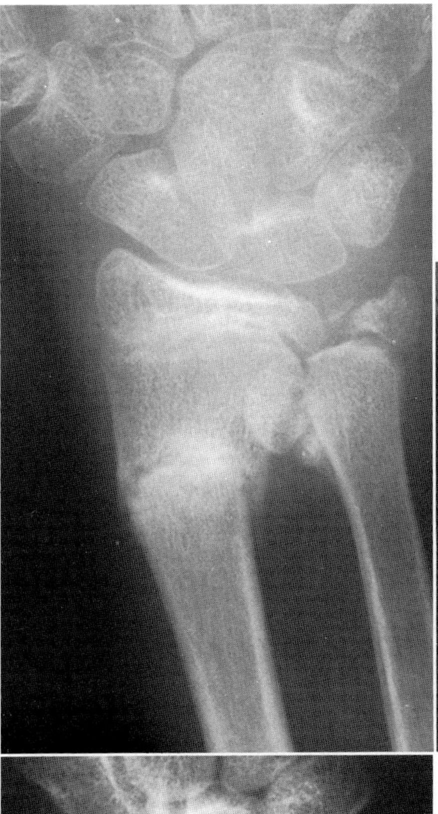

B

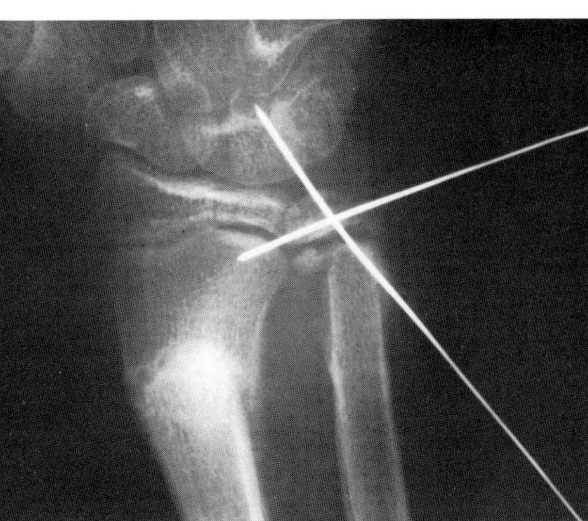

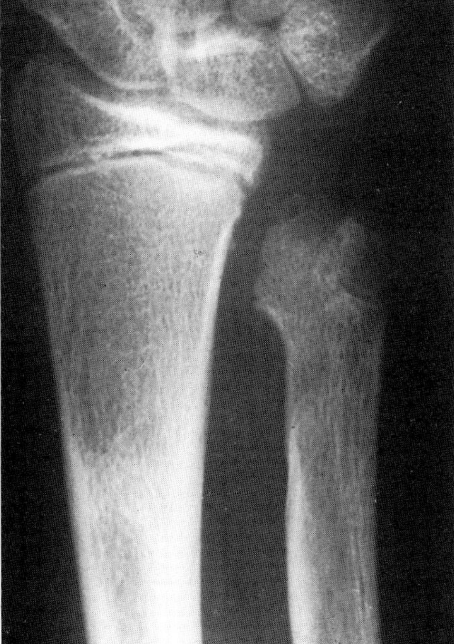

C

Fig. 11-6. A, A 3-month-old Galeazzi-equivalent lesion consisting of a distal radial fracture and a type IV distal ulnar epiphyseal injury. Initial closed reduction was unsuccessful and resulted in a disabling malunion characterized by complete loss of pronation and supination. **B,** Osteotomy and replacement of the ulnar head were necessary to restore a functional radioulnar joint. **C,** Three years after surgery an inevitable growth arrest of the ulna is apparent, but see **D** and **E.**

Continued.

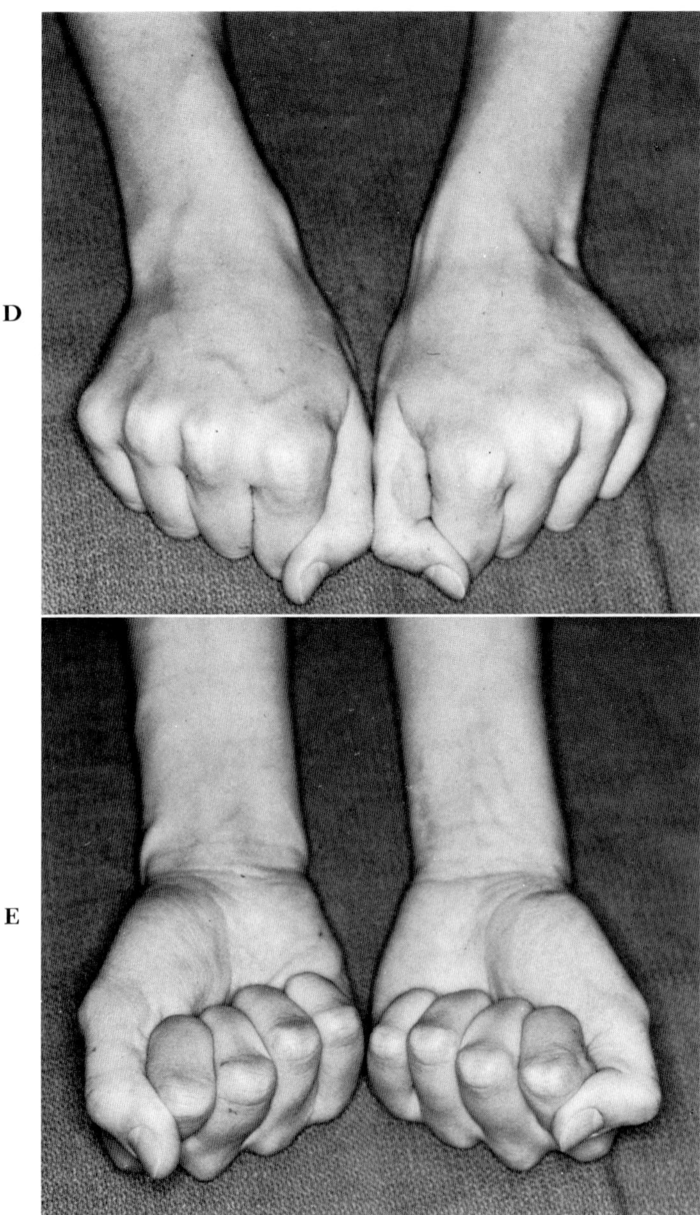

Fig. 11-6, cont'd. D and **E,** The injured wrist (on the right) demonstrated normal rotation and minimal deformity. Although satisfactory function was salvaged, primary open reduction would have been a superior method of treatment.

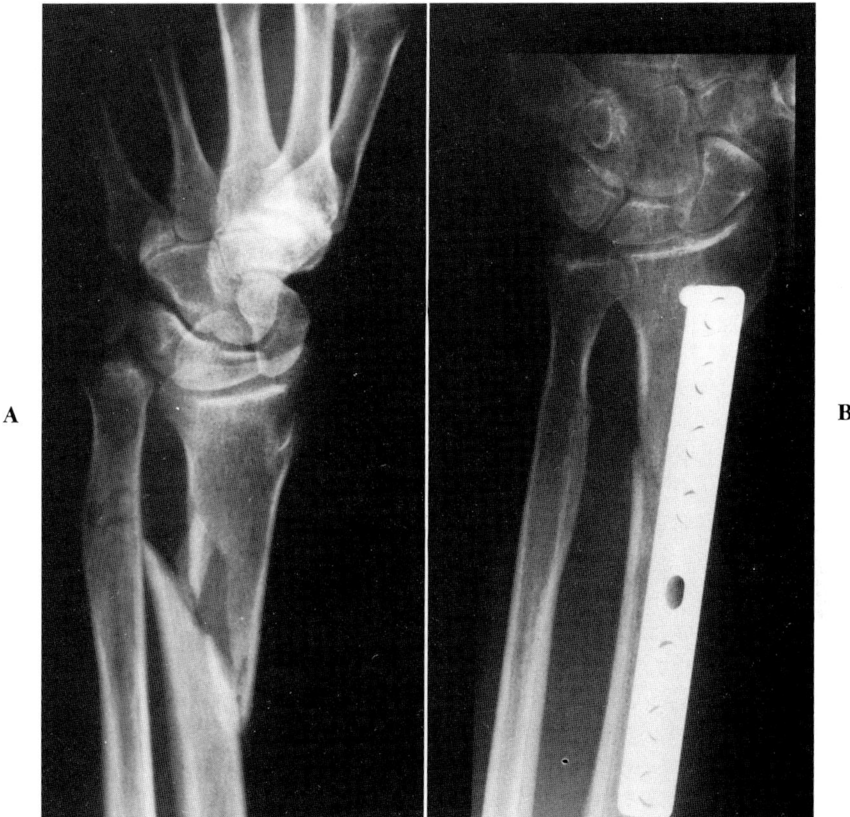

Fig. 11-7. A, An adult Galeazzi injury with noticeable displacement of the radial diaphyseal fracture and the distal radioulnar joint. **B,** Despite a 4-week delay in treatment, anatomic reduction and rigid plate fixation of the radius results in spontaneous relocation of the radioulnar joint and restitution of skeletal stability.

Distal third diaphyseal fractures

Fractures of the radius: the Galeazzi fracture (Fig. 11-7). Increasing experience with diaphyseal fractures of the distal end of the radius has led to basic concepts that rational management should incorporate. First, closed reduction and cast immobilization of even minimally displaced fractures consistently results in malunion or nonunion of the radius. Uncomplicated fracture healing requires precise open reduction and stable fixation.[2,9,16,19,20,24] Second, these fractures invariably occur with serious disruption of the distal radioulnar joint, and persistent subluxation of this articulation is a major cause of functional derangement. Maximum recovery depends on restoration of joint and bone stability as well.

An anterior exposure is preferable to provide access to the flat surface of the radius, which is ideally suited to plate fixation. Sequential reflection of the pronator quadratus, flexor pollicis longus, and flexor digitorum superficialis muscles by judicious periosteal stripping exposes the fracture site. Subperiosteal dissection, in contrast to extraperiosteal division, preserves muscle integrity thereby enhancing vascularity of the fracture and promoting rapid union.[29] Preservation of periosteal-muscle continuity also facilitates postoperative mobilization of the fingers and thumb.

After an accurate reduction narrow self-compressing (DCP) plates designed for 3.5 or 4.5 mm cortical screws[20] are preferred for rigid fixation. At least two and preferably three screws must securely engage both the distal and proximal fragments. Compression is achieved by eccentric placement of screws through the holes of the plate. The oval configuration of these holes permits insertion of cancellous screws, which are usually necessary to achieve a firm purchase in the metaphyseal bone at the distal end of the plate, and it also allows placement of angled lag screws, which augment stability of oblique fractures. Although bone grafting is seldom necessary, it should be considered for extensively comminuted fractures and in cases of delayed treatment.

After fracture reduction but before plate fixation, stability of the distal radioulnar joint must be carefully assessed by palpation and intraoperative radiography. Usually the distal ulnar dislocation spontaneously reduces with anatomic positioning of the radial fracture. Infrequently, disruption and displacement of the triangular fibrocartilage complex is responsible for a mechanical block to radioulnar reduction.[1,4] A grossly unstable joint with roentgenographic demonstration of a large displaced avulsion fracture of the ulnar styloid should alert the examiner to the probability of this pathologic condition and the need for open reduction. Extraction of interposed tissues with the repair of ruptured ligaments and Kirschner wire fixation of the avulsion fracture restores joint congruity, and temporary transarticular pin fixation provides additional stability. It needs to be emphasized that an unstable distal ulna, regardless of the cause, should not be resected at the time of primary fracture treatment. Excisional arthroplasty eliminates the stabilizing influence of an intact ulnar and is prone to result in plate loosening, delayed union, or nonunion of the radius. Symptomatic instability is preferentially treated after fracture union is completed.

All Galeazzi injuries should be protected for 6 weeks with a cast that incorporates the humeral epicondyles and maintains the forearm in full supination. Effective immobilization ensures fracture union as well as soft-tissue healing sufficient for preservation of radioulnar stability.

Fractures of the ulna: nightstick fractures. Because of the high ratio of cortical to cancellous bone of the distal ulnar diaphysis, healing of the isolated ulnar fractures is characteristically slow. The strut effect of the parallel radius may also cause continuous distraction of these fractures and contribute to a prolonged healing time. Roentgenographic union often requires 2 or 3 months, and the incidence of nonunion ranges from 0.8% to 12%.[23] Slightly displaced fractures are generally stable and unite with minimal immobilization. Below-elbow casts,[10] functional bracing,[26] and short-term splinting[23] have been employed successfully for these injuries. In contrast, fractures demonstrating 50% or more displacement of their cortices cause a serious disruption of the adjacent periosteum and interosseous membrane that results in a prominent loss of stability.[10] These unstable injuries may eventually heal with long arm cast immobilization but, in our experience, accurate reduction and rigid fixation is a more predictable method of successful treatment (Fig. 11-8).

Open reduction is accomplished by exposure along the subcutaneous border of the ulna, and stable fixation is obtained by application of narrow self-compressing plate to the dorsal aspect of the fracture. A dorsally affixed plate provides continuous compression on the tension side of the fracture thereby expediting union, and it avoids disturbance of the critical ulnar neurovascular bundle. Postoperatively, a protective splint, which the patient frequently removes for active exercises, is employed until roentgenographic union is apparent.

Open fractures. Caution is advised in the immediate plating of distal forearm fractures in the presence of open wounds. Although skin disruption usually results from a displaced bone fragment within the wound and is not associated with extensive soft-tissue damage, it does increase the risk of infection.[5,9,14] Open fractures should be managed by an initial débridement and irrigation, prophylactic antibiotics, primary or secondary skin closure, splinting, and delayed plating. Temporary external fixation is not necessary for isolated diaphyseal fractures that are sufficiently stabilized by the intact adjacent bone. Deferment of internal fixation—even for several

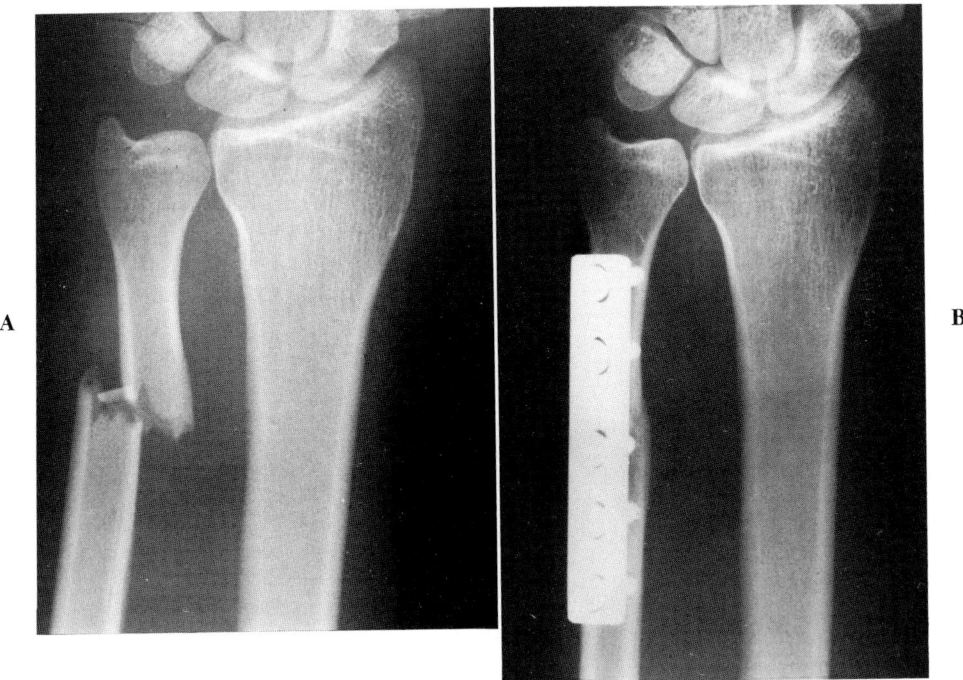

Fig. 11-8. A, A 27-year-old baseball catcher was struck with a bat and incurred this unstable fracture of the distal ulnar diaphysis. **B,** Open reduction and rigid fixation allowed restoration of the interosseous space and after 6 weeks resulted in uncomplicated union. Four months after the operation, he returned to competition and played one season with the plate intact.

Continued.

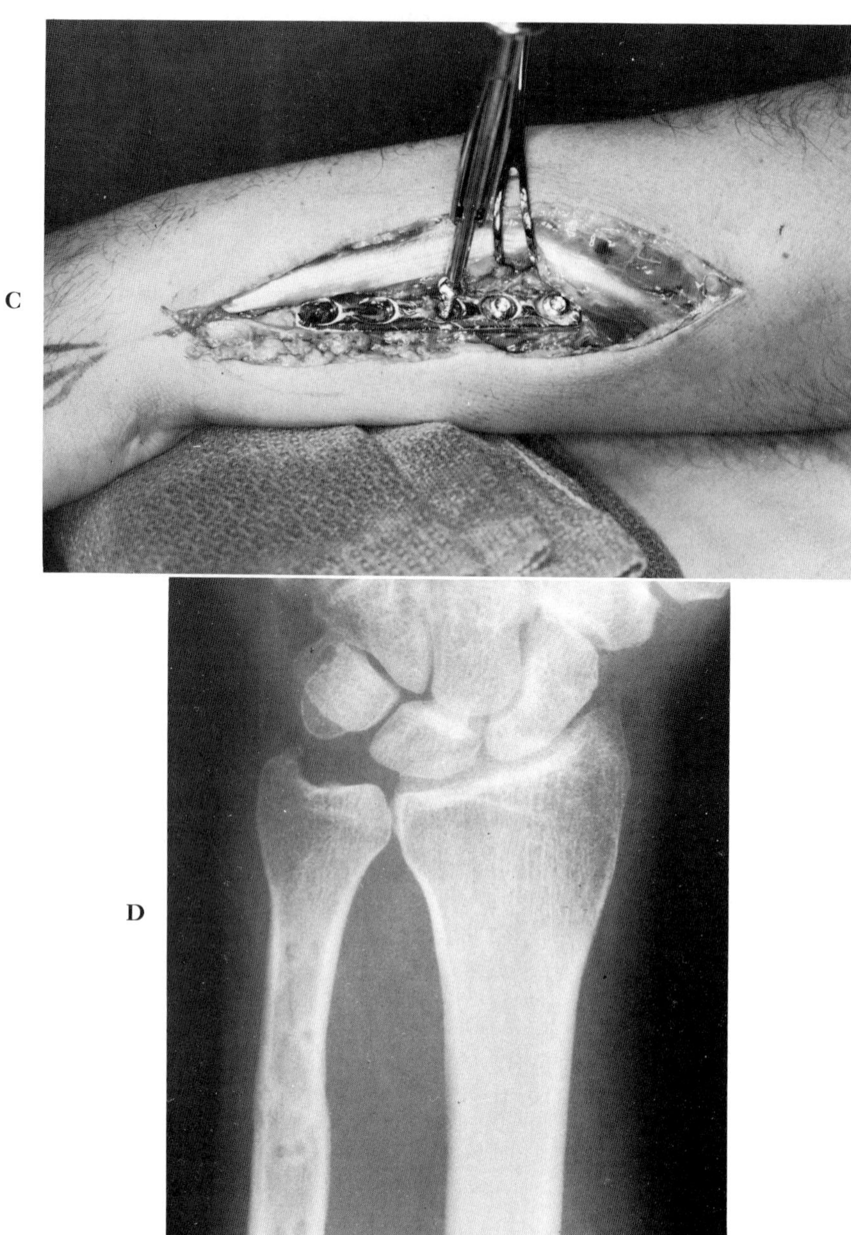

Fig. 11-8, cont'd. **C,** Fourteen months after its application (during the "off" season), the plate was removed, and, **D,** 4 months thereafter, when the athlete returned to spring training, the healed ulna demonstrated reconstitution of its cortices and osteogenesis within its screw holes. Refracture was prevented by complete healing and rehabilitation after both insertion and extraction of the plate.

weeks—until the wound conditions are optimal minimizes the risk of a disastrous complication without compromising the results of treatment. In his experience with 28 open diaphyseal fractures treated by delayed plating, Anderson[2] reported uncomplicated healing and an excellent recovery of function in all cases.

Refracture of the plated forearm. Stress shielding of a rigid plate results in considerable osteopenia, and as long as the plate is present, the underlying bone remains weakened and vulnerable to injury.[28,30] Refracture is prone to occur at the end of the plate where a sharp transition from atrophied to normal bone exists or at the previous site of fracture where osteoporosis is most prominent. Removal of the plate permits restitution of normal skeletal strength and is therefore advisable once the fracture is completely united. However it is important to recognize that the majority of reported refractures have occurred after hardware extraction.[2,9,15,20] This paradoxical situation is attributed to prematurity in either removal of the plate or returning to strenuous activity without protection. Refractures must be promptly diagnosed and treated; undisplaced injuries usually unite with long arm cast immobilization for 6 to 8 weeks, whereas displaced fractures require replating and bone grafting.

Clearly the athlete, who is constantly exposed to violent trauma, is at a high risk for refracture after both plate application and removal. Rational management of the plated forearm requires careful consideration of many factors: the type of fracture, the rigidity of fixation, the rapidity and thoroughness of healing as well as the patient's age, extent of rehabilitation and level of competition. Although it is impossible to establish absolute principles of aftercare for patients who are always vulnerable to injury, the following guidelines are proposed: first, after a technically sound plating, a minimum of 4 months is generally required for complete healing at the fracture site as well as rehabilitation of the forearm. Return to competition should be permitted only when the roentgenograms illustrate obliteration of the fracture and the patient demonstrates near-normal levels of strength and mobility of the injured extremity. Also the plated forearm must always be protected against further trauma. Leather gauntlets and soft rubber casts are usually permissable at all levels of competition, whereas plastic splints and even fiberglass or plaster casts are often allowed in the professional ranks. Second, the plate is optimally removed between 1 and 2 years after its application. Müller et al.[20] in their vast experience have rarely encountered refracture of a healed bone when the plate was left intact for more than a year. Obviously removal should be electively planned to cause the least interference with the athlete's career. Third, after plate extraction, the forearm must be protected for at least 6 weeks with a splint or removable cast that permits active exercises but prevents deleterious passive forces. Again, contact sports should be avoided for at least 4 months. Experimental studies[3,28] indicating that bone at the site of extracted plates and screws requires several months for maturation and strengthening commensurate with strenuous activities are substantiated by clinical experience[15] demonstrating that refracture is most likely to occur within 3 months after plate removal.

Employing these criteria for management of the plated forearm we have encountered no instance of refracture among 19 patients returning to contact sports or heavy labor.

SUMMARY

Fractures of the distal radius or ulna rarely occur without concomitant injury to the adjacent bone and soft tissues. Prompt recognition of the magnitude of injury and restoration of anatomic relationships of these parallel bones are the basis for optimal management. In addition to uncomplicated fracture union, maximum recovery is largely dependent on preservation of the interosseous space, stability of the radioular joint, congruity of the radiocarpal joint, and, in the younger patient, integrity of the epiphyseal plate. The key to prevention of reinjury is thorough healing and rehabilitation of the injured extremity.

REFERENCES

1. Alexander, A.H., and Lichtman, D.M.: Irreducible distal radioulnar joint occurring in a Galeazzi fracture—case report, J. Hand Surg. 6:258-261, May 1981.
2. Anderson, L.D., et al.: Compression-plate fixation in acute diaphyseal fractures of the radius and ulna, J. Bone Joint Surg. (Am.) 57:287-297, April 1975.
3. Burstein, A.H., et al.: Bone strength: the effect of screw holes, J. Bone Joint Surg. (Am.) 54:1143-1156, Sept. 1972.
4. Cetti, N.E.: An unusual cause of blocked reduction of the Galeazzi injury, Injury 9:59-61, 1977.
5. Chapman, N.W., and Mahoney, M: The role of early internal fixation in the management of open fractures, Clin. Orthop. (138):120-131, Jan.-Feb. 1979.
6. Chapman, R.D., et al.: Complications of distal radial fractures: pins and plaster treatment, J. Hand Surg. 7:509-512, Sept. 1982.
7. Cooney, W.P., Linscheid, R.L., and Dobyns, J.H.: External pin fixation for unstable Colles' fractures, J. Bone Joint Surg. (Am.) 61:840-845, 1979.
8. DePalma, A.F.: Comminuted fractures of the distal end of the radius treated by ulnar pinning, J. Bone Joint Surg. (Am.) 34:651-662, 1952.
9. Dodge, H.S., and Cady, G.W.: Treatment of fractures of the radius and ulna with compression plates: a retrospective study of one hundred and nineteen fractures in seventy-eight patients, J. Bone Joint Surg. (Am.) 54:1167-1176, Sept. 1972.
10. Dymond, I.W.D.: The treatment of isolated fractures of the distal ulna, J. Bone Joint Surg. 66B:408-410, May 1984.
11. Ellis, J.: Smith and Barton's fractures: a method of treatment, J. Bone Joint Surg. (Br.) 47:724-727, 1965.
12. Gartland, J.J., Jr., and Werley, C.W.: Evaluation of healed Colles' fractures, J. Bone Joint Surg. (Am.) 33:895-907, Oct. 1951.
13. Green, D.P.: Pins and plaster treatment of comminuted fractures of the distal end of the radius, J. Bone Joint Surg. (Am.) 57:304-310, April 1975.
14. Gustilo, B.R., and Anderson, J.T.: Prevention of infection in the treatment of one thousand and twenty-five open fractures of long bones, J. Bone Joint Surg. (Am.) 58:453-458, June 1976.
15. Hidaka, S., and Gustilo, R.B.: Refractures of bones of the forearm after plate removal, J. Bone Joint Surg. 66A:1241-1243, Oct. 1984.
16. Hughston, J.C.: Fracture of the distal radial shaft: mistakes in management, J. Bone Joint Surg. (Am.) 39:249-264, April 1957.
17. Lidström, A.: Fractures of the distal end of the radius: a clinical and statistical study of end results, Acta Orthop. Scand. 41 (suppl.):1-118, 1959.
18. Melone, C.P., Jr.: Articular fractures of the distal radius, Orthop. Clin. North Am. 15:217-236, April 1984.
19. Mikić, Z.K.: Galeazzi fracture-dislocations, J. Bone Joint Surg. (Am.) 57:1071-1080, Dec. 1975.
20. Müller, M.E., et al.: Manual of internal fixation: technique recommended by the AO-Group, ed. 2, New York, 1979, Springer-Verlag.
21. Palmer, A.K., Glisson, R.R., and Werner, F.W.: Ulnar variance determination, J. Hand Surg. 7:376-379, July 1982.

22. Palmer, A.K., and Werner, F.W.: The triangular fibrocartilage complex of the wrist—anatomy and function, J. Hand Surg. **6**:153-162, March 1981.

23. Pollock, F.M., et al.: The isolated fracture of the ulnar shaft, J. Bone Joint Surg. (Am.) **65**:339-342, March 1982.

24. Reckling, F.W.: Unstable fracture-dislocation of the forearm (Monteggia and Galeazzi lesions), J. Bone Joint Surg. (Am.) **64**:857-863, July 1982.

25. Salter, R.B., and Harris, W.R.: Injuries involving the epiphyseal plate, J. Bone Joint Surg. (Am.) **45**:587-622, April 1963.

26. Sarmiento, A., et al.: Treatment of ulnar fractures by functional bracing, J. Bone Joint Surg. (Am.) **58**:1104-1107, Dec. 1976.

27. Thomas, F.B.: Reduction of Smith's fracture, J. Bone Joint Surg. (Br.) **39**:462-470, Aug. 1957.

28. Uhthoff, H.K., and Dubuc, F.L.: Bone structure changes in the dog under rigid internal fixation, Clin. Orthop. (81):165-170, Nov.-Dec. 1971.

29. Whiteside, L.A., and Lesker, P.A.: The effects of extraperiosteal and subperiosteal dissection. II. On fracture healing, J. Bone Joint Surg. **60A**:26-30, Jan. 1978.

30. Woo, S.L.-Y., et al.: A comparison of cortical bone atrophy secondary to fixation with plates with large differences in bending stiffness, J. Bone Joint Surg. **58A**:190-195, March 1976.

12. Flexor and extensor tendon injuries

John F. Mosher

There are only three common tendon injuries about the hand and wrist in sports.

Common:
1. Extensor mechanism—mallet deformity
2. Extensor mechanism—boutonnière or pseudoboutonnière deformity
3. Flexor mechanism—avulsion of the flexor digiti profundus (football finger)

Less common:
1. Extensor mechanism over metacarpal head
   a. Longitudinal split in extensor *tendon*
   b. Longitudinal split in *sagittal band*
      mechanism
   c. Tooth wound
2. Extensor carpi ulnaris dislocation
3. Synovitis of the flexor carpi ulnaris (racket player's pisiform)

Synovitis of any tendon may occur, such as De Quervain's disease of the first dorsal compartment. They seem however to be relatively infrequently related to sport and are not covered here.

THE MALLET DEFORMITY

There are three types of disorders that give the appearance of a mallet finger[10] or thumb.[2]

1. Extensor tendon avulsion
   a. Without bone fragment (75%)
   b. With bone fragment (25%)
2. Fracture subluxation of distal joint
3. Epiphyseal plate fracture

All three are the result of a longitudinally directed force. In the adult the force can produce an extensor tendon avulsion or a fracture subluxation of the DIP joint.

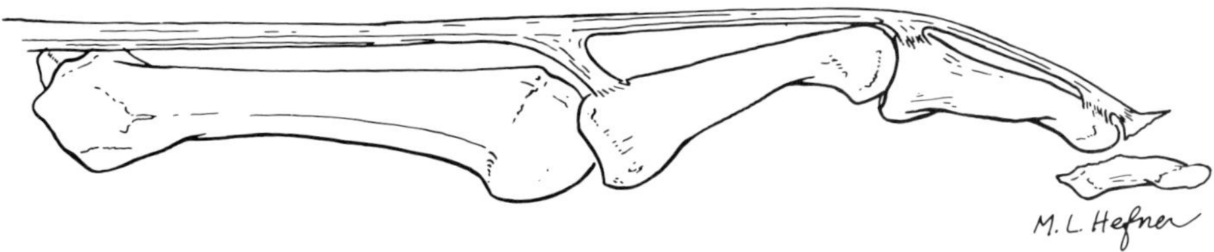

Fig. 12-1. This fracture dislocation mallet deformity caused by a violent extension injury to the distal joint is primarily a joint injury and differs from the more trivial flexion mallet finger, which is an extensor tendon injury.

Pathosis of extensor tendon avulsion

Subcutaneous rupture
1. Without bone fragment—produced by trivial trauma
2. With bone fragment—off dorsal lip of distal phalanx and produced by sudden forceful flexion of greater than 90 degrees

Both of these lesions occur when the distal joint is forceably flexed while the middle joint is held in extension. With the extensor tendon avulsion type of injury the mechanism of injury is sudden flexion and the joint is not subluxated.

Fracture subluxation of the distal joint (Fig. 12-1). This lesion is caused by a severe trauma to the distal phalanx driving the distal joint into extension and shearing off a dorsal articular fragment of the distal phalanx (usually greater than a third of the articular surface). Volar subluxation of the joint results.

Epiphyseal plate fracture of distal phalanx. Either the flexion or the extension mechanism can result in a growth plate injury in the growing athlete. Most commonly it is a Salter II type of fracture. A Salter III injury may occur but rarely with joint subluxation.

Coincident with the mallet finger the PIP joint may be injured. A zigzag buckling occurs with these linked interphalangeal joints and a flexion DIP injury will be associated with hyperextension PIP injury and vice versa an extension fracture avulsion DIP injury with a flexion PIP injury.

Treatment

The mallet finger is probably compatible with continued competition in a splint depending on the hand requirement of the sport. For instance, this would be an incapacitating injury for the throwing hand.

I agree with the thought expressed by Wehbé and Schneider[9] that surgery is rarely indicated for a mallet injury regardless of the type. Since almost any good splint regimen will produce a satisfactory result, I favor the "stack"[1] splint because of its simplicity. It is necessary that the distal joint be protected in full extension 24 hours per day, and the program for the stack splint has been well outlined by Crawford.[1] For sport activity a splint can be applied dorsally with tape to allow more exposure of the tactile pulp. The splint regimen should be continued 24 hours per day for at least 6 weeks and then at night for perhaps another 4 to 6 weeks. If after 6 weeks an extension lag develops when the splint is removed, the finger should be returned to full-time splinting for at least another 2 weeks.

The epiphyseal plate fracture should be treated with a similar splint program but can be totally discontinued at 5 or 6 weeks. The greatly angulated epiphyseal fracture may avulse the nail from the matrix bed and thus present as an open fracture. This injury demands surgical cleansing of the finger, and the nail should be replaced under the eponychial fold as the fracture is reduced. Infection is a definite possibility, and the finger should be assessed for this problem during the first week.

EXTENSOR TENDON INJURIES AT PROXIMAL INTERPHALANGEAL JOINT

Injuries to the extensor mechanism at the PIP joint are usually the result of the same longitudinally directed forces that produce the mallet deformity. Sudden forced flexion of an actively extended PIP joint causes a disruption of the central slip mechanism. Initially only a minimal extension lag may be noticed because there is usually a partial central slip disruption. This untreated condition may progress to a more severe extension loss as more of the extensor tendon fibers are disrupted and eventually may lead to the heralded boutonnière deformity.

Following are the only indications for immediate repair of the central slip:

1. Open injury with central slip laceration or avulsion
2. Closed injury with displaced fragment of central slip insertion (usually subsequent to joint dislocation)

Even though the mild central slip injury is quite common and resultant problems are surprisingly few, close attention should be paid to this injury. The joint (PIP only) should be splinted in full extension if the roentgenogram does not show any dorsal subluxation on the full-extension lateral view.

Recommendation program

1. Splint PIP joint in full extension when not competing.
2. Tape joint to reduce flexion and buddy tape for sport.
3. Repeat the exam for extension lag.
4. Continue this regimen until there is full active range of motion without pain or swelling.

Surgery for the established boutonnière deformity should not be necessary for the well-attended athlete. The injury should not progress to that stage.

Pseudoboutonnière deformity is the result of injury to the volar plate side of the PIP joint (hyperextension injury) causing volar scarring and a flexion contracture. The extension splinting program should also be instituted for this injury.

AVULSION OF FLEXOR DIGITORUM PROFUNDUS

Whereas the previous deformities rarely require surgical intervention, avulsion of the flexor digitorum profundus requires urgent surgical attention.

This injury is seen most frequently in U.S. football but can be seen in any tackling sport. It is caused by a violent pull against the isolated flexed DIP joint. The ring finger is by far the most commonly victim. The usual mechanism is a Jersey tackle. Many reasons for the preponderance of injuries to the ring finger have been advanced.[6] Manske and Lester[7] have shown that the flexor profundus insertion on the ring finger is weaker than that to any other finger.

Although there is sudden pain, there is little noticeable loss of function, only the loss of flexion of the distal joint. This may account for the late reporting of the injury by the player.

The diagnosis is made by the loss of active flexion of the distal finger joint (especially ring finger) with intact passive flexion.

If the player does not require skilled hand function, he may return to the game with the hand in a padded fist position. The hand should be protected at all times until a surgical decision is reached. If there is only one more game, the finger is not badly swollen, and the player is important to the game (and the game to the player), I believe one can delay surgery (8 to 10 days) without jeopardizing the result. If any of the above requirements are not met, immediate reattachment of the profundus is advised.

The terminal portion of the profundus tendon is flattened and split into halves similar to the superficialis before its insertion. For this reason I advocate placing a grasping type of suture into each slip of insertion, passing each double tail through the distal phalanx, and tying the two separate sutures over the nail (Fig. 12-2).

Avulsion of the flexor digitorum profundus has been divided into 3 types:[6]

  I. Retraction into the palm

  II. Retraction to the PIP joint (most common type)

  III. Large bony fragment off volar aspect of distal phalanx may be articular fragment

Types I and III are more violently disruptive injuries. They are likely to present with the more swollen ecchymotic finger and thus be candidates for the more urgent surgery.

Late avulsion of flexor digitorum profundus

Late is the time beyond which reattachment of the tendon of the flexor digitorum profundus is not advised. This may be as early as 8 to 10 days in the more violent injuries (types I and III) or as late as 3 to 6 weeks in the type II injury. DIP fusion, tenodesis (with free tendon graft), or tendon graft through intact flexor digitorum sublimis may be indicated. If the distal joint does not hyperextend and is stable and painless, no reconstruction may be necessary. The coiled distal stump in the palm may be painful with an irritant bursa, and this may require excision.

EXTENSOR MECHANISM OVER THE METACARPAL HEAD

Injuries over the metacarpal head are usually the result of a punch, inadvertent or advertent.

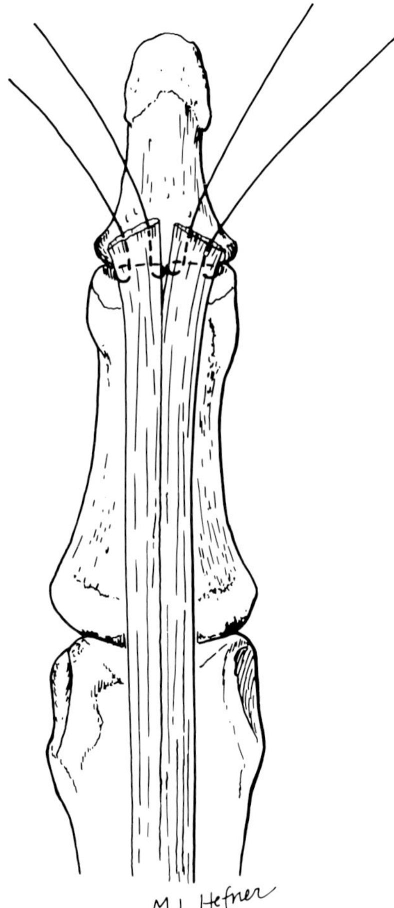

Fig. 12-2. Near its insertion the flexor digitorum profundus tendon splits into two flat tendons. A grasping type of suture is placed in each half.

Tooth wound—recommendation

1. Surgical cleansing
2. Penicillin and synthetic penicillin prophylaxis for 7 days
3. Daily observation

Because of the sagittal band attachments the tendon does not retract at this level and later repair is not necessary. Infection will usually develop within 24 hours.[3] With daily observation and prophylactic antibiotics, this injury may be compatible with return to play in a matter of days in a protective soft dressing.

Split extensor mechanism[5]

A split extensor or mechanism is usually the result of a punch injury to something other than a tooth. There are two types.

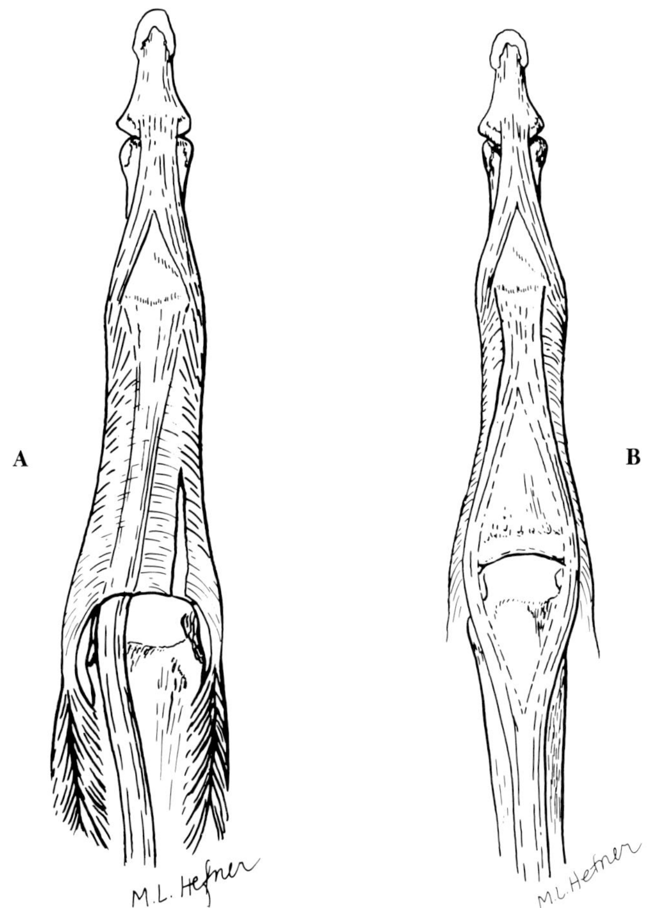

Fig. 12-3. A, Split in the sagittal band mechanism extending into the intrinsic mechanism. **B,** Split in the extensor tendon substance.

Longitudinal split in the sagittal band mechanism. With flexion of the metacarpophalangeal joint the extensor tendon subluxates to one side of the joint (Fig. 12-3, *A*).

Split in the extensor tendon itself (Fig. 12-3, *B*). The split portions slip to either side of the metacarpal head with metacarpophalangeal flexion. It is a rare injury. The middle finger is most frequently involved. These injuries are probably quite common but not reported. Pain and a bursa-like swelling may develop over the metacarpal head. In the sagittal band injury the subluxating tendon may eventually fix in a position in the valley between the metacarpal heads and limit metacarpophalangeal extension and deviate the finger.

I have operated upon only two such injuries in athletes. One was the longitudinal split in the tendon with 3 months of persistent pain and swelling with metacarpophalangeal flexion. The second was a split sagittal band with progressive extensor subluxation, pain, and finger deviation. Both repairs were simple longitudinal repair of the defect followed by limiting strong fist flexion for 8 weeks. Other methods have been described.[5]

RECURRENT DISLOCATION OF THE EXTENSOR CARPI ULNARIS TENDON

The extensor carpi ulnaris (ECU) tendon occupies the sixth dorsal tunnel or compartment. This tendon is held tight to the dorsal groove of the ulna by a tendon sheath that is separate from the extensor retinaculum, which passes distal to the ulnar styloid. This ECU tendon sheath may be torn by sudden supination, flexion, and ulnar deviation of the wrist, and the ECU tendon may dislocate out of the groove. It will then reduce with pronation. This tendon dislocation may produce a painful "click" over the distal dorsal ulna, especially with club (golf, baseball, lacrosse) or racket sports.

This rare painful lesion may respond to temporary decreased activity. Reconstruction of the sheath with a slip of extensor retinaculum[8] has been described.

LESIONS OF THE FLEXOR CARPI ULNARIS TENDON MECHANISM

"Racket player's pisiform"[4] is attributable to minor degrees of subluxation of the pisiform or chondromalacia of the articular cartilage. This sesamoid bone set in the dorsal fibers of the flexor carpi ulnaris tendon has important ligamentous attachments to the fifth metacarpal, hamate, and triquetral bones. The abductor digiti quinti arises from this bone. It is closely related to the ulnar nerve on its radial side.

Pain on the ulnar aspect of the proximal palm should lend to careful exam of the inferior radioulnar joint, the triangular fibrocartilage complex, the hook of the hamate, the tendon of the flexor carpi ulnaris and the PLSO triquetral joint. Increased pain on resisted flexion and ulnar deviation of the wrist, joint tenderness over the pisiform, increased pain on pisiform grinding, and abnormal laxity of the pisiform are important localizing signs. Roentgenograms, including carpal tunnel views and arthrography, will probably not define the pathologic condition. Surgical excision of the pisiform has been described as curative for this condition.

SUMMARY

There are only *three common tendon* injuries to the hand and wrist in sport. Conservative care is most important in the extensor tendon injuries, and surgery is rarely indicated. Avulsion of the flexor digitorum profundus is, however, an injury that needs early surgery.

REFERENCES

1. Crawford, G.P.: The molded Polythene splint for mallet deformities, J. Hand Surg. **9A:**231, Mar. 1984.
2. Din, K.M., and Meggilt, B.F.: Mallet thumb, J. Bone Joint Surg. [Br.] **65B:**606, 1983.
3. Goldstein, E., et al.: Infections following closed fist injury: a new perspective, J. Hand Surg. **2:**97, Mar. 1977.

4. Helal, B.: Racquet player's pisiform, The Hand **10**:87, 1978.
5. Kettelkamp, D.B., Flatt, A.E., and Moulds, R.: Traumatic dislocation of the long finger extensor tendon, J. Bone Joint Surg. **53A**:229, 1971.
6. Leddy, J.P., and Lesker, P.A.: Avulsion of the ring finger flexor digitorum profundus tendon: an experimental study, The Hand **10**:52, 1978.
8. Palmer, A.K., and Eckhardt, W.A.: Recurrent dislocation of extensor carpi ulnaris tendon, J. Hand Surg. **6**:629, Nov. 1981.
9. Wehbé, M.D., and Schneider, L.H.: Mallet fractures, J. Bone Joint Surg. **66A**:658, June 1984.
10. Zancalli, E.: Structural and dynamic bases of hand surgery, ed. 2, Philadelphia, 1979, J.B. Lippincott Co.

13. Carpal injuries

Robert J. Neviaser

Injuries to the carpus are relatively common. They encompass a wide variety of problems, but this discussion concentrates on fractures and dislocations. The inter-carpal ligament injuries are discussed in Chapters 14 and 15.

FRACTURES OF THE CARPUS

The scaphoid is probably the most commonly fractured of the carpals. It can be seen either as an isolated fracture or less commonly in association with a perilunate dislocation. Other carpals that are fractured with some frequency are the hamate and the triquetrum. There is evidence to indicate that Kienböck's disease or osteonecrosis of the lunate may be the result of microfractures and repeated trauma. This entity, however, is not discussed here.

Fracture of the scaphoid

As already mentioned, scaphoid fractures can occur either as an isolated fracture or less commonly associated with perilunate dislocation. The frequency of this fracture is related to the scaphoid traversing both carpal rows and serving as a link between them. Because of its position, excessive dorsiflexion of the wrist allows the scaphoid to abut against the dorsal lip of the radius and the radial styloid. With further forceful extension of the wrist, especially in radial deviation, a fracture will occur.

The physical findings are usually characteristic. There is tenderness over the dorsal radial aspect of the wrist at the radioscaphoid articulation and in the anatomic snuffbox. There may be volar radioscaphoid tenderness as well. This, combined with the history of a fall on the outstretched hand, should raise the index of suspicion for the presence of a fracture of this kind. Routine roentgenograms may not show the fracture if obtained immediately after injury. Initial appropriate treatment should include splinting of the hand and wrist and a second roentgenogram in 7 to 14 days. After the hyperemia of injury has produced resorption around the fracture site, the fracture may be more visible (Fig. 13-1). An anteroposterior roentgenogram of the wrist in ulnar deviation may show the fracture to advantage. With a stable fracture, which most of these are, treatment by casting is usually effective. There are many preferences for types of casting. An effective means is to incorporate the thumb and

122

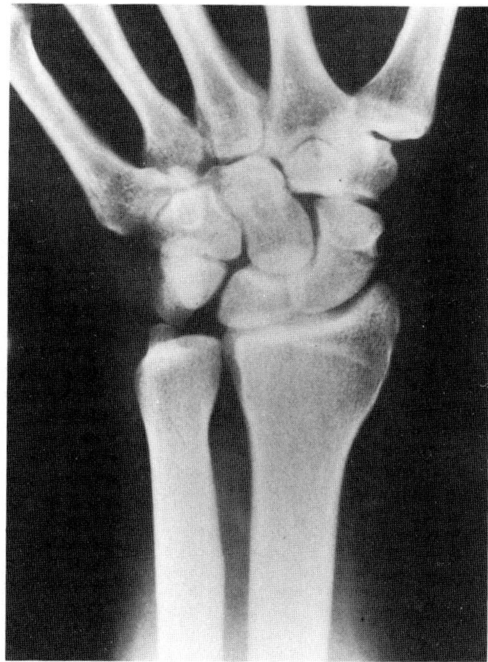

Fig. 13-1. A scaphoid fracture that has become evident on an anteroposterior roentgenogram taken 2 weeks after injury. Ulnar deviation of the wrist is also helpful in demonstration of the fracture.

wrist in an above-elbow plaster that controls rotation of the forearm but allows some flexion and extension, a Munster type of thumb spica. This should be continued until the fracture heals.

When a scaphoid fracture is healed is a difficult question. A minimum of 6 weeks, but more commonly 3 or more months, is often required. Because of the peculiar nature of the blood supply of this small bone,[2,8] healing may be prolonged. It also may be associated with osteonecrosis of the proximal pole. This finding may not prove to be of clinical significance if the fracture heals and revascularization then occurs.

If the fracture fails to unite within 6 months, consideration should be given to bone grafting. After this time an established diagnosis of nonunion of the carpal scaphoid can be made. In the expected absence of extensive intercarpal or radiocarpal arthrosis, bone grafting from the volar approach, as described by Russe,[7] is the preferred technique. This should produce a high rate of union of the carpal scaphoid. Alternative techniques such as carpal implants, arthrodesis, and resection arthroplasty are rarely indicated. They have a greater role as salvage procedures with extensive intercarpal changes where simply obtaining union of the scaphoid would be insufficient to address the problems of a posttraumatic arthrosis.

Unstable scaphoid fractures as isolated entities are unusual. Because the carpal scaphoid is surrounded by cartilage on virtually all sides, it is uncommon to find a

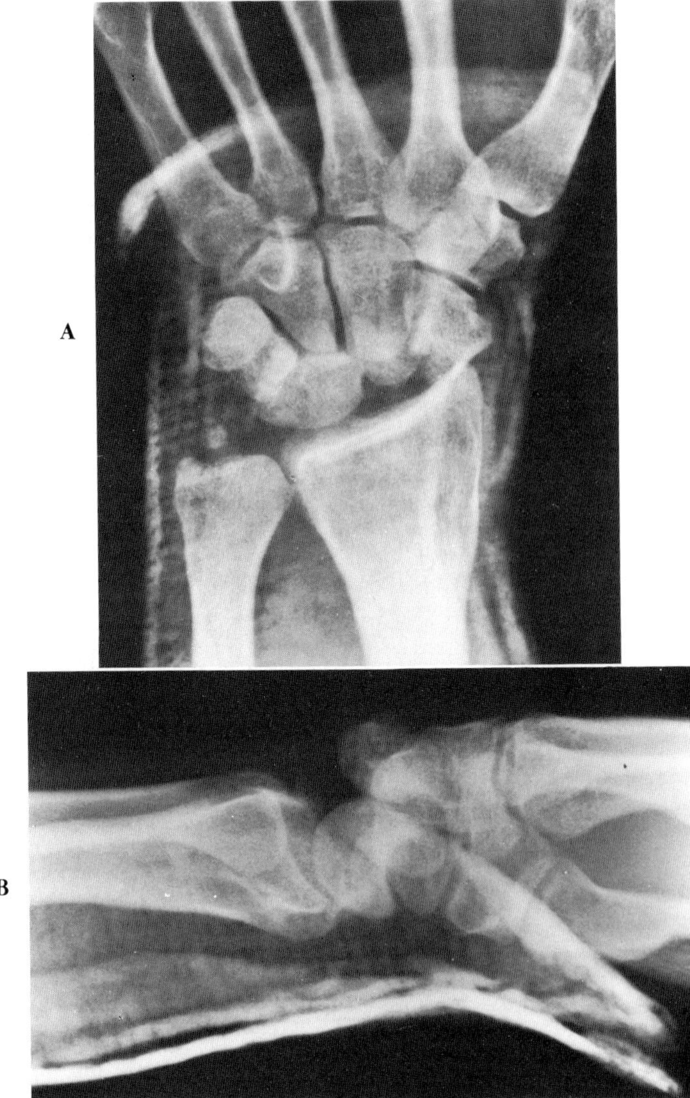

Fig. 13-2. A, Anteroposterior roentgenogram of a dorsal transscaphoid perilunate dislocation. **B,** Direction of dislocation is more readily identified on the lateral roentgenogram. The lunate and proximal pole of the scaphoid remain in articulation with the radius.

completely displaced or unstable fracture without associated perilunate dislocation. Motion at the fracture site with gapping of the fragments or significant residual displacement on acute injury is an indication for open reduction. Attention must be paid to the intercarpal relationships associated with fractures of the scaphoid. Occasionally ligamentous disruption will cause an intercarpal collapse pattern. This must be recognized as an indication for early open reduction and pinning.

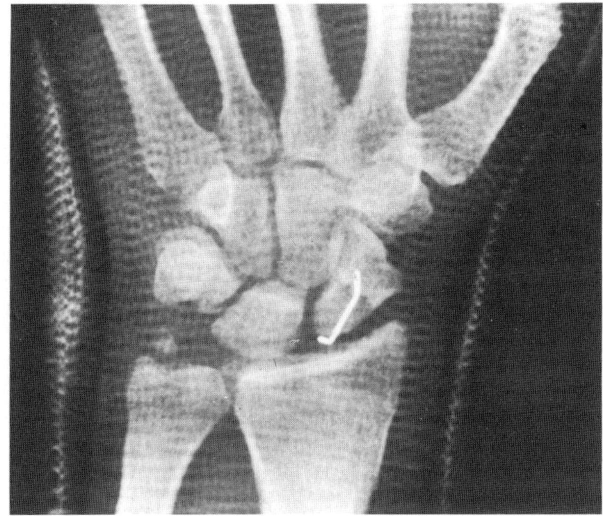

Fig. 13-3. The residually displaced fracture of the scaphoid after reduction of the dislocation has been fixed internally with a staple.

Transsscaphoid perilunate fracture-dislocations

The mechanism of injury in transcaphoid perilunate fracture-dislocations is similar to that of the isolated scaphoid fracture but obviously requires a greater force or more violent injury to produce. The dislocation is usually dorsal (Fig. 13-2) though on a rare occasion a volar transscaphoid perilunate dislocation[9] can occur. Closed reduction of the dislocation is usually readily accomplished. The difficulty with this injury is the common residual displacement of the fracture fragments. When this exists, and it almost inevitably does, the operation of open reduction and internal fixation is indicated (Fig. 13-3). If this is not undertaken in the acute phase, the rate of the nonunion can be expected to be extremely high. There are various techniques for internal fixation, and it is not the intent of this discussion to advocate any one in particular.

There is controversy whether bone grafting is necessary at the time of fixation of an acute displaced scaphoid fracture. As a general rule, secure fixation has proved to be adequate without bone grafting. Immobilization after operation or a closed reduction can lead to further complications if not properly done. It is not necessary to maintain the wrist in severe flexion because intercarpal stability is quite satisfactory in a neutral or only minimally flexed position of the wrist. Keeping the wrist in severe flexion for 6 weeks leads to persistent intercarpal subluxation at the capitolunate articulation, which can result in severe difficulty with posttraumatic instability problems.

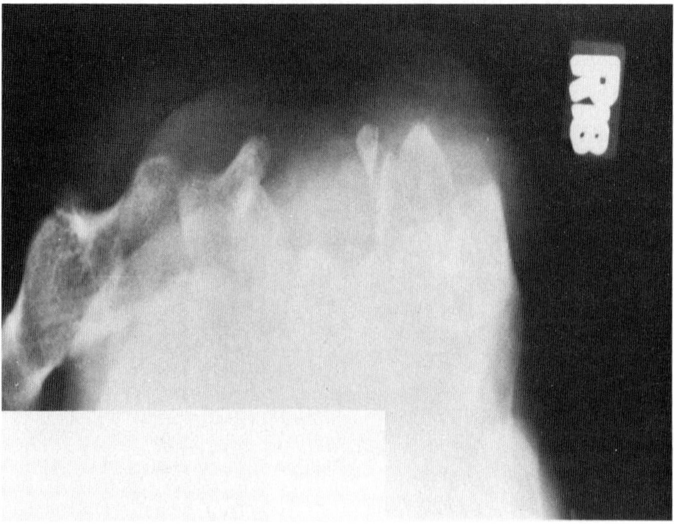

Fig. 13-4. The carpal tunnel view clearly demonstrates a fracture of the hook of the hamate.

Other carpal fractures

The triquetrum is the next most commonly fractured of the carpal bones. Fortunately it is rarely if ever a significant injury. The small dorsal chip fracture that is often seen on wrist roentgenograms usually arises from the dorsal surface of the trapezium. Simple immobilization for comfort until the acute phase has subsided is all that is required. This rarely proves to be a clinically significant disability in the long term.

Another carpal bone that is fractured with some frequency is the hook of the hamate. This is often seen in golfers who strike the ground behind the ball with the club with great force. This applies direct pressure to the hook of the hamate, and the patient complains of pain at the ulnar side of the base of the palm. This fracture is extremely difficult to see from routine anteroposterior, lateral, and oblique roentgenograms. For this reason it is frequently missed.[6] It can be associated with an ulnar nerve palsy because of the proximity of the hook of the hamate to the canal of Guyon. A carpal tunnel view is extremely important in establishing the diagnosis (Fig. 13-4). In acute cases short-arm cast immobilization incorporating the ring and small fingers to prevent persistent traction on the hook of the hamate by the hypothenar musculature is necessary. Fortunately, when not diagnosed until a nonunion is established, the fracture is often not disabling. Occasional discomfort with direct pressure may be the only symptom noticed by the patient. No therapy is indicated with the nonunion of the hook of the hamate unless the fracture is disabling; then excision of the hook of the hamate is the preferred procedure.[6]

DISLOCATIONS

Dislocations of the carpus are discussed under three general headings: lunate dislocations, perilunate dislocations, and other dislocations. In situ subluxation of various carpal bones and carpal collapse patterns are not discussed in this section as isolated entities. They are referred to only as complications of the overt dislocations of the carpals.

In situ carpal instability patterns, perilunate dislocations, and lunate dislocations have been thought to be part of a continuum of the same mechanism of injury.[4] Certainly the same mechanism appears to be responsible for the production of the various instability patterns.[1,3] Whether a lunate dislocation is a result of a spontaneously reduced dorsal perilunate dislocation is not known. It is not an unreasonable contention, however, since an attempt at reducing a dorsal perilunate dislocation often will result in replacement of all the carpals except for the lunate, which is then dislocated volarward.

Perilunate dislocations

The mechanism of injury of perilunate dislocations is probably a dorsiflexion of the wrist after a fall on the outstretched hand. The strong palmar radiocarpal and intercarpal ligaments rupture allowing the carpus to dislocate from the radiocarpal joint and around the lunate (Fig. 13-5, *A*). It is sometimes difficult to interpret the anteroposterior roentgenogram, but the key to diagnosis is the shape of the lunate as well as the relationship of the various carpals. As long as the lunate retains its normal quadrilateral appearance and the other relationships are distorted, one can suspect that a perilunate dislocation has occurred. The majority of these are dorsal perilunate dislocations, though, of course, there is the rare instance of the volar perilunate dislocation. On the lateral view the key to establishing the diagnosis is again the position of the lunate. One will find the lunate articulating with the radius at the lunate fossa, but the head of the capitate will not be found seated in the lunate cup on the distal end of the latter (Fig. 13-5, *B*). Occasionally the lunate can be tilted volarward by the pressure of the head of the capitate on its dorsal lip.

There may be associated median nerve symptoms that are best treated, of course, by reduction of the dislocation. The reduction is carried out under adequate anesthesia with traction and dorsiflexion of the hand and wrist. Pressure is applied volarward over the lunate to prevent subsequent conversion to a lunate dislocation, and with continued traction, the hand and wrist are palmar flexed. Reduction is usually accomplished rather readily and is fairly stable. It is therefore unnecessary to maintain the wrist in severe palmar flexion, which will create further problems with the median nerve and can result in a persistent midcarpal subluxation. Immobilization of the hand, wrist, forearm, and elbow are necessary.

It is extremely important to observe these patients with follow-up roentgenograms frequently in the first 10 to 14 days. The usual occurrence is that a pattern of dorsal intercalated segmental instability (DISI)[3] will occur with in situ rotation of the scaphoid (Fig. 13-6). This scapholunate dissociation is an indication for immediate

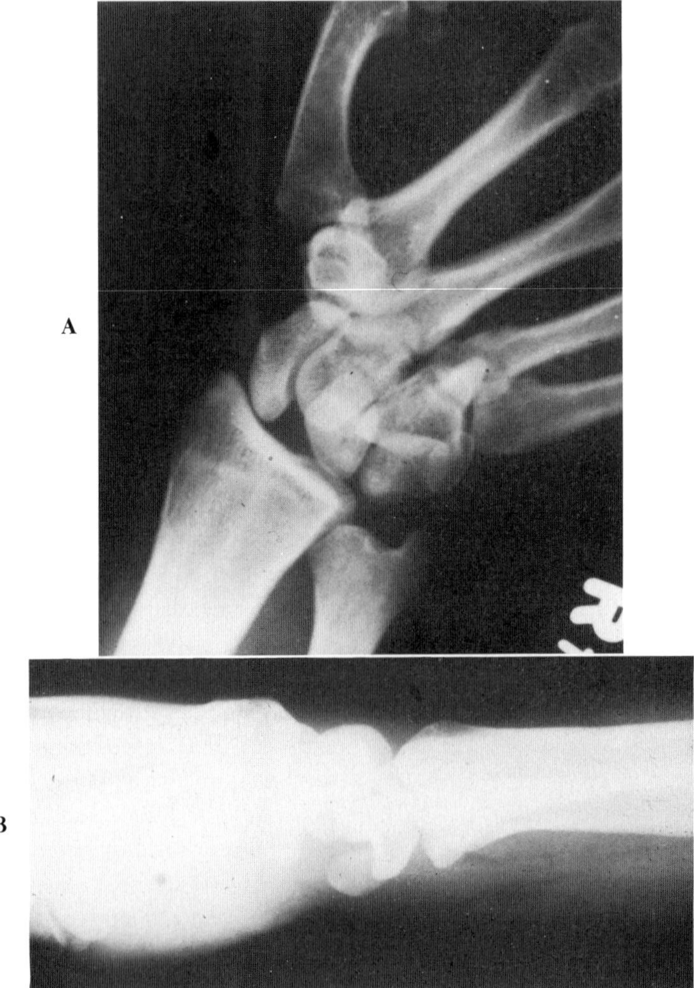

Fig. 13-5. A, Perilunate dislocation seen in the anteroposterior roentgenogram. The key is determining the shape of the lunate, which here retains its normal quadrilateral appearance. **B,** The lateral roentgenogram gives confirmatory evidence that the lunate remains located whereas the other carpals have become dislocated.

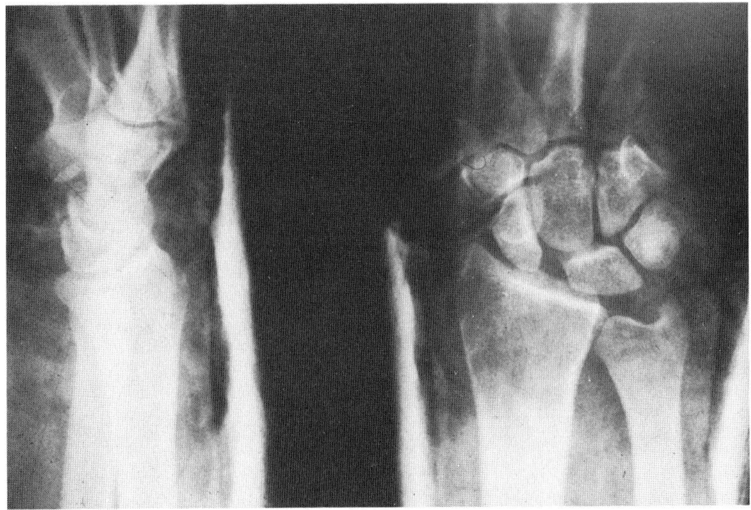

Fig. 13-6. *Left,* The reduced perilunate dislocation has left the lunate tilted dorsally and the scapholunate angle has increased. *Right,* The space between the lunate and scaphoid is wider than normal, confirming rupture of the supporting ligaments. This requires operative intervention.

open reduction with derotation and pinning of the scaphoid and lunate, and repair or reconstruction of the ligaments. The technique for this is described elsewhere. Failure to recognize this complication will result in a long-term poor functional result.

Lunate dislocation

Lunate dislocation can occur either volarly or dorsally. The mechanism of injury is the same for this as it is for most dislocations and fracture-dislocations. Whether it is a continuum of a spontaneously reduced perilunate dislocation or not is subject to debate, though many observers do believe that there is a definitive relationship. Associated median nerve symptoms with the acute injury are also common. It is best treated by closed reduction.

Roentgenographic evaluation is similarly difficult, but if one concentrates on the shape and position of the lunate, the diagnosis becomes easier. On the anteroposterior projection, the lunate will assume a triangular shape in contradistinction to its normal quadrilateral configuration (Fig. 13-7, *A*). On the lateral, the remainder of the carpals will generally be well aligned with the radius, but the half-moon-shaped lunate will have displaced volarly and no longer be in articulation with the lunate fossa of the radius (Fig. 13-7, *B*). The distal cup of the lunate will generally be facing palmarward.

Closed reduction is most successful when performed under adequate anesthesia. With traction on the hand and wrist and placement of the wrist in dorsiflexion, direct pressure over the lunate palmarward often will allow this small bone to slip back into its normal position in the lunate fossa. Once reduced these lesions are quite stable,

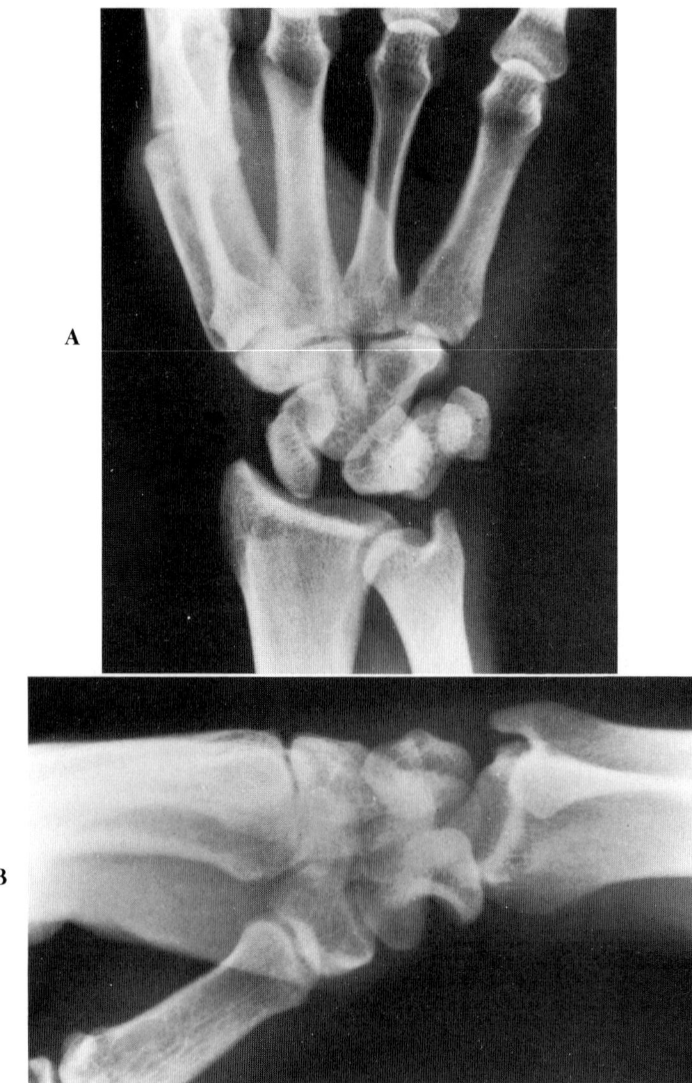

Fig. 13-7. A, Anteroposterior roentgenogram of a lunate dislocation. The configuration of the lunate is triangular indicating that it is dislocated while the remaining carpals are aligned. **B,** Lateral roentgenogram confirms the volar dislocation of the lunate.

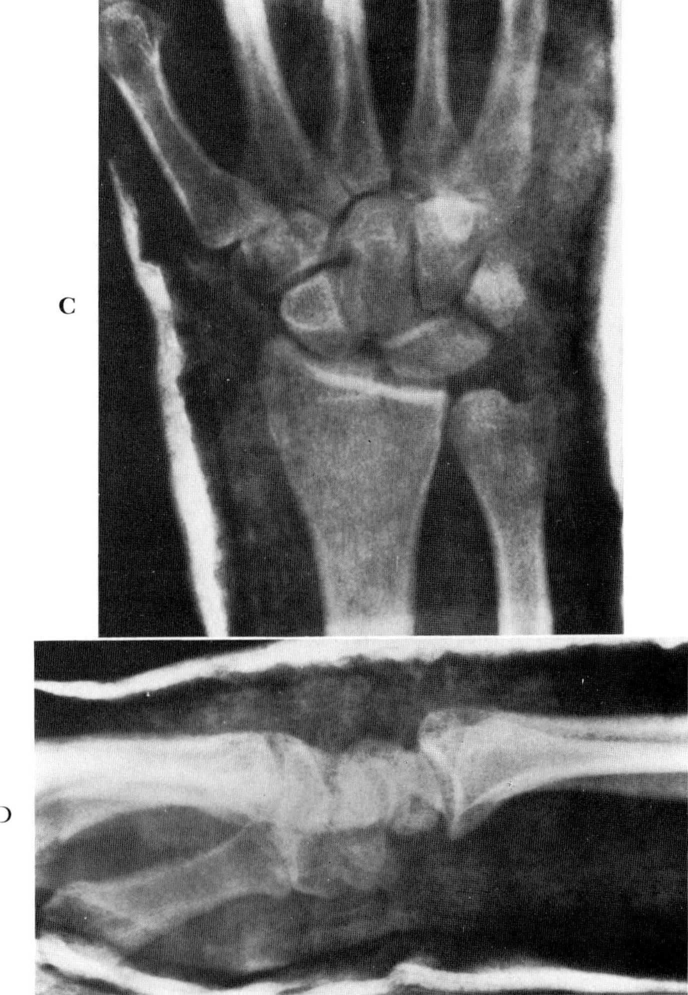

Fig. 13-7, cont'd. C, Anteroposterior roentgenogram showing the increased scapholunate angle after reduction of the dislocation. **D,** Lateral roentgenogram showing an increased scapholunate angle after reduction of the lunate dislocation.   *Continued.*

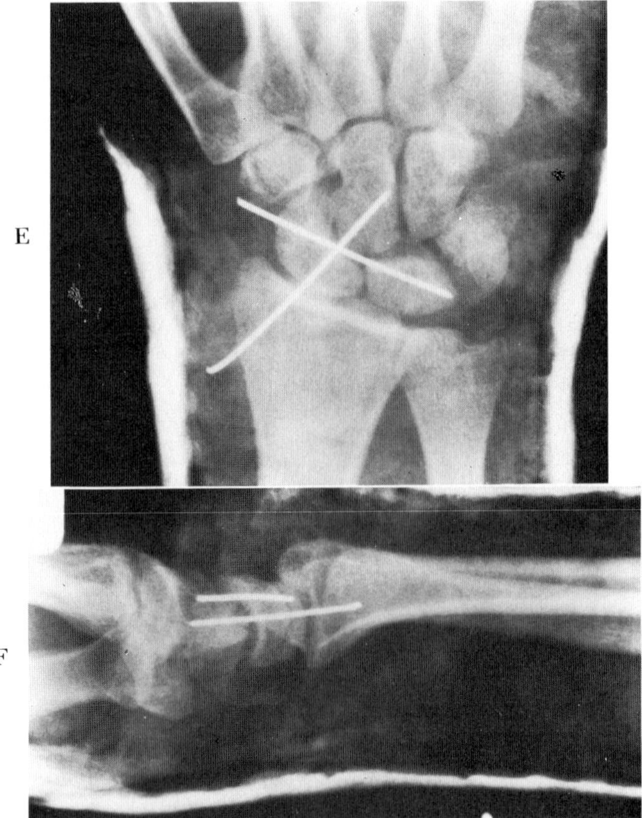

Fig. 13-7, cont'd. E, Anteroposterior roentgenogram after open reduction, derotation of the carpals, and pinning of the scapholunate ligaments repaired. **F,** Lateral roentgenogram of the same case postoperatively. The scapholunate angle has been reduced.

and severe flexion of the wrist is not justified. The early complication of intercarpal instability is also common with lunate dislocations and close roentgenographic assessment over the first 10 to 14 days after reduction is necessary to avoid missing the diagnosis (Fig. 13-7, *C* and *D*). If it occurs, open reduction of the rotated carpals must be accomplished and ligamentous repair or reconstruction is also indicated (Fig. 13-7, *E* and *F*).

If median nerve symptoms persist after perilunate or lunate dislocations, carpal tunnel release is justified. Fortunately, the symptoms usually subside once reduction is effected and the wrist is immobilized with the hand elevated.

Other carpal dislocations

All the carpal bones have been reported as having been dislocated individually. Obviously each must be treated according to its particular needs. Open reduction is frequently required, but if closed reduction is successful, close observation in the early phases for carpal instability patterns must be undertaken.

SALVAGE PROCEDURE FOR CARPAL INJURIES

Long-standing scapholunate dissociation after carpal dislocations, long-standing scaphoid nonunions with periscaphoid arthrosis, and old fracture-dislocations of the wrist with persistent midcarpal subluxations are often not amenable to simple open reduction and fixation of the original problems. The reason for this, of course, is that extensive intercarpal degenerative changes have occurred and they would result in persistent pain even if the original lesions were corrected. Once these severe, degenerative conditions have been established, the treatment options include radiocarpal arthrodesis, intercarpal arthrodesis, and arthroplasty. In the latter group are included replacement arthroplasty and resection arthroplasty such as proximal row carpectomy. Each observer has his favorite technique, but it is important to realize that the complication rate with arthrodesis is much higher than generally appreciated. In addition, arthrodesis often requires prolonged immobilization and, of course, severely limits wrist motion.

Implant arthroplasty, except in isolated instances, has not yet defined its proper role in the treatment of posttraumatic disorders. Total wrist arthroplasty, though promising, cannot be advocated at this time for a wide variety of disorders. Proximal row carpectomy, however, has stood the test of time and is a most satisfactory procedure for those patients who wish to retain wrist motion and have a satisfactory grip.[5] It has had an unsatisfactory reputation for a long period of time despite reports of successful series. Motion, of course, is retained through varying degrees, depending on the underlying original diagnosis. The degree of motion compares favorably to that with scaphotrapezial trapezoidal arthrodesis and other intercarpal fusions. It is, of course, far better than that with formal wrist arthrodesis. The complication rate of proximal row carpectomy is low. It must be emphasized, however, that this, as are the arthrodeses, is a salvage procedure and should not be considered a primary reconstructive operation.

REFERENCES

1. Dobyns, J.H., and Linscheid, R.L.: Fractures and dislocations of the wrist. In Rockwood, C.A., and Green, D.P., editors: Fractures in adults, ed. 2, Philadelphia, 1984, J.B. Lippincott Co.
2. Gelberman, R.H., et al.: The vascularity of the scaphoid bone, J. Hand Surg. **5:**508, 1980.
3. Linscheid, R.L., et al.: Traumatic instability of the wrist: diagnosis, classification, and pathomechanics, J. Bone Joint Surg. **56A:**1612, 1972.
4. Mayfield, J.K.: Mechanism of carpal injuries, Clin. Orthop. (149):45, 1980.
5. Neviaser, R.J.: Proximal row carpectomy for posttraumatic disorders of the carpus, J. Hand Surg. **8:**301, 1983.
6. Nisenfeld, F.G., and Neviaser, R.J.: Fracture of the hook of the hamate—a diagnosis easily missed, J. Trauma **14:**612, 1974.
7. Russe, O.: Fracture of the carpal navicular: diagnosis, nonoperative treatment and operative treatment, J. Bone Joint Surg. **42A:**759, 1960.
8. Taleisnik, J., and Kelly, P.J.: The extraosseous and intraosseous blood supply of the scaphoid bone, J. Bone Joint Surg. **48A:**125, 1966.
9. Woodward, A.H., Neviaser, R.J., and Nisenfeld, F.G.: Radial and volar perilunate transscaphoid fracture-dislocation, South. Med. J. **68:**926, 1975.

14. Ligament injuries about the wrist

James H. Dobyns

If one concentrates upon the forearms, wrists, and hands in Michelangelo's famous painting of the creation of Adam, one can see two primary postures of the wrist and hand. There is the active, prehensile, and directorial hand of God in the act of bringing life to the resting, passive hand of Adam. Wrist function, demonstrated in those two positions, is important in three ways:[2,5] (1) spatial orientation of the hand, (2) mechanical augmentation of the finger range (digit flexion aided by wrist extension and digit extension aided by wrist flexion), (3) torque transmission from the forearm. The usual injuries of the hand, some 90% or more, are incurred in the extended wrist position with the outthrust hand supporting the body weight as occurs during a fall.[2] This results in compression and shear forces along the dorsum of the wrist and tensile stresses along the palmar surface. Each injury is part of a continuum, a pattern that is common in the upper limb. It is unusual to have only a single problem after a significant stress.

The determinants of the type of injury include the type of three-dimensional loading, the magnitude and the duration of the forces, the position of the wrist and hand at impact, and the biomechanical properties of the natural materials such as bones and ligaments.[2,5]

ANATOMY: BIOMECHANICS

A brief review of wrist anatomy follows.[2,7,10] Three joints are normal: the midcarpal joint, the radiocarpal joint, the distal radioulnar joint. These often communicate, and most of the fenestrations are probably attritional and traumatic, since they are not seen in the infant. The capsular envelope has certain intracapsular thickenings; the strongest are on the palmar aspect, which has to bear tremendous tensile stresses. The former volar radiocarpal ligament is now called the volar radioscaphocapitate (radiocapitate) ligament. There is also a volar radiolunotriquetral (radiotriquetral) ligament, which is very strong. There is a weaker volar radioscapholunate ligament. There is a similar ligament complex connecting the carpus to the ulnar side of the radius and also to the ulna. The strongest of these ligaments are the ulnolunate, the ulnotriquetral, and the triangular fibrocartilage complex.[8] There are also important interconnecting ligaments between certain of the carpal bones. The ones that

134

have received the most attention so far are the scapholunate interosseous ligament and the lunotriquetral interosseous ligament. On the dorsum of the wrist, ligaments are weaker than on the volar aspect, often to the point of being attenuated or anomalous. Most likely to be present are the radiotriquetral band of the triangular fibrocartilage and the dorsal radiolunotriquetral (radiotriquetral) ligament. Ligamentous injuries of the wrist are to be discussed, but this will not include dislocations, which are discussed in another presentation. However, in both dislocations and lesser ligamentous injuries, these are the biomechanics concerned.[2,4-7] The ligaments are the constraints to the excursion and the translation of the carpal bones. At limiting angulations, there is tensile loading on one side, compression loading on the other side. The forces are dissipated by physiologic lengthening of the tissues and by tissue compliance. When these physiologic responses are exceeded, failure of the materials involved results in fracture of bone, disruption of cartilage, and disruption of ligament. The fundamental biomechanical concept involving the wrist is that of the intercalated segment, nicely elucidated by Landsmeer in anatomic studies.[4] The proximal carpal row is an intercalated segment that has no direct control by musculotendinous units, is stable only in tension, and falls into a low-energy position in compression. The stops or check to carpal collapse are the ligaments and the scaphoid itself, which spans both carpal rows. If all the stops and checks are working, the angle between the scaphoid and the lunate is about 45 degrees and there is collinear alignment of radius, lunate, capitate, and third metacarpal. The two major collapse positions are the zigzag patterns of any link system and in the wrist are called "dorsiflexed intercalated segment instability (DISI)" for the dorsiflexion instability pattern and "volar (palmar) flexed intercalated segment instability (VISI or PISI)" for the palmar-flexion pattern.[2] Biomechanical considerations include the kinematic control of the proximal carpal row induced by the scaphoid when palmar flexion is the stance of the wrist, and induced by the triquetrum when dorsiflexion is the wrist stance. The lunate is the most protected carpal bone. It has no tendinous insertions but is well guarded by bone and well supported by ligament constraints. Such ligaments, as are present, attach to bone and to articular cartilage margins. When the interosseous ligaments tear, there is a great deal of force exerted to distract the carpal bones. There is little healing reaction seen clinically. With the larger extrinsic ligaments, there is more of a vascular response and a better healing tendency, though often with lengthening. The classic instance of ligamentous disruption in the wrist is the perilunate dislocation. The many varieties of perilunate dislocation and fracture-dislocation result from the addition of deviation and torque to the fundamental hyperextension. Rather than dislocations, subluxation is discussed in this presentation; the common ones are scapholunate dissociation[6] and lunotriquetral dissociation.[9] There are others that are not so common; in fact, the current excitement in the wrist injury field is in working out the pathomechanics, making an early diagnosis, and finding proper treatments for these other injuries such as radioulnar instability, ulnar translation, dorsal and palmar translation, and proximal row instability.[2] To identify these problems, one starts with the history. There is usually significant single-episode trauma, though the cause may be repetitive stress or there may have been ancient injury or disease and a relatively trivial, recent injury. For diagnosis there is much reliance on x rays and the methods currently used are (1) standard posteroanterior and lateral roentgenograms; (2) motion study roentgenograms (that is, radial deviation and ulnar deviation posteroanterior views, flexion and extension lateral views with or without grip stress), and (3) stress views with the stress created either actively by the patient or passively by the investigator. Finally, there are three special studies of great value—the scan, tomography (particularly the trispiral tomogram), and arthrography.[2]

SCAPHOLUNATE DISSOCIATION

The wrist injury that is most common is scapholunate dissociation[6] (Fig. 14-1), the ligament analog of scaphoid fracture. The symptoms are central wrist pain and tenderness 2 to 3 cm distal to Lister's tubercle. Roentgen findings include the dramatic scapholunate gap, which is now so well known that the diagnosis is often mistakenly discounted when the gap is not present. There is a whole spectrum of scapholunate problems, some of which do not have a gap and some of which do not have a scapholunate angle change.[2,5] The classic or advanced scapholunate dissociation does have a scapholunate gap on the posteroanterior view with an angle change between scaphoid and lunate on the lateral view in excess of 70 degrees. In addition an arthrogram will show radiocarpal to midcarpal dye flow with the dye flowing through the scapholunate interval. The treatment, currently the most popular, is that of stabilizing the unstable scaphoid by fusion of its distal pole to the trapezium and the trapezoid but only after the scaphoid proximal pole is reduced in its relation to the scaphoid sulcus of the radius.[11] Others still repair the ligaments.[2,6] Since tendon grafts don't heal very well in a joint fluid environment, it is better to repair the ligament itself, which has better quality and better vascularity than a tendon graft. Reattachment is to the bone from which the ligament is stripped, usually the scaphoid. Augmenting with a tendon graft or a capsular flap may be needed, and very infrequently some other sort of carpal fusion may be required.[2]

It is important to hold ligament repair and reconstruction long enough that the repair heals and the whole capsular-ligamentous apparatus shrinks. We now have many cases of scapholunate dissociation treated by ligament repair, occasionally with tendon graft augmentation, that have maintained correction and maintained a clinical improvement pattern.[2,6] Others report similar results with scaphotrapezium-trapezoid fusion. Some favor scapholunate fusion.

LUNOTRIQUETRAL DISSOCIATION

The second most common of the intercarpal problems is the lunotriquetral sprain (Fig. 14-2), which also comes in a variety of clinical presentations: acute, semiacute, chronic, and sometimes those with arthritic changes.[9] It too has a standard group of clinical findings. It has a regular group of roentgenographic findings, which are not so dramatic in the early stages as in scapholunate dissociation. The lunotriquetral joint is less mobile and less stressed than the scapholunate joint, and so it may take longer for

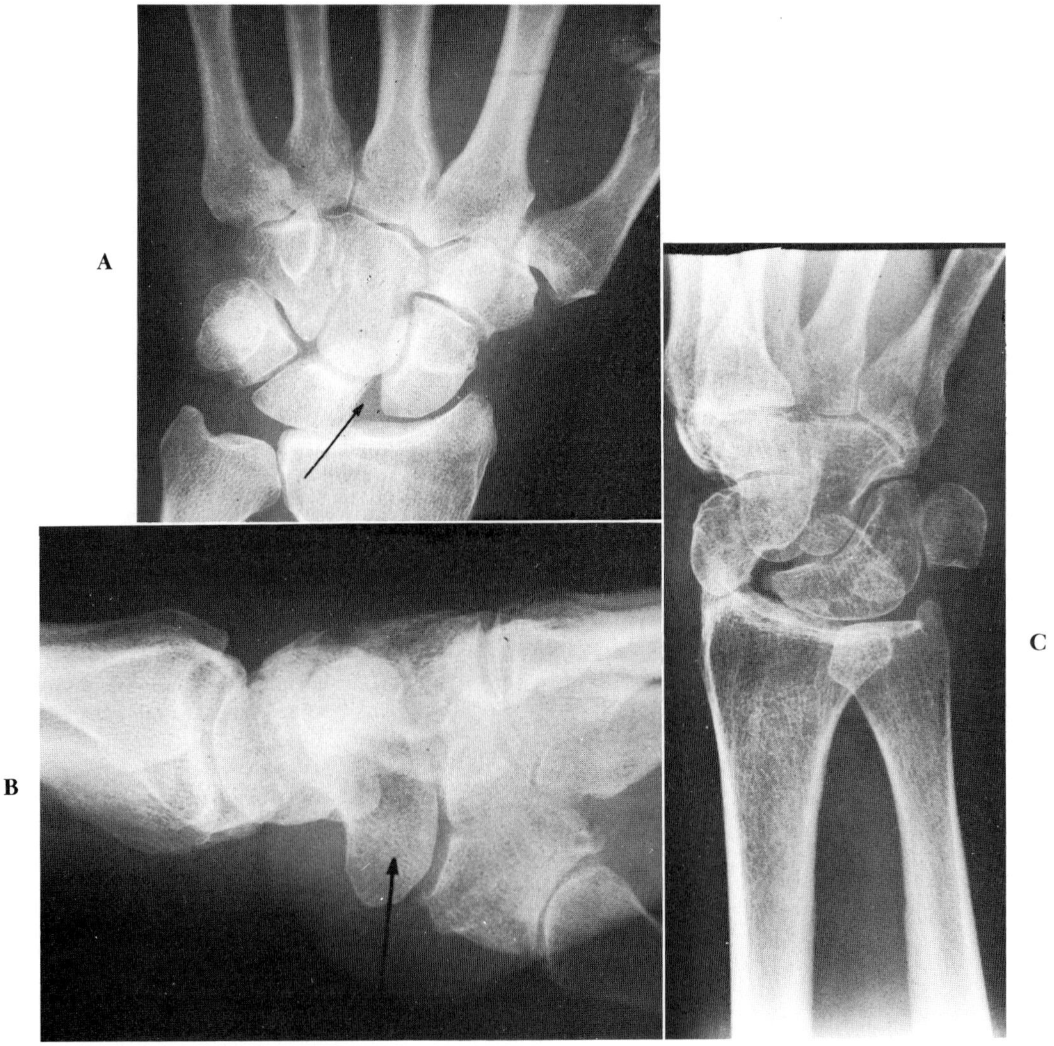

Fig. 14-1. Scapholunate dissociation. **A,** This posteroanterior view of a wrist shows the classic scapholunate gap, *black arrow*, with rotated (volarflexed) scaphoid and overlap of capitate by the opposite rotation (dorsiflexion) of the lunate. **B,** This roentgenographic lateral view of the same wrist as in **A** shows the classic increase of the scapholunate angle (near 90 degrees here). *Black arrow*, Distal end of the volarflexed scaphoid; the mild dorsiflexion of the lunate can be seen. **C,** Oblique view of the wrist in another instance of scapholunate dissociation shows that a severely unstable scaphoid may overlap or even "catch" upon the dorsal radius. This also demonstrates why the proximal scaphoid is dorsally prominent in this condition.

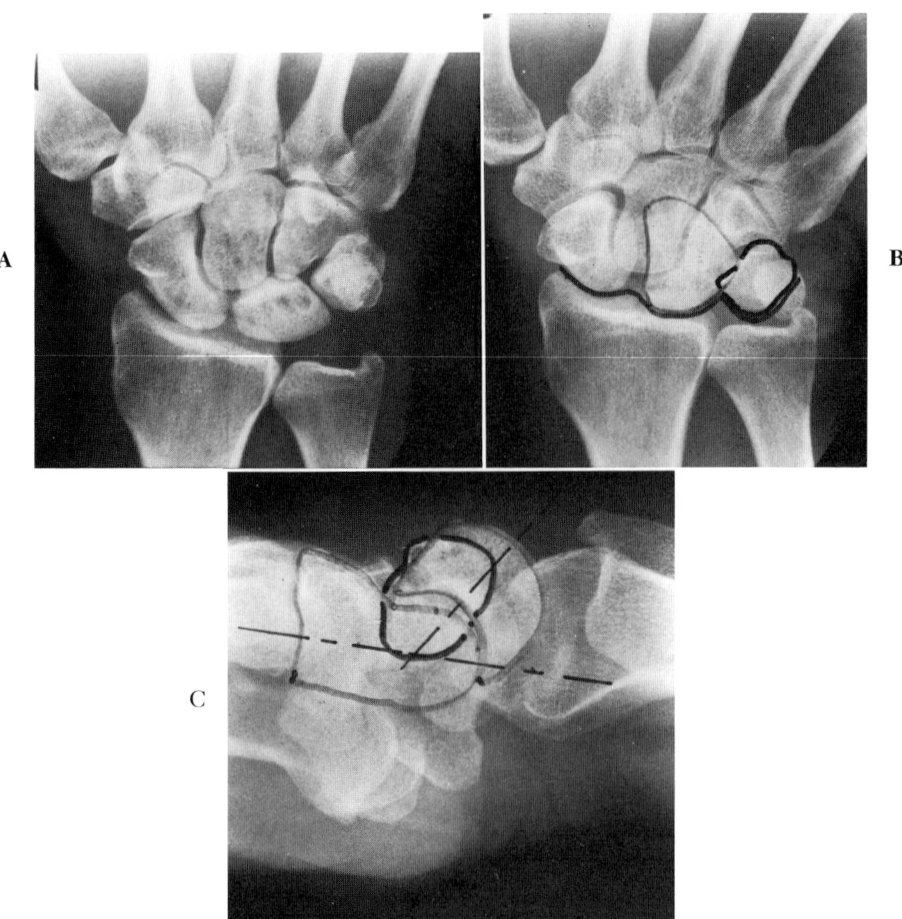

Fig. 14-2. Lunotriquetral dissociation. **A,** This posteroanterior roentgenographic view of a wrist is normal except for variations in bone density in the carpals and a break in the smooth-arc outline of the distal subchondral bone of the proximal carpal row. The break occurs between lunate and triquetrum. **B,** With compression, views of the same wrist show noticeable overlap of the distal carpals by the lunate and scaphoid, but they are not accompanied by the triquetrum (a dissociative type of VISI, or volar intercalary segment instability). **C,** Lateral view of the same wrist shows the severe VISI position with capitate well volar to the flexing scaphoid and lunate.

roentgenographic and arthritic changes to present. A wrist may look normal after an injury, but in days to weeks a VISI (volar intercalary segment or volar flexion instability pattern) may develop with the lunate slightly dorsally translocated and flexed over the capitate; the capitolunate angle is usually in excess of 15 degrees. Some such patients may be treated adequately with splinting. Sometimes there is a fracture to be seen, particularly if tomograms are used to identify it. Some patients may have a fracture of the volar pole of the lunate, avulsing support ligaments with it and eventually developing an extreme volar flexion instability. Other patients may show triquetral or lunate margin fractures where ligament avulsion has occurred. When lunotriquetral dissociation has progressed far enough, these roentgenographic findings may be seen: an overlap of proximal and distal carpal rows, a loss of the smooth arc of the proximal carpal row, and change of angle between lunate and triquetrum. Even in extreme capitolunate angulation the scaphoid accompanies the lunate because this most common of the VISI collapse patterns is a dissociative collapse with loss of bonding between the triquetrum and the lunate. The scaphoid and the lunate are still moving together, and they both flex on the capitate. Surgery may be needed and several different stabilizing procedures seem to work relatively well. Some are treated simply by ligament repair and reconstruction. Lunotriquetral fusion is also used. Results are comparable, with improved wrist comfort after technical success with any of these procedures.[9]

INSTABILITY OF THE DISTAL ULNA

The final group of instabilities for discussion today are at the distal radioulnar joint (Fig. 14-3), triangular fibrocartilage, and ulnocarpal complex, all of which function together. The causes of injury are diverse, but a triangular fibrocartilage injury is more common in an ulna-plus (ulna longer than radius) wrist, which gives increased loading to the triangular fibrocartilage complex. As that complex gives way, the distal ulna and the carpus come closer together with development of an impingement syndrome.[1,2,3,8] The roentgenographic changes are first narrowing and then subchondral sclerosis of the ulnocarpal area. Arthrographic studies reveal a dye leak between radiocarpal and distal radioulnar joints.

The surgical premise here is that there is a need to unload the ulnocarpal area, change the bearing surfaces in the distal radioulnar joint, and tighten the ligamentous constraints of the ulnocarpal ligament system. This is accomplished by osteotomy and shortening of the ulna. One may also repair the triangular fibrocartilage complex at the same time. Results of this procedure have been good as assessed by return to work statistics. This procedure has advantages over excision of the distal ulna in that it maintains the interosseous space, maintains distal radioulnar stability, improves ulnocarpal stability, and minimally alters forearm kinematics. The higher the level of performance the more important are these advantages, since they may permit rehabilitation to a near-normal level.[1,2]

Ligament injury with or without associated bone injury is a common problem at the wrist.[2,5] Levels of healing that might prove satisfactory in single joints often prove

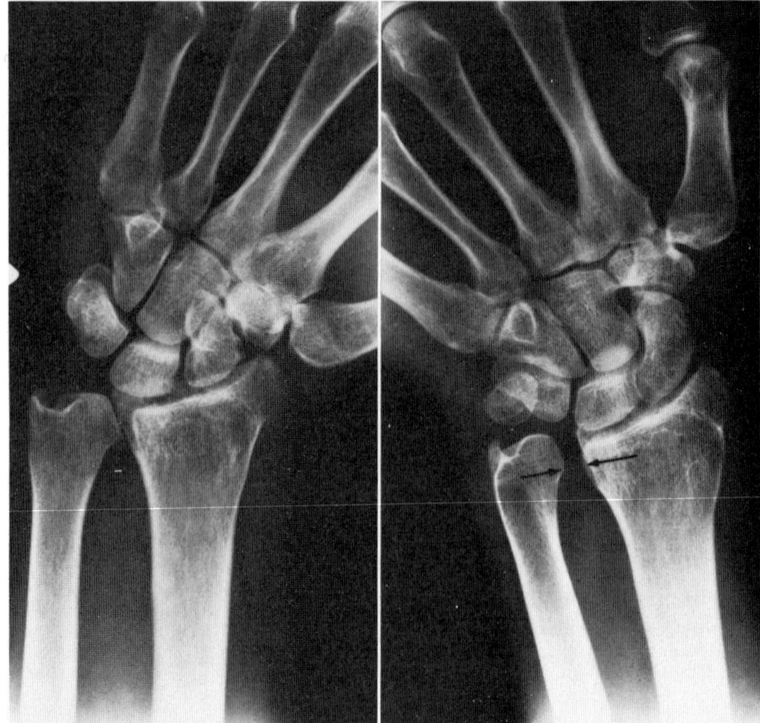

Fig. 14-3. Instability of the distal end of the ulna. Such instability of the ulna often affects both the ulnocarpal and distal radioulnar joints, which are associated with the distal end of the ulna. Although injury may involve the distal ulna alone, it often occurs in association with a distal radius injury. A typical case is revealed in the accompanying roentgenogram, which shows evidence of prior radial fracture. Furthermore, the two views (posteroanterior views in radial deviation and ulnar deviation) show the effect of stress and position on the unstable ulna (radioulnar separation and ulnocarpal impingement are much more obvious on the ulnar deviation view).

inadequate in this multibone, multijoint, interrelated, linkage system. This is particularly true when peak performance stresses are regularly applied. In athletes it is vital to suspect, make, and manage the proper diagnosis, adequately and early. If this is not done or is proving inadequate, surgical repair or protective reconstruction is advisable.

REFERENCES

1. Darrow, J.C., Jr., et al.: Distal ulnar recession for disorders of the distal radioulnar joint, J. Hand Surg. 10A(4):482-491, July 1985.
2. Dobyns, J.H., and Linscheid, R.L.: Fractures and dislocations of the wrist. In Rockwood, C.A., Jr., and Green, D.P., editors: Fractures, Philadelphia, 1975, J.B. Lippincott Co.
3. Dobyns, J.H., Sim, F.H., and Linscheid, R.L.: Sports stress syndromes of the hand and wrist, Am. J. Sports Med. 6(5):236-254, 1978.

4. Landsmeer, J.M.F.: Studies in the anatomy of articulation. I. The equilibrium of the "intercalated" bone, Acta Morphol. Neerl. Scand. 3:287-303, 1961.
5. Linscheid, R.L., et al.: Instability patterns of the wrist, J. Hand Surg. 9(5):682-686, Sept. 1983.
6. Linscheid, R.L., Dobyns, J.H., and Bryan, R.S.: Traumatic instability of the wrist: diagnosis, classification and pathomechanics, J. Bone Joint Surg. 54A(8):1612-1632, Dec. 1972.
7. Mayfield, J.K., Johnson, R.P., and Kilcoyne, R.F.: The ligaments of the human wrist and their functional significance, Anat. Rec. 186:417-428, 1976.
8. Palmer, A.K., and Werner, F.W.: The triangular fibrocartilage complex of the wrist—anatomy and function, J. Hand Surg. 6:153-162, March 1981.
9. Reagan, D.S., Linscheid, R.L., and Dobyns, J.H.: Lunotriquetral sprains, J. Hand Surg. 9A(4):502-514, July 1984.
10. Taleisnik, J.: The ligaments of the wrist, J. Hand Surg. 1:110-118, 1976.
11. Watson, H.K., Goodman, M.L., and Johnson, T.R.: Limited wrist arthrodesis. II. Intercarpal and radiocarpal combinations, J. Hand Surg. 6:223-233, May 1981.

15. Complex joint injuries of the hand

Charles P. Melone, Jr.

Because of their continual exposure to violent trauma, the small joints of the hand are prone to sports injuries. Particularly prevalent among athletes are complex joint injuries, defined in this chapter as those requiring open treatment for preservation of the articular surfaces. This group includes the following:

1. Dislocations irreducible by closed manipulation
2. Unstable fracture-dislocations
3. Displaced articular fractures
4. Complete collateral ligament disruptions

Basic to all complex injuries is a profound articular disruption that is likely to result in contracture or instability. Optimal treatment must accurately restore joint congruity and stability and yet permit early joint motion. After repair the interphalangeal joints are preferentially immobilized in slight flexion for no longer than 4 weeks and the metacarpophalangeal joints are positioned in acute flexion for a similar period. Because of their limited periarticular soft-tissue support and an exaggerated tendency for redisplacement, the carpometacarpal joints generally require 6 weeks of protection. After discontinuance of postoperative immobilization a program of supervised rehabilitation, usually requiring 6 weeks, is essential to restore a satisfactory level of function and lessen the risk of reinjury. Thus an athlete who suffers a complex joint injury of the hand generally requires a 3-month period of recovery before resuming competition. The use of a protective device is also advisable until such time as the articular swelling and stiffness have completely resolved.

This chapter categorizes these complex injuries according to the level and type of joint disruption and describes techniques of diagnosis and treatment that have proved successful for the majority of cases.

DISTAL INTERPHALANGEAL (DIP) JOINT INJURIES
Mallet fractures

Rational management of distal phalangeal articular fractures is based on the size and displacement of the dorsal fracture fragment as viewed on the lateral roentgenograms. Fragments constituting less than 25% of the articular surface heal satisfacto-

142

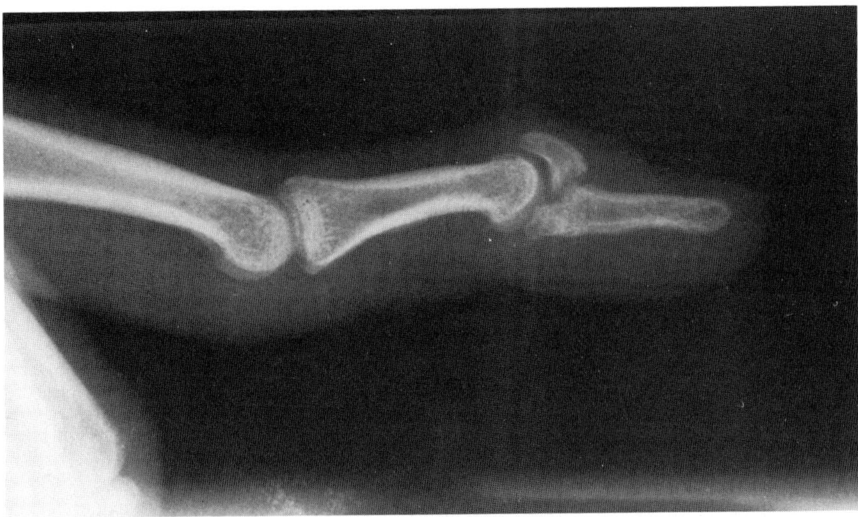

Fig. 15-1. A displaced mallet fracture treated with extension splinting and resulting in mal-union with dorsal prominence and palmar subluxation of the distal phalanx. Arthrodesis was necessary to eradicate painful arthritis.

rily with 4 weeks of extension splinting. In contrast, splinting of larger fragments with displacement greater than 2 mm frequently leads to a troublesome malunion and is prone to result in an arthritic joint that requires arthrodesis (Fig. 15-1).

Serious mallet fractures that typically demonstrate displacement of a fragment constituting between 30% and 50% of the articular surface and that often result in palmar subluxation of the distal phalanx require open reduction for restoration of joint congruity (Fig. 15-2). Intraosseous wiring coupled with temporary transarticular Kirschner wire fixation provides a method of secure fixation for these fractures.[2,10] This technique avoids further fragmentation and provides compression at the fracture interface thereby accelerating the healing process. Fracture union is usually achieved in 4 weeks, at which time the transarticular wire is removed and active motion of the joint is started.

A preliminary review of 30 mallet fractures demonstrating prominent displacement or joint subluxation and treated with intraosseous wire fixation supports the opinion that prompt open reduction and internal fixation is a superior method of treatment for these injuries.[2,8,20] In the majority of these cases a congruous joint and a near-normal range of painless motion have been restored, and on follow-up as long as 9 years none of the cases has required reconstructive surgery.

Articular condylar fractures

Condylar fractures frequently involve both the middle and proximal phalangeal heads. In most cases one condyle is excessively compressed and displaced proximally (Fig. 15-3, *A*). Even minimal displacement indicates instability that must be recog-

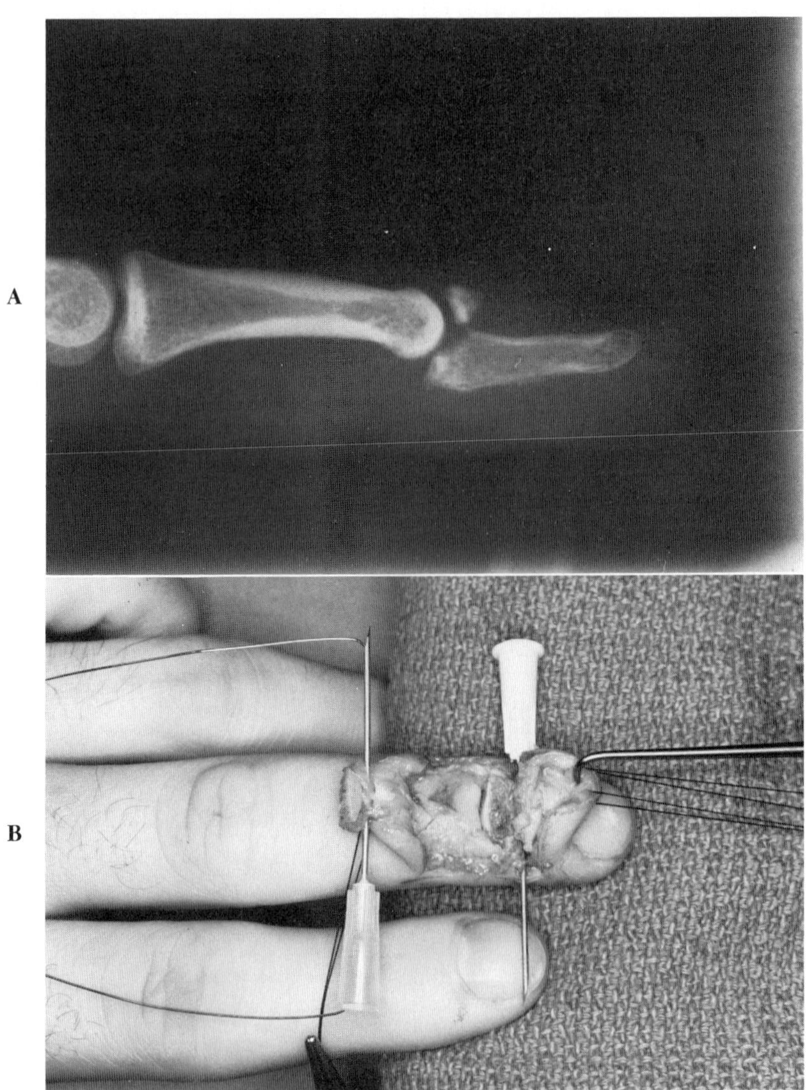

Fig. 15-2. A, A mallet fracture with major articular disruption. Treatment by open reduction and intraosseous wire fixation. **B,** Dorsal H incision provides excellent exposure of the joint and the displaced articular fragment, which is reflected proximally. The extensor mechanism, the collateral ligaments, and the nail bed are not disturbed. The use of a No. 20 hypodermic needle facilitates passage of a 26-gauge monofilament wire at the juncture of the displaced fragment and the attached extensor tendon and then distally through the palmar aspect of the distal phalanx.

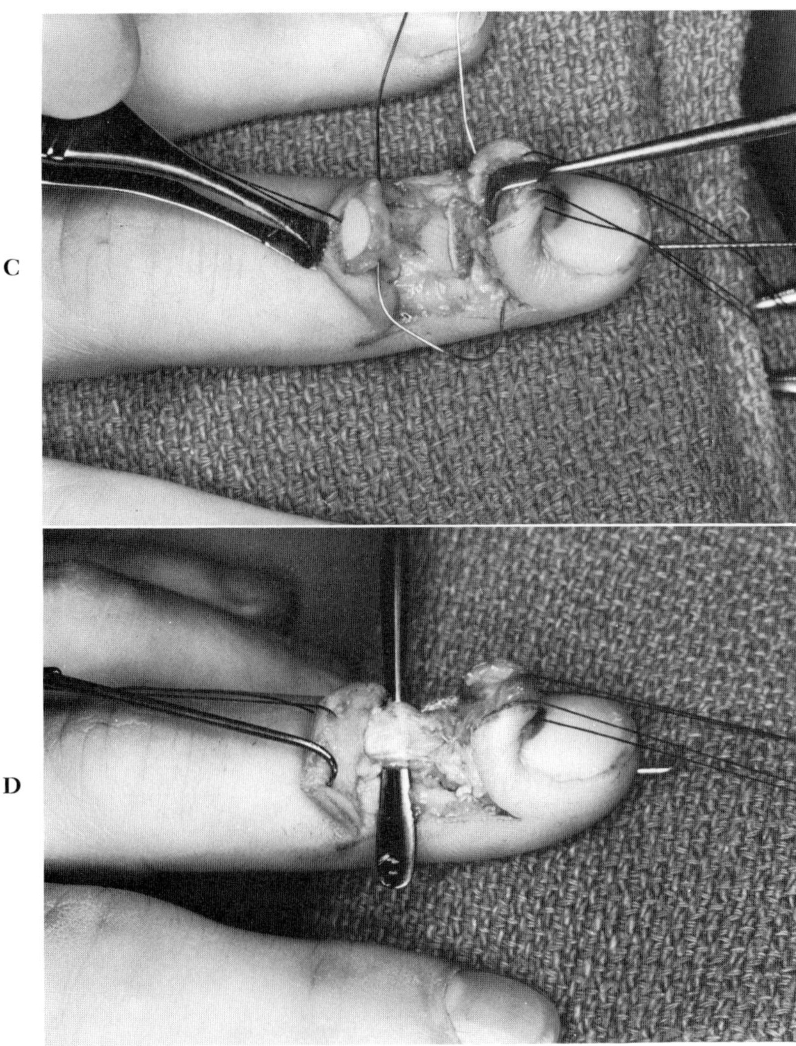

Fig. 15-2, cont'd. C, Before a reduction of the articular fragment, palmar displacement of the distal phalanx is corrected and the joint is fixed with a 0.035-gauge Kirschner wire. **D,** After an anatomic reduction, the intraosseous wire is tightened so that articular congruity and continuity of the extensor mechanism can be restored.
                                                    Continued.

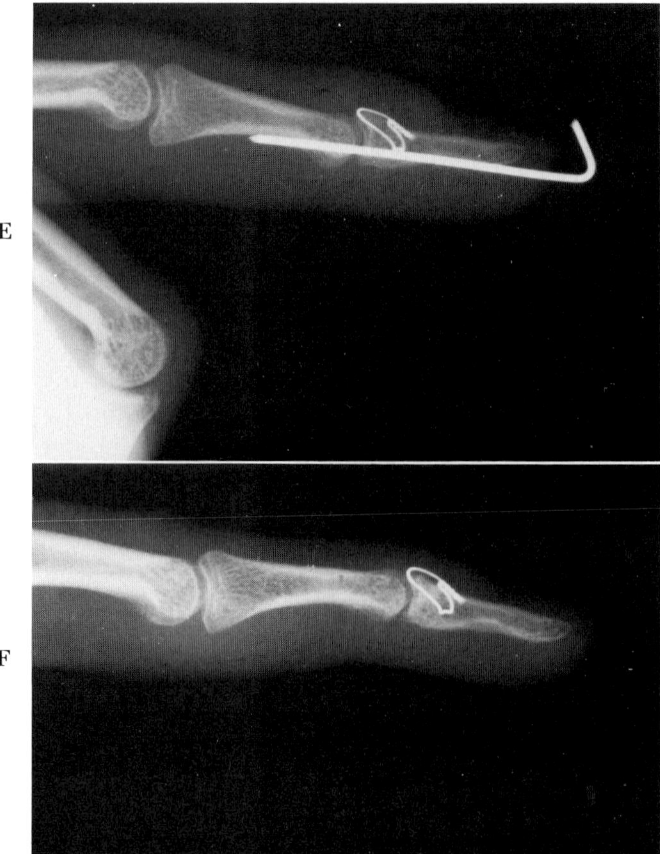

Fig. 15-2, cont'd. E and **F,** Postoperative roentgenograms demonstrating an accurate reduction and 6 months later preservation of the articular surface.

nized and corrected by open reduction. Neglected injuries result in a considerable loss of interphalangeal joint motion as well as a disabling angular deformity characterized by overlapping of the injured digit and the adjacent one.

Because of their oblique plane, these fractures are often suitable for rigid fixation with small screws. After an anatomic reduction, interfragmental compression is achieved with 1.5 or 2 mm cortical screws (Fig. 15-3, *B*). Although technically demanding, this method permits early active joint motion thereby facilitating rapid recovery. Importantly, interfragmental compression with corrective osteotomy has also been used to salvage malunited condylar fractures treated as late as 3 months after injury. Obviously excessive comminution precludes screw fixation, and in such cases the employment of fine Kirschner wires has proved to be a satisfactory method of fracture stabilization.[12,20]

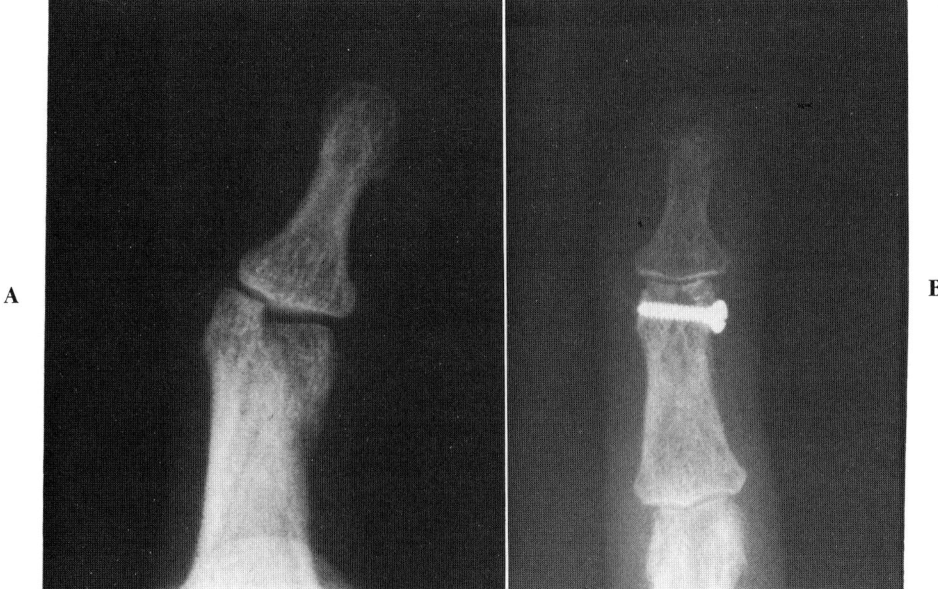

Fig. 15-3. A, Displaced condylar fracture of the distal interphalangeal joint causing articular disruption and a characteristic angular deformity. After reduction, interfragmental compression is achieved with a 1.5 mm screw, **B.**

PROXIMAL INTERPHALANGEAL (PIP) JOINT INJURIES
Dorsal fracture-dislocations

In contrast to the obvious bayonette deformity of a simple dislocation, the fracture-dislocation is characterized by a subtle dorsal prominence of the middle phalanx, which on casual observation is easily overlooked. Nonetheless a high-quality lateral roentgenogram clearly demonstrates the magnitude of injury. The palmar articular surface of the middle phalanx is fractured and separated from the rest of the middle phalanx, which is dislocated dorsally (Fig. 15-4).

Stability of the fracture-dislocation depends on the size of the palmar fragment.[6,13,22] If the fragment is less than one third of the joint surface, a stable reduction can usually be achieved by closed manipulation and maintained by an extension block splint.[13] However, if the articular fragment constitutes more than one third of the joint surface, it comprises the major attachment of the key collateral ligament–volar plate complex and results in a profound loss of joint stability. Despite attempts at closed reduction, the middle phalanx is repeatedly redisplaced dorsally because it has been stripped of its ligament restraints, which remain affixed to the palmar fragment. Injuries with sizable articular fragments and instability demonstrable when the joint moves through a functional arc of motion require open treatment for restoration of joint congruity and stability.

Comminution of the palmar fragment and the time of repair are major factors

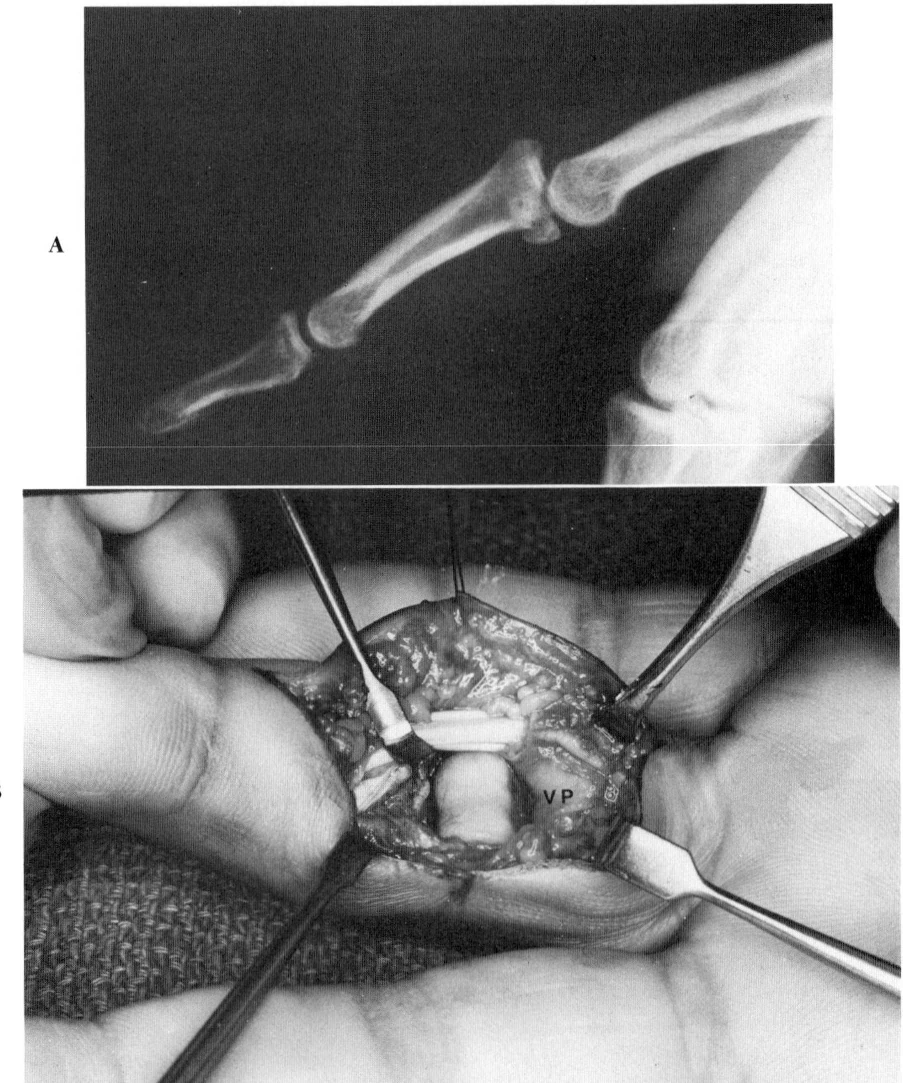

Fig. 15-4. Fracture-dislocation of the proximal interphalangeal joint treated by volar plate advancement. **A,** The lateral roentgenogram illustrates the comminuted palmar articular fragment and dorsal displacement of the middle phalanx. **B,** Through a palmar approach, the flexor tendons are retracted and the volar plate, *VP*, with its attached articular fragments (held with the forceps) is separated from the collateral ligaments and reflected proximally. The prominent articular condyles of the proximal phalanx and distally the fractured and displaced middle phalanx are clearly visible.

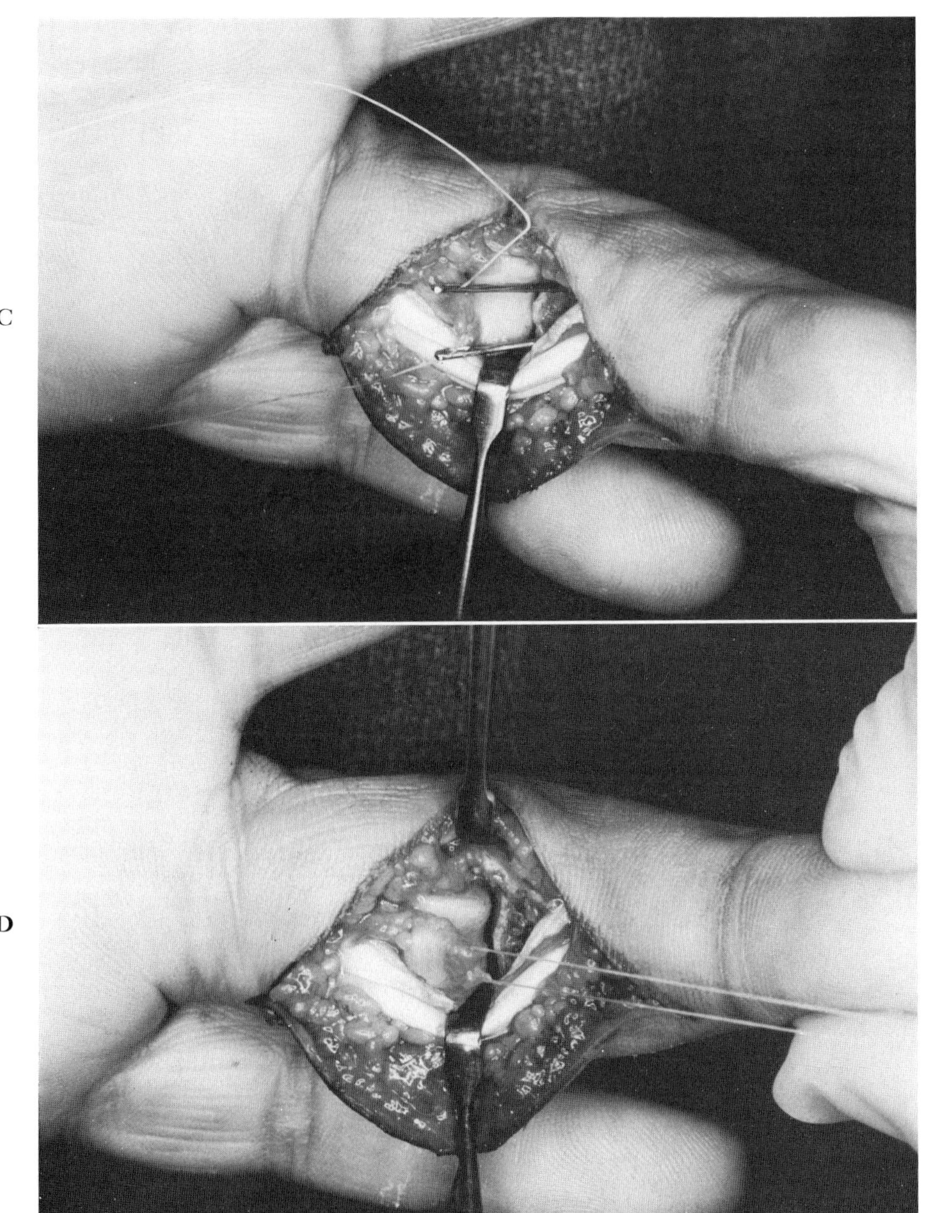

Fig. 15-4, cont'd. C, After excision of the comminuted fragments, the volar plate is advanced by sutures to a trough at the base of the reduced middle phalanx. **D,** Employing Keith needles at the margins of the trough, the sutures are passed to the dorsum of the digit and then tied over a small piece of cotton.   *Continued.*

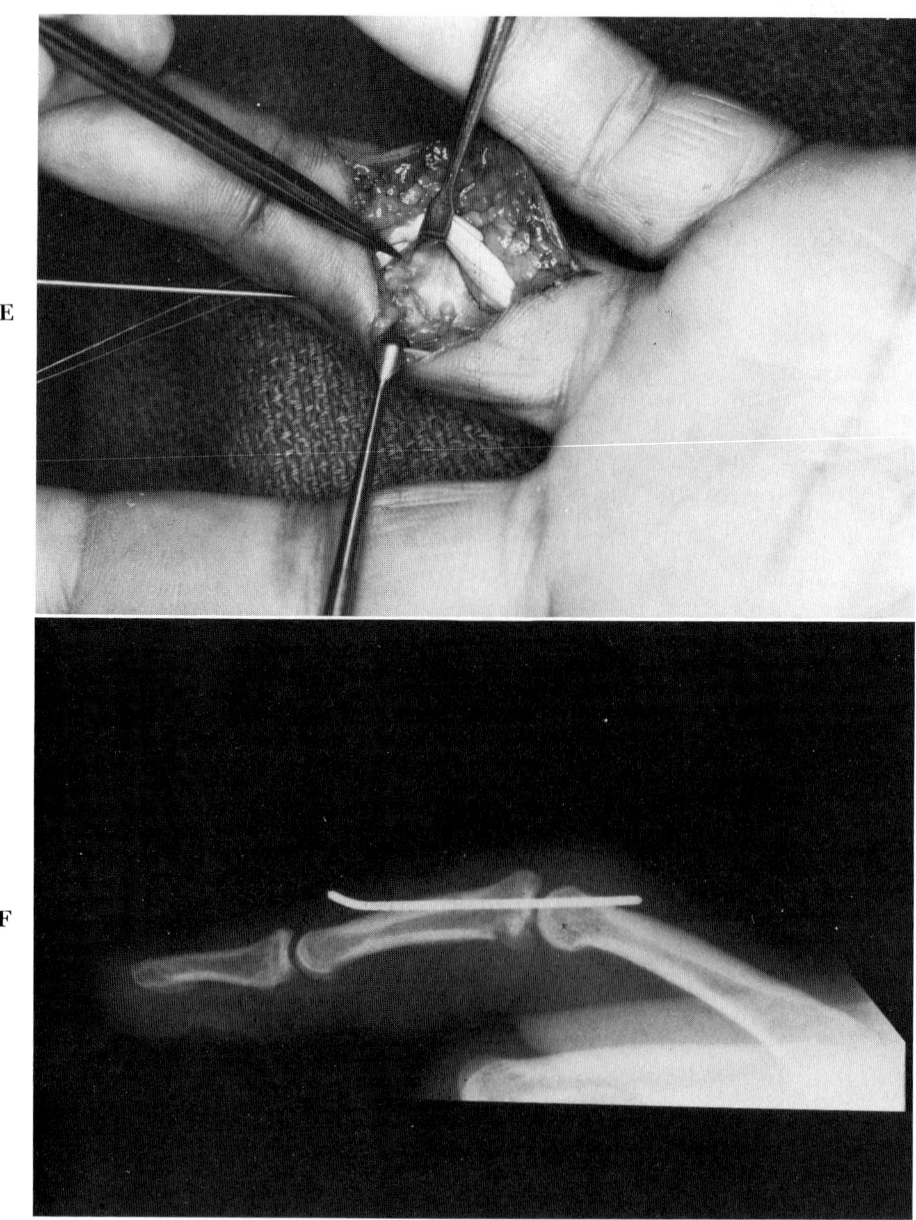

Fig. 15-4, cont'd. E, Securely anchored in the trough, the volar plate is also sutured to the collateral ligaments, so that the key restraint to dorsal displacement is restored and the entire palmar aspect of the joint is resurfaced. **F,** Temporary transarticular fixation in a position of mild flexion maintains a congruous reduction.

influencing the choice of treatment. Acute injuries with minimal fragmentation are optimally treated by open reduction and internal fixation with either fine Kirschner wires[12,20,22] or a circlage wire technique similar to that employed for the mallet fracture. Temporary transarticular fixation provides additional security.

More frequently the palmar fragment is excessively comminuted and unsuitable for precise reduction and fixation. In these cases the volar plate arthroplasty, skillfully performed, restores joint stability and a smooth articular surface (Fig. 15-4).[6] Through a palmar approach to the joint the comminuted fragments are excised and the volar plate is advanced distally and secured in a trough at the base of the reduced middle phalanx. A symmetric and stable reduction requires preservation of the full width of the volar plate and fixation of the repaired joint in a position of mild flexion for 3 weeks.

Treatment of chronic fracture-dislocation depends on the extent of articular destruction. If the damage is confined to the palmar surface of the middle phalanx, volar-plate arthroplasty[6] or an open-wedge osteotomy at the base of the middle phalanx[12,22,23] has been employed for salvage of a functional joint. Both procedures rely on remodeling of the articular contours for joint restitution and a satisfactory recovery of mobility. Chronic injuries complicated by diffuse and painful arthritis require either implant arthroplasty or arthrodesis.

Collateral ligament injuries

The majority of collateral ligament injuries of the PIP joint are partial ruptures and can be successfully managed by splinting and early motion. However complete ruptures resulting in an obvious angular deformity or gross instability as determined by gentle passive stress testing or subluxation on the stress roentgenogram are preferentially treated by prompt repair.[12,17] Accurate coaptation of the disrupted ligament ends ensures optimal healing and minimizes the problems of prolonged swelling and stiffness, residual instability, and recurrent injury, which are commonly associated with conservative treatment. For chronically unstable injuries, treated initially by splinting or being previously neglected, secondary repair or tendon graft reconstruction is necessary to restore joint stability (Fig. 15-5). Successful grafting must duplicate the normal configuration of the collateral ligament to restore lateral stability and reinforce the dorsal and palmar margins of the joint to provide rotatory stability.

Palmar dislocations

The most profound collateral ligament injury of the PIP joint occurs with disruption of the extensor mechanism and results in palmar displacement of the middle phalanx (Fig. 15-6).[19] A violent force applied to the flexed joint disrupts initially the collateral ligament near its proximal attachment and then the central slip at its insertion. Usually a concomitant tear extends proximally between the central slip and the lateral band adjacent to the disrupted collateral ligament.[14,16] The ipsilateral condyle of the proximal phalanx, lacking its ligament restraint, protrudes through this tear and

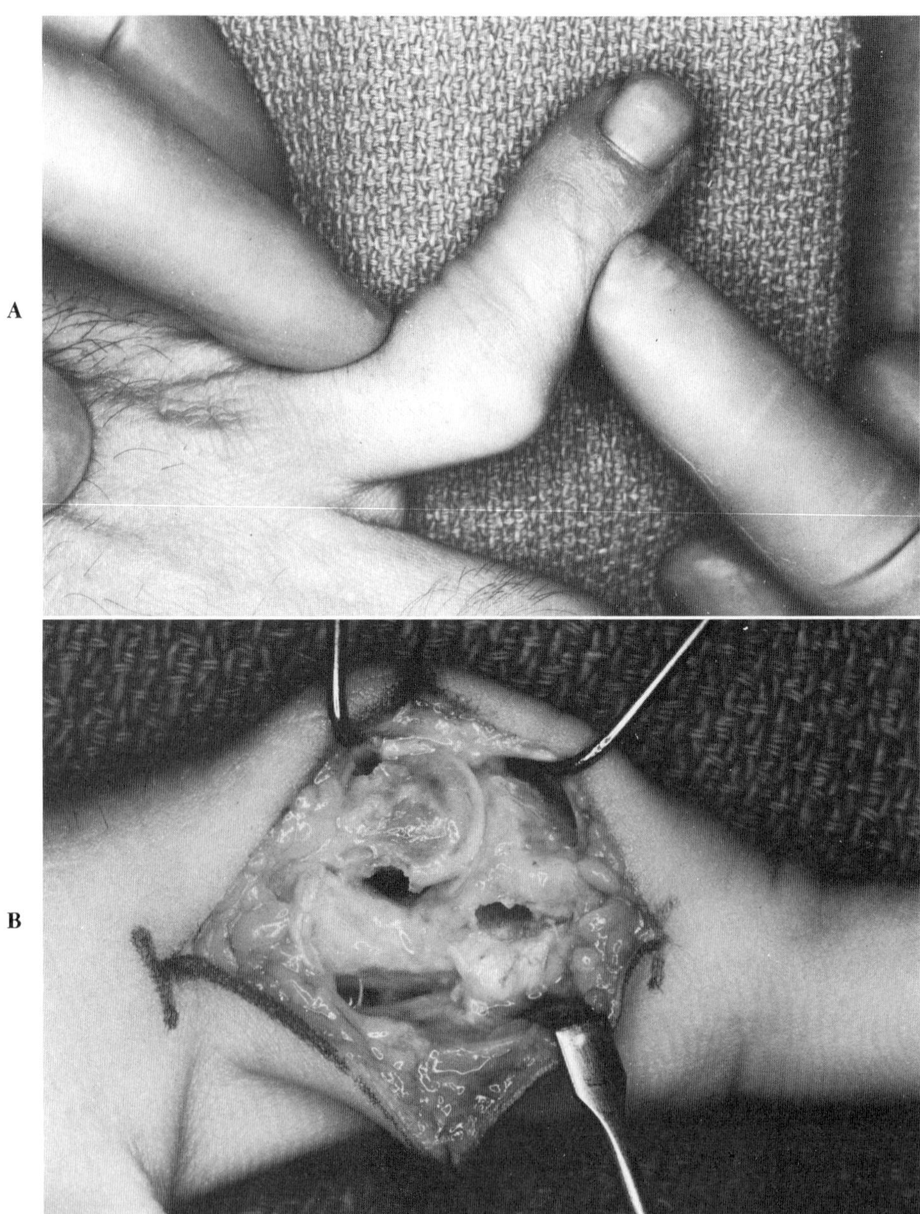

Fig. 15-5. A, Tendon graft reconstruction was necessary for this radial collateral ligament disruption of the proximal interphalangeal joint resulting in chronic instability. **B,** Vertical tunnels are burred proximally near the origin of the irreparable ligament and distally through the middle phalanx at the ligament's insertion.

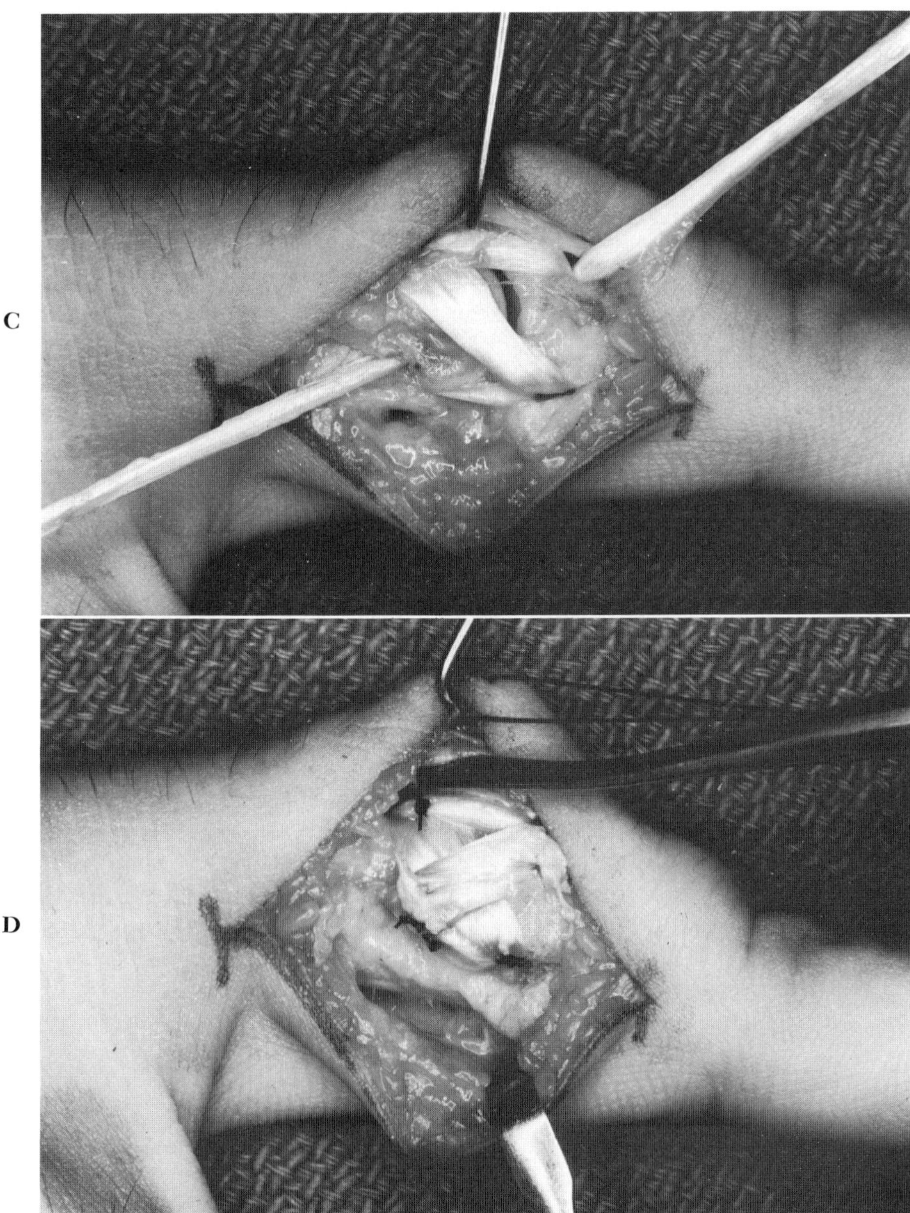

Fig. 15-5, cont'd. C, A plantaris tendon graft is passed through the tunnels duplicating the configuration of the proper collateral ligament. **D,** The graft is then anchored to the dorsal and palmar aspects of the joint so that both rotatory and lateral stability are restored. *Continued.*

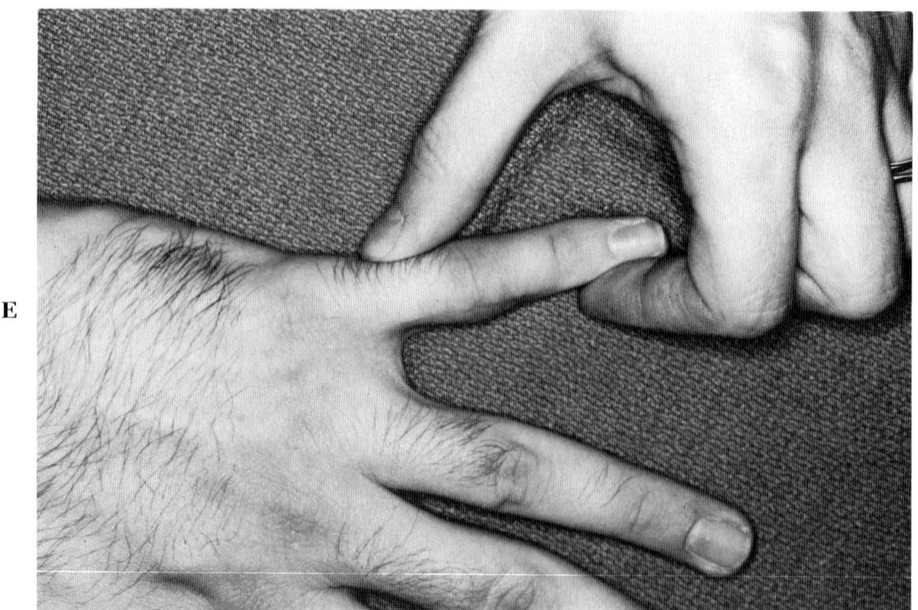

E

Fig. 15-5, cont'd. E, Stability of the joint is demonstrated postoperatively.

causes palmar displacement of the lateral band. Interposition of the lateral band between the proximal and middle phalanges results in a complex dislocation as well as a seemingly paradoxical deformity: the tethering effect of the entrapped lateral band causes the injured joint to angulate in the direction of its greatest instability. Thus a palmar dislocation resulting in disruption of the radial collateral ligament and entrapment of the adjacent lateral band demonstrates radial deviation of the joint. Without recognition and prompt correction of this unique pathologic condition, the injured joint demonstrates a predictable sequence of events: persistent instability, progressive contracture, and ultimately the development of a disabling boutonnière deformity.

Occasionally the lateral band can be dislodged from the joint by closed manipulation, and a successful reduction is accomplished.[16,20] However in the majority of cases a stable reduction requires open treatment, which is also preferred as a more predictable method of achieving precise healing of the severely disrupted soft tissues. Under direct visualization the lateral band is atraumatically repositioned dorsally, the joint is relocated and temporarily pinned, and the collateral ligament and extensor mechanism are accurately repaired. After 4 weeks of immobilization, the transarticular pin is removed and active exercises are started.

METACARPOPHALANGEAL (MCP) JOINT INJURIES
Dorsal dislocation of the metacarpophalangeal joint

Dorsal dislocation of the MCP joint is frequently irreducible by closed manipulation because of entrapment of the volar plate between the base of the proximal

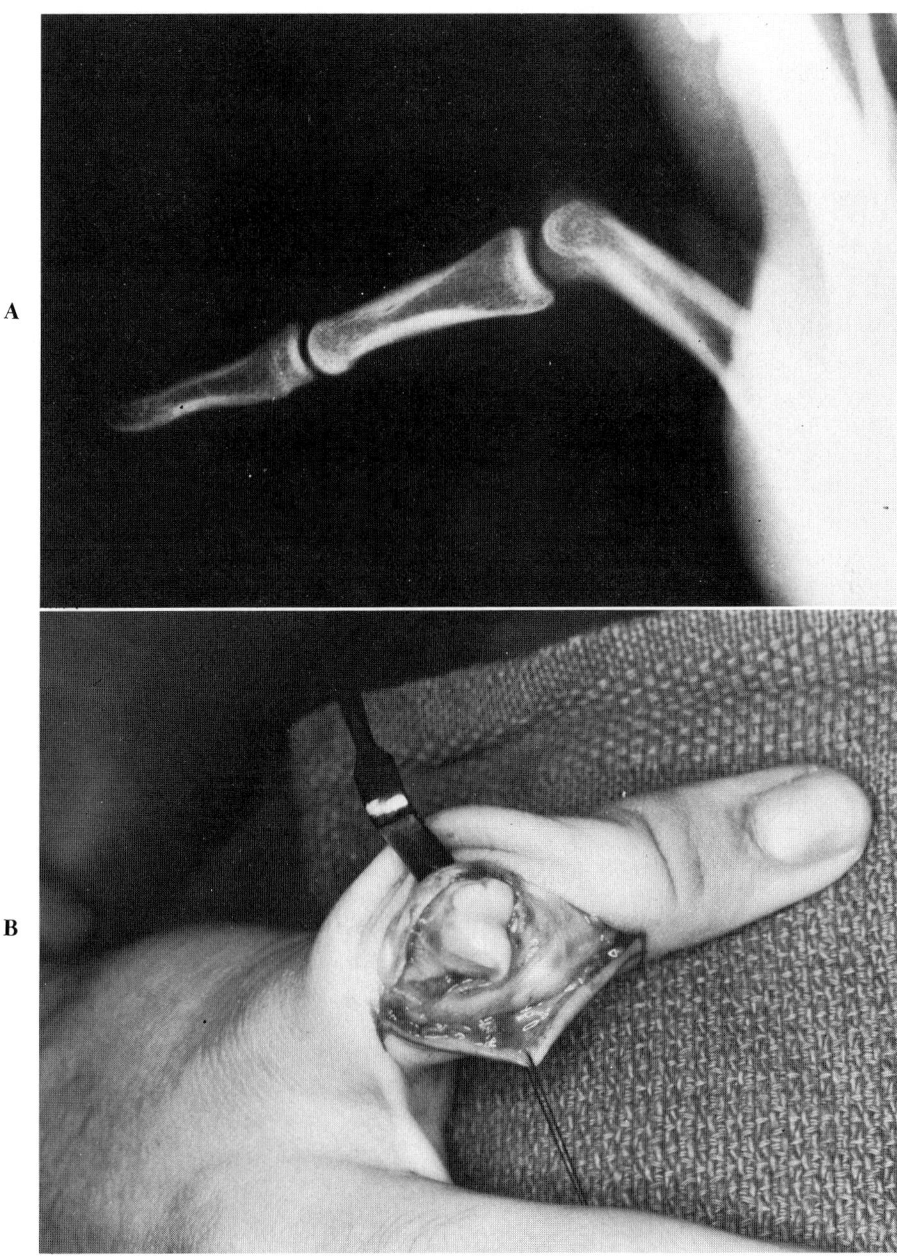

Fig. 15-6. A, Palmar displacement of the middle phalanx resulting from disruption of the radial collateral ligament and the extensor mechanism at the proximal interphalangeal joint level. **B,** Displacement and interposition of the radial lateral band between the prominent proximal phalangeal condyles and the middle phalanx prevents reduction by closed manipulation.

Continued.

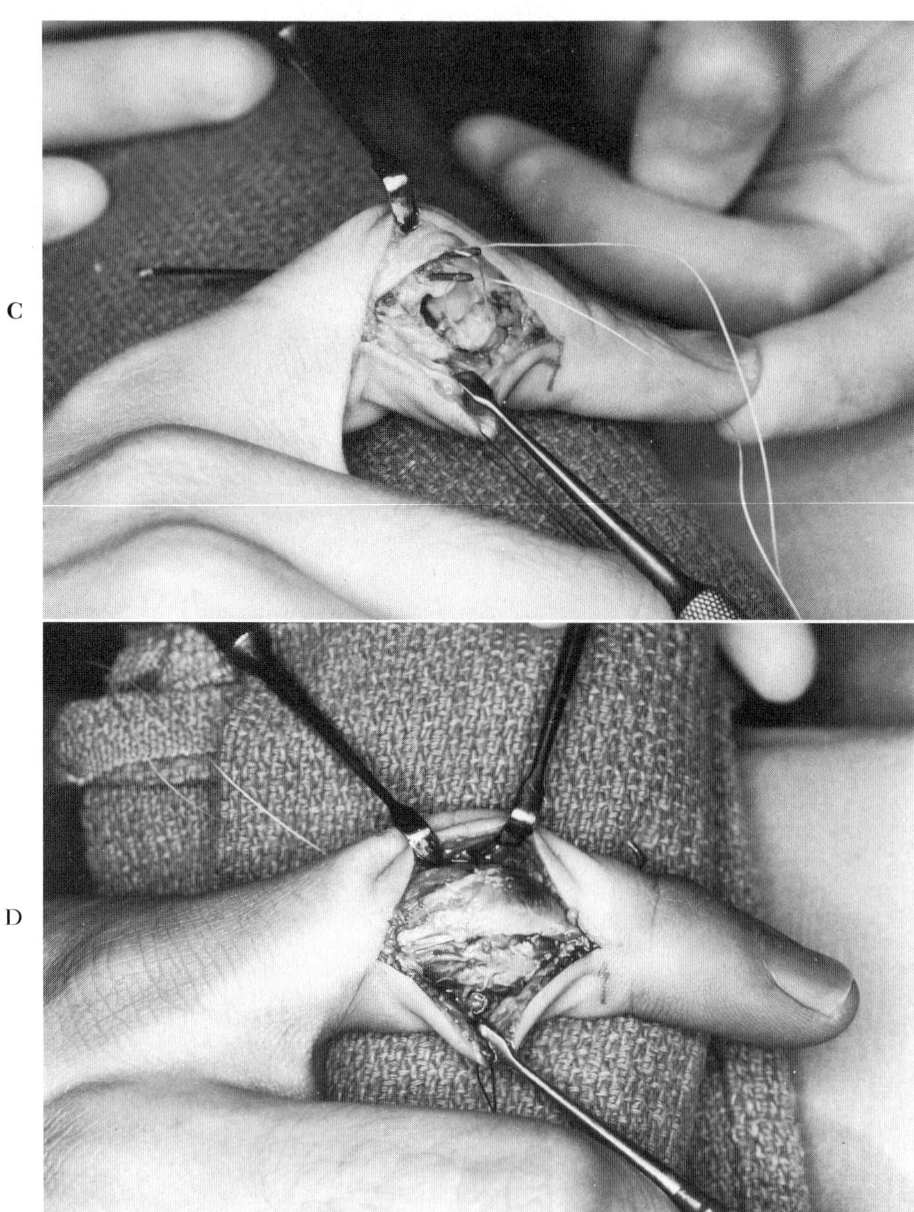

Fig. 15-6, cont'd. C, Dorsal relocation of the lateral band permits reduction of the joint and reattachment of the collateral ligament to its origin. **D,** After transarticular pin fixation, the central slip and the lateral band are precisely repaired.

phalanx and the metacarpal head.[1,3,7,9,20] The complex dislocation commonly involves the index finger and less often the little finger and thumb and displays characteristic features (Fig. 15-7): the proximal phalanx is fixed in a bayonette position, asymmetrically displaced dorsal to the metacarpal head; the metacarpal head is excessively prominent in the palm causing dimpling and occasionally disruption of the

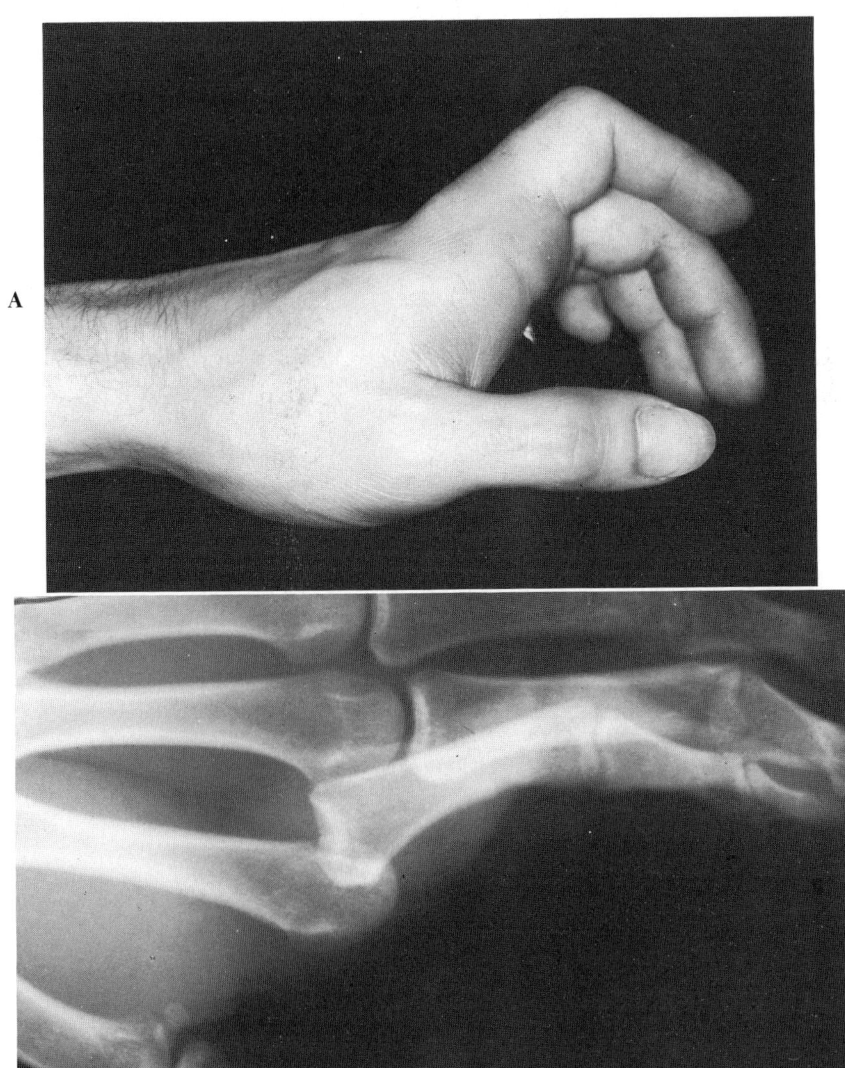

Fig. 15-7. A and **B,** Characteristic features of the complex dislocation of the index-finger metacarpophalangeal joint. There is an asymmetrical bayonette configuration of the proximal phalanx and metacarpal head with loss of their articular contact and ulnar deviation of the digit. In this case the prominent metacarpal head has caused disruption of the palmar skin.

Continued.

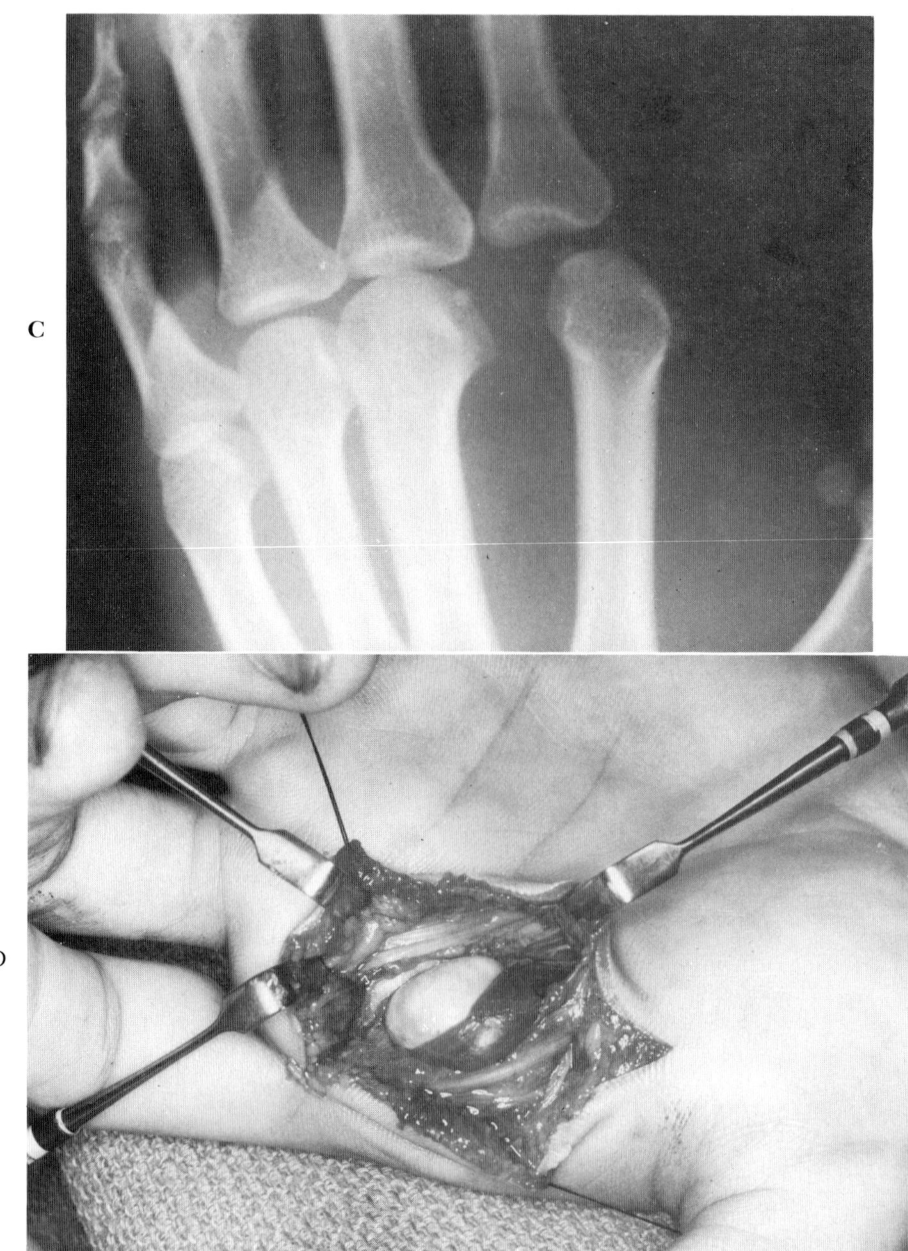

Fig. 15-7, cont'd. C, The posteroanterior roentgenogram demonstrates a widened joint space with interposition of the sesamoids. **D,** A palmar incision demonstrating the vulnerability of the radial digital nerve overlying the lumbrical and incarceration of the metacarpal head.

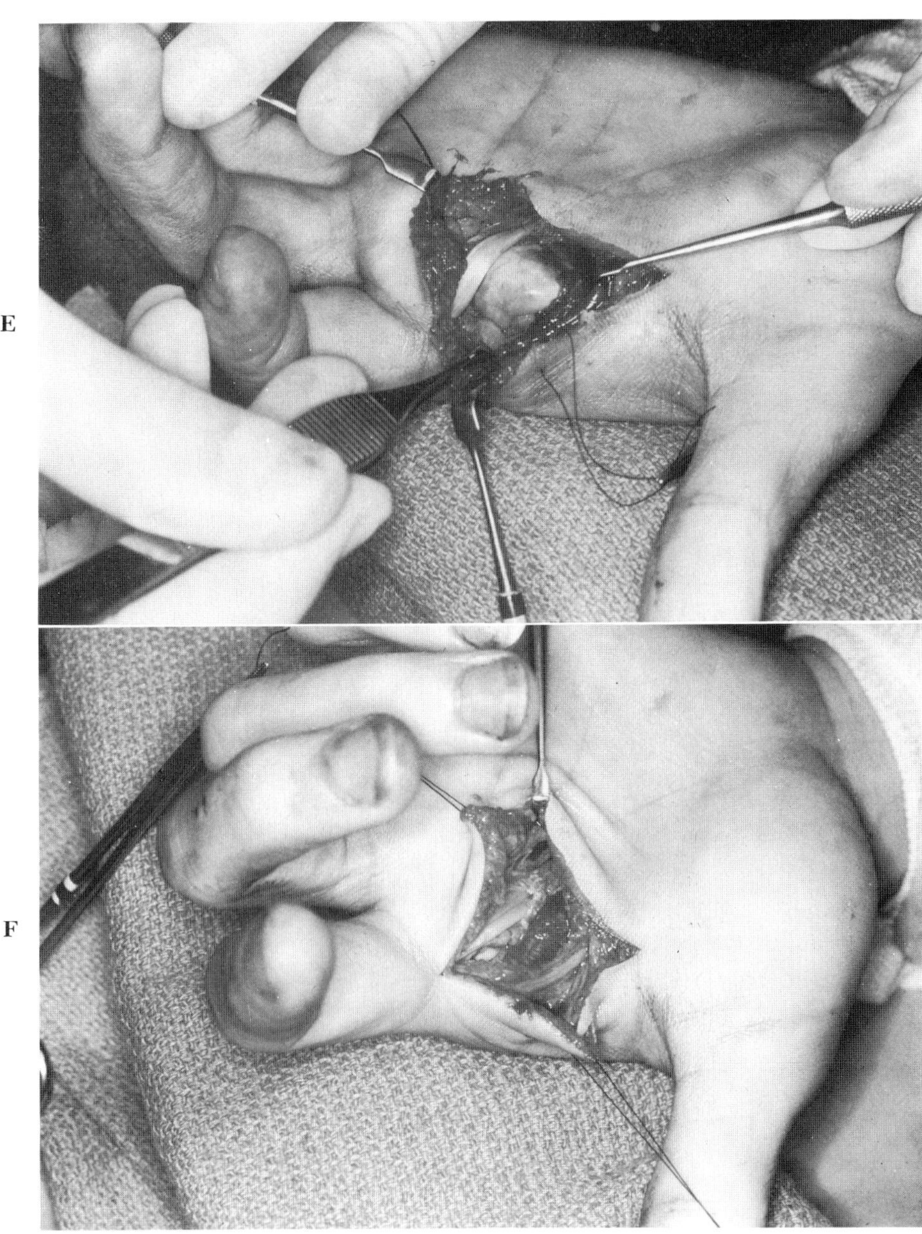

Fig. 15-7, cont'd. E, Incision of the A1 pulley relaxes the flexor tendons and releases confinement of the metacarpal. The volar plate (held with the forceps) is extracted from the joint. **F,** A stable reduction is achieved.

palmar skin; and on the roentgenogram the sesamoids, embedded in the substance of the displaced volar plate, may be observed in a widened joint space. In some cases the roentgenograms may also demonstrate concomitant osteochondral fractures of the dorsal aspect of the metacarpal head. These fractures result from a shearing force transmitted by the displaced phalanx and can be distinguished from the sesamoids by their larger size and irregular shape (Fig. 15-8).

Reduction is accomplished through an incision extending from the midpalm to the base of the dislocated digit. Immediately beneath the skin the radial digital nerve of the index finger or the ulnar digital nerve of the little finger is vulnerable to injury and must be protected. The metacarpal head is observed protruding and incarcerated between the taut extrinsic flexor tendons and the intrinsic muscles. Incision of the proximal annular pulley of the flexor mechanism releases confinement of the metacarpal bone and permits removal of the entrapped volar plate from the joint. Occasionally an additional incision between the volar plate and the adjacent intermetacarpal ligament is necessary to complete the reduction. After extraction of the volar plate the joint is invariably stable, and active motion with extension block splinting is begun immediately.

In those cases with osteochondral fractures a dorsal approach is used to expose both the fracture and the displaced volar plate (Fig. 15-8).[3] Incision of the volar plate permits reduction of the dislocation, and the fracture fragment is either excised or reduced and fixed with fine wires. A dorsal approach is also necessary for chronic dislocations in which the contracted joint capsule and collateral ligaments must be released so that reduction is achieved.

Collateral ligament injuries

There is a clear consensus that disruption of the ulnar collateral ligament of the thumb MCP joint requires repair so that joint stability is preserved (Fig. 15-9).[4,11,15,18,21] Wide separation of the torn ends of the ligament and in many cases interposition of the adductor aponeurosis between these ends—the lesion described by Stener[21]—prevents ligament approximation with conservative management. Reflection of the adductor aponeurosis is necessary to enable precise coaptation of the ligament.

Differentiation of a complete ligament disruption requiring surgery from a partial injury that can be successfully managed by casting or splinting is a topic of considerable controversy.[4,15,18] In my experience in managing over 200 injuries with adequate follow-up, physical stress testing with stress roentgenography, facilitated by a local anesthetic, has been an accurate method of determining the need for surgery. A 30-degree or more difference in laxity between the injured and uninjured thumbs as demonstrated with comparative stress examinations coupled with 30% or more subluxation of the joint as measured on the stress roentgenogram confirms complete ligament disruption and should be considered an indication for repair (Fig. 15-9).

For the majority of cases treated within several months of injury direct repair or ligament advancement to bone results in an excellent recovery. Tendon graft recon

Text continued on p. 165.

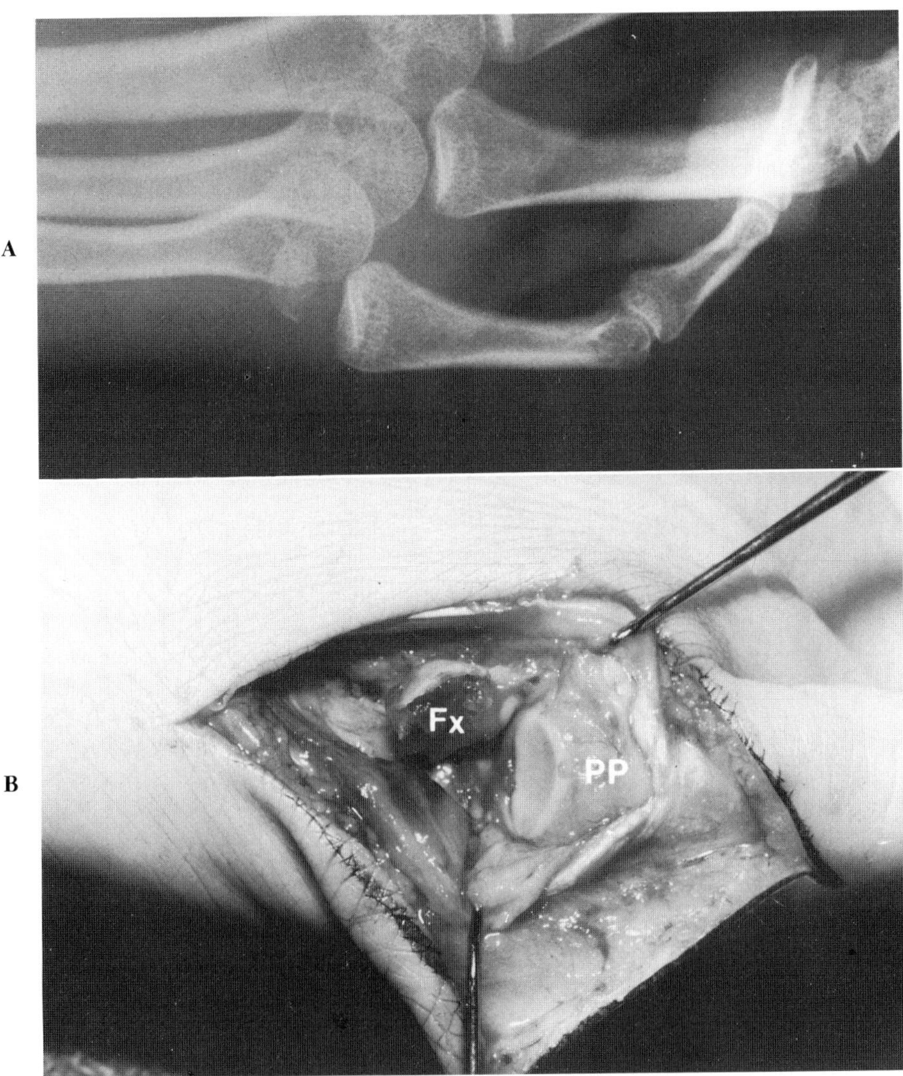

Fig. 15-8. **A** and **B,** Complex dislocation of the little finger with a large osteochondral fracture, *Fx,* of the metacarpal head and dorsal displacement of the proximal phalanx, *PP. Continued.*

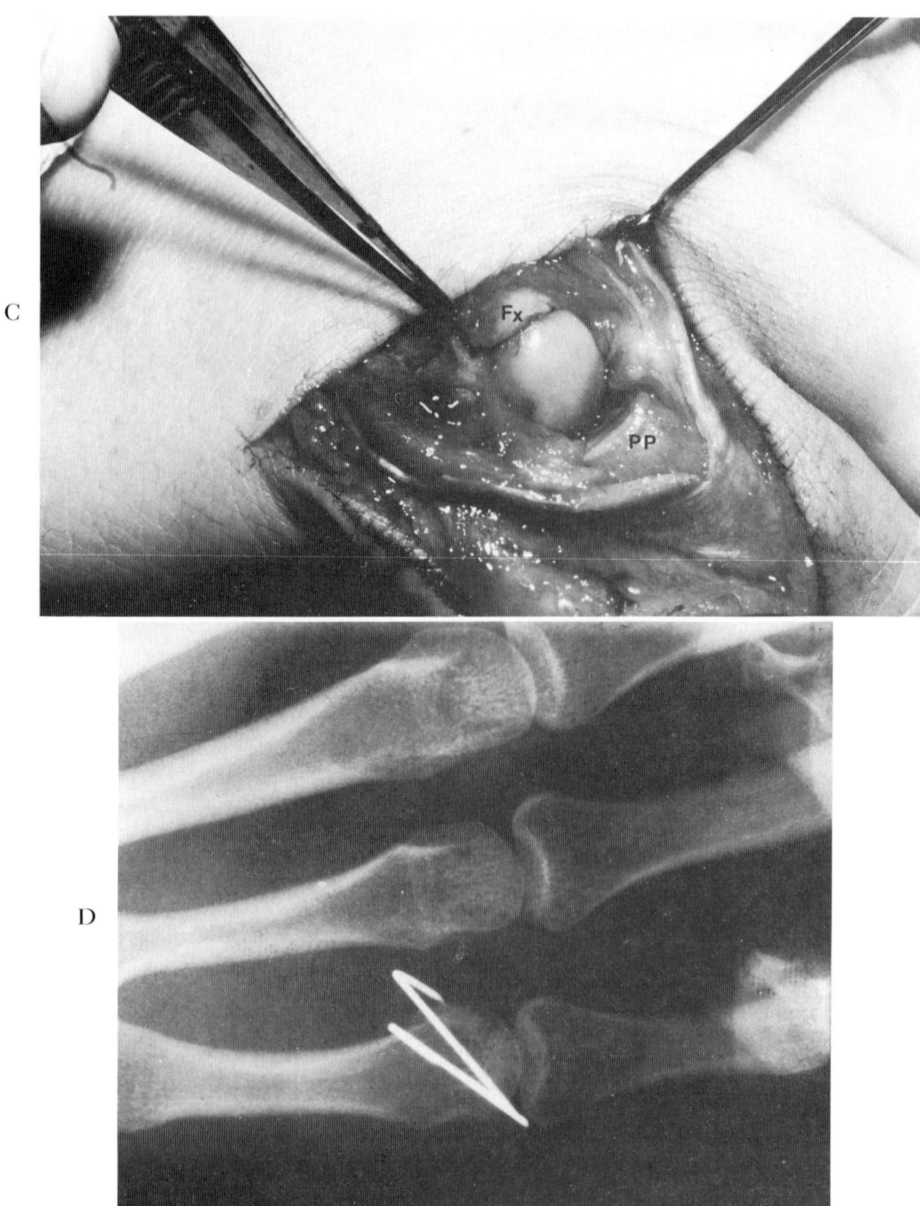

Fig. 15-8, cont'd. C and **D,** Through a dorsal approach the volar plate has been incised, the joint has been reduced, and the fracture fragment replaced and fixed with fine Kirschner wires.

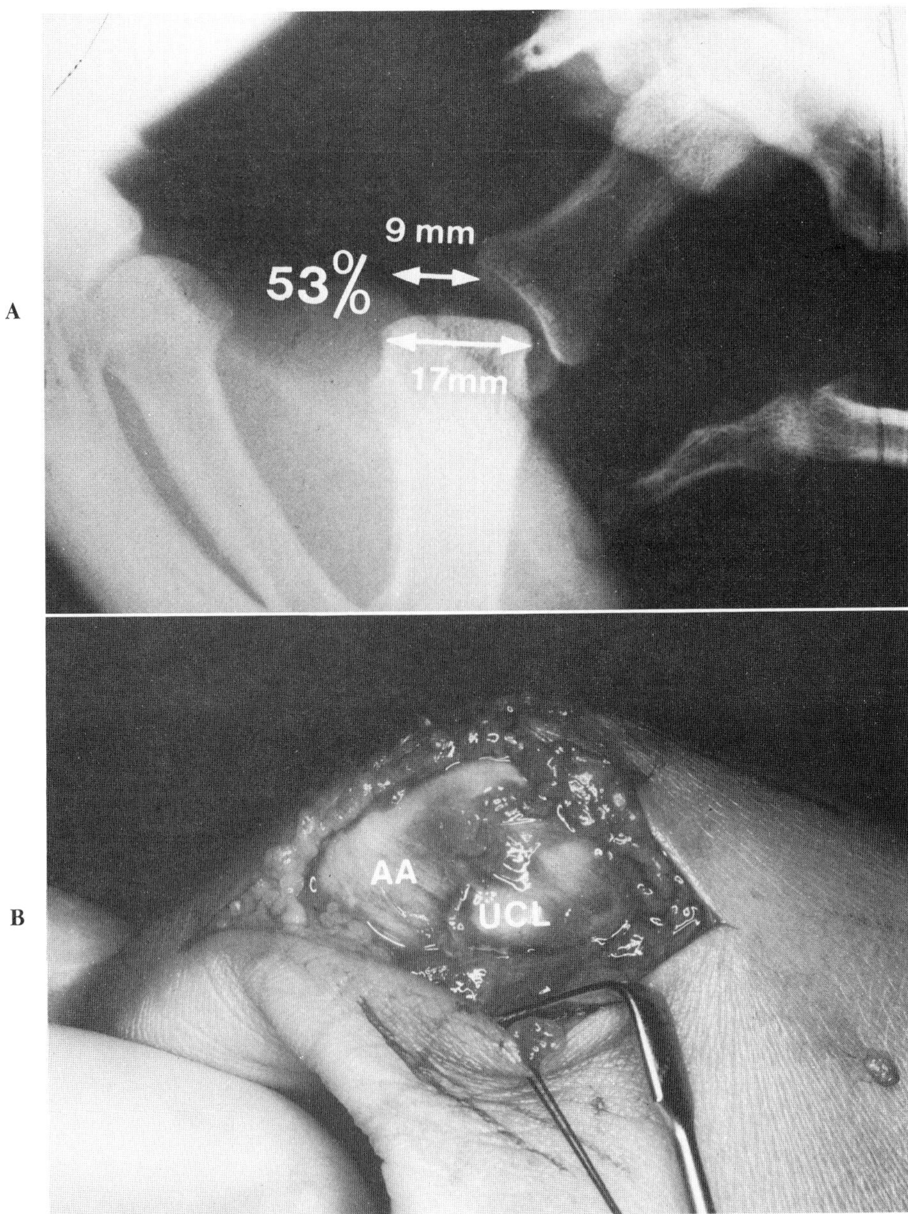

Fig. 15-9. A, Complete rupture of the ulnar collateral ligament of the thumb metacarpophalangeal joint detected by standardized stress roentgenography. Displacement of the proximal phalanx is measured in millimeters and recorded as a percentage of the width of the articular surface. A 30% or more shift of the phalanx indicates subluxation resulting from a serious ligament disruption. **B,** As in this case, pronounced subluxation is invariably associated with wide displacement of the ulnar collateral ligament, *UCL,* and interposition of the adductor aponeurosis, *AA.*

Continued.

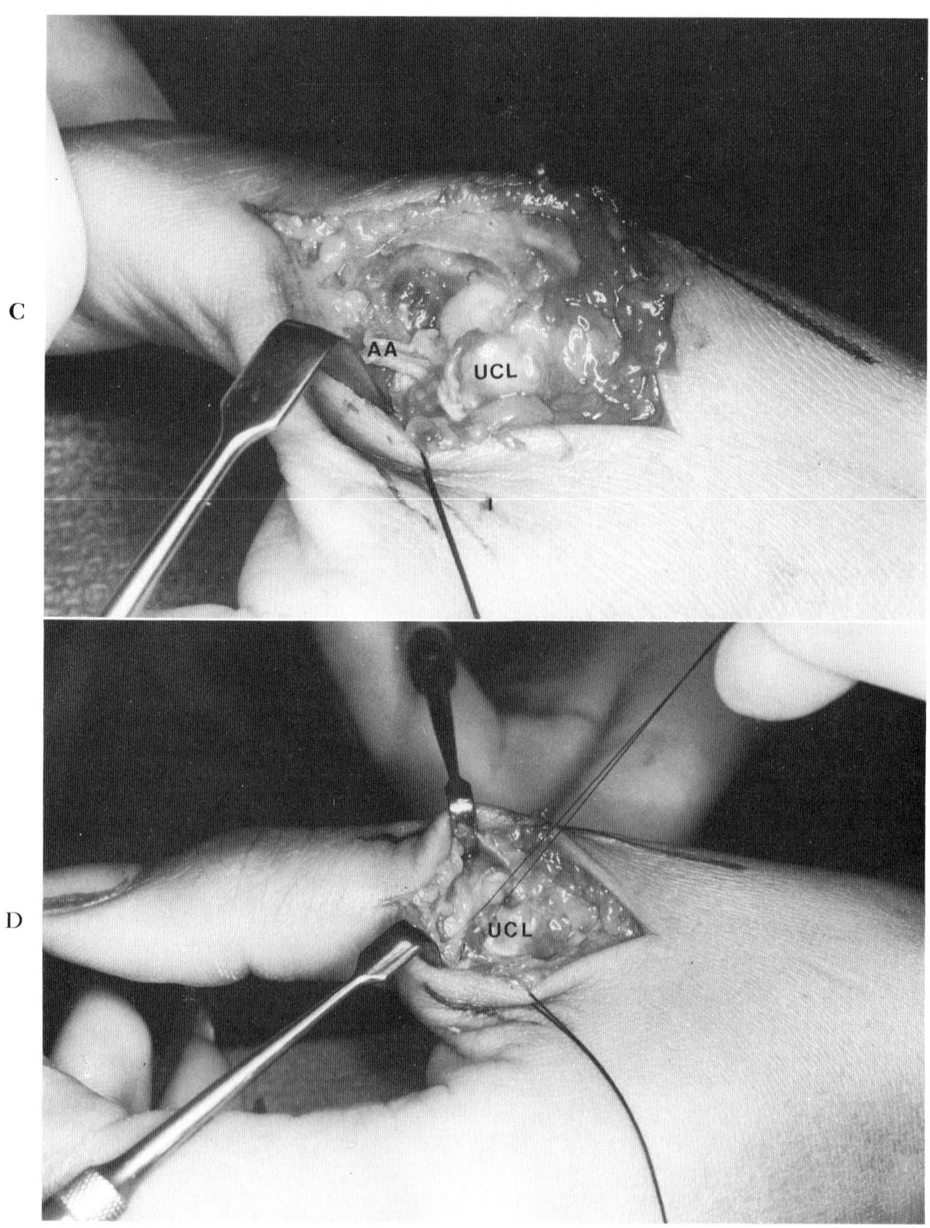

Fig. 15-9, cont'd. C and **D,** Restoration of joint stability requires reflection of the adductor aponeurosis for precise coaptation of the ligament ends.

struction is reserved for cases with irreparable ligament damage and arthrodesis is indicated principally in situations complicated by arthritis.

Most radial collateral ligament injuries of the MCP joint do not result in serious instability and can be treated successfully by 4 weeks of continuous immobilization or buddy splinting to an adjacent digit. However an obvious deformity or joint subluxation demonstrated with stress roentgenography indicates pronounced instability resulting from complete disruption and displacement of the ligament (Fig. 15-10). In these cases a prompt repair, before scarring and contraction of the ligament, assures the maximum recovery of stability and mobility.[5] The joint is exposed by a curved dorsal skin incision, with the prominence of the metacarpal head being avoided, followed by a longitudinal splitting of the extrinsic extensor tendon and lateral retraction of the extensor hood. Disturbance of the sagittal (shroud) fibers of the hood is prone to cause imbalance or subluxation of the extensor mechanism and should be avoided.

Epiphyseal injuries

In the adolescent athlete a violent force, instead of rupturing the collateral ligament, disrupts the potentially weakest part of the joint: the epiphysis. A rotatory or angular deformity of an injured digit in a young patient with a tender swollen MCP joint should arouse suspicion of an epiphyseal fracture, usually at the base of the

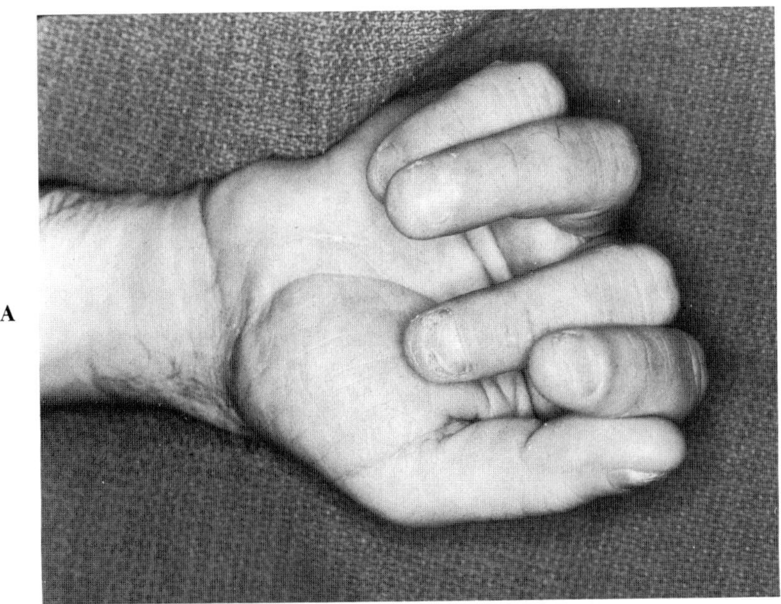

Fig. 15-10. A, Acute radial collateral ligament injury of the ring-finger metacarpophalangeal joint resulting in gross instability and an obvious clinical deformity.   *Continued.*

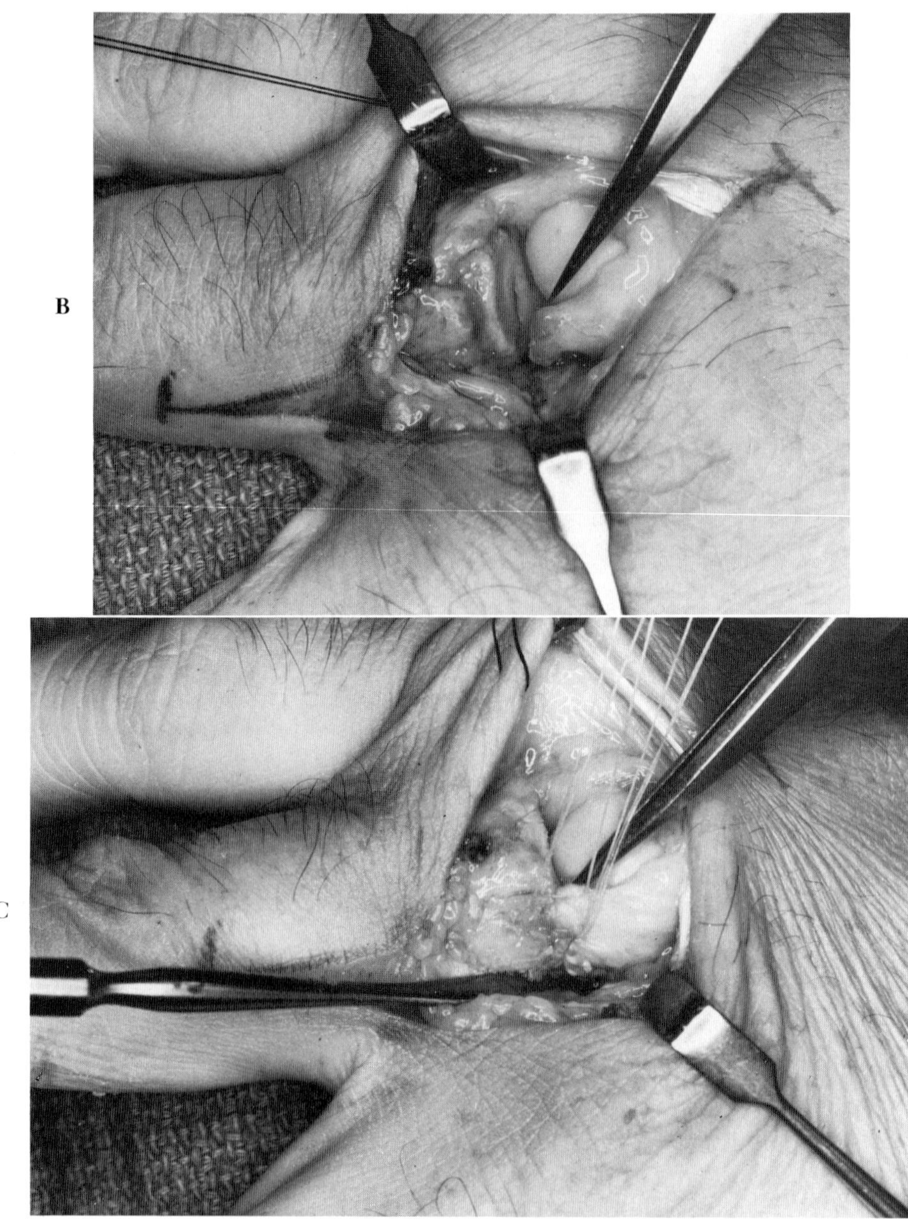

Fig. 15-10, cont'd. B, Exposure of the joint demonstrates a distal rupture and displacement of the ligament into the joint. **C,** Prompt end-to-end repair ensures preservation of stability and maximum recovery of mobility.

A   B   C

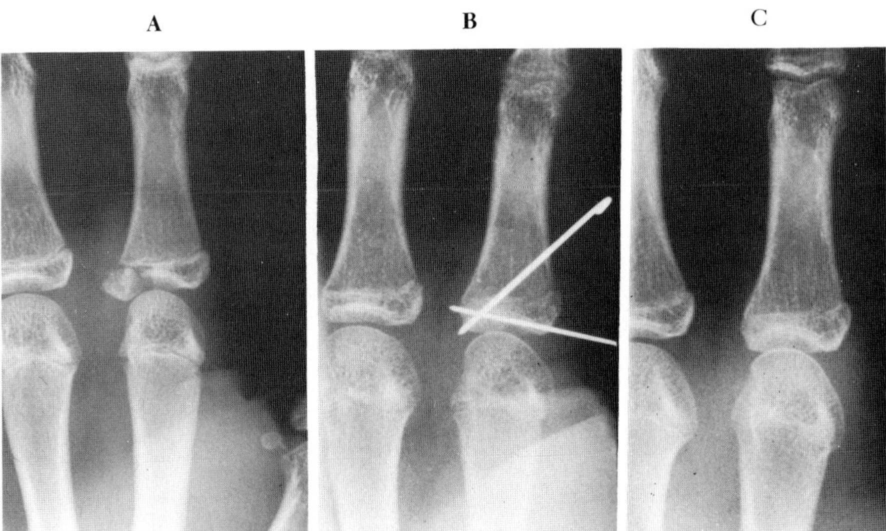

Fig. 15-11. A, Displaced epiphyseal fracture of the proximal phalanx with articular disruption. **B,** Open reduction and internal fixation with fine Kirschner wires. **C,** Preservation of the joint surface and normal growth are demonstrated postoperatively.

proximal phalanx. The extent of injury must then be accurately assessed with roentgenograms. Fractures causing articular displacement require a meticulous open reduction and internal fixation for restoration of joint stability and congruity as well as preservation of the growth plate (Fig. 15-11).

CARPOMETACARPAL (CMC) JOINT INJURIES

Although carpometacarpal disruptions of the thumb are usually obvious, those of the fingers are less apparent. This is largely attributable to the difficulty encountered in roentgenographic interpretation of these joints, which require multiple views and frequently comparison studies of the opposite hand for an accurate assessment. Also the ring and little-finger metacarpals, like the forearm bones, function as a mobile unit and are prone to concomitant injury, occasionally at distant levels. Thus a dislocation of the little finger CMC joint should increase one's suspicion of injury to not only the ring finger's CMC joint, but also its metacarpal shaft or metacarpophalangeal joint. Recognition of the extent of injury requires an end-to-end evaluation of both bones.

In my experience with more than 40 CMC injuries including 25 Bennett fracture-dislocations, prompt closed reduction with transarticular pin fixation and 6 weeks of cast immobilization have consistently resulted in stability and excellent mobility. The injury that has most frequently required open treatment is the fracture-dislocation of the base of the little-finger metacarpal, commonly termed the mini- or reverse Bennett fracture (Fig. 15-12). Because of the restraint imposed by the intermetacarpal

A   B

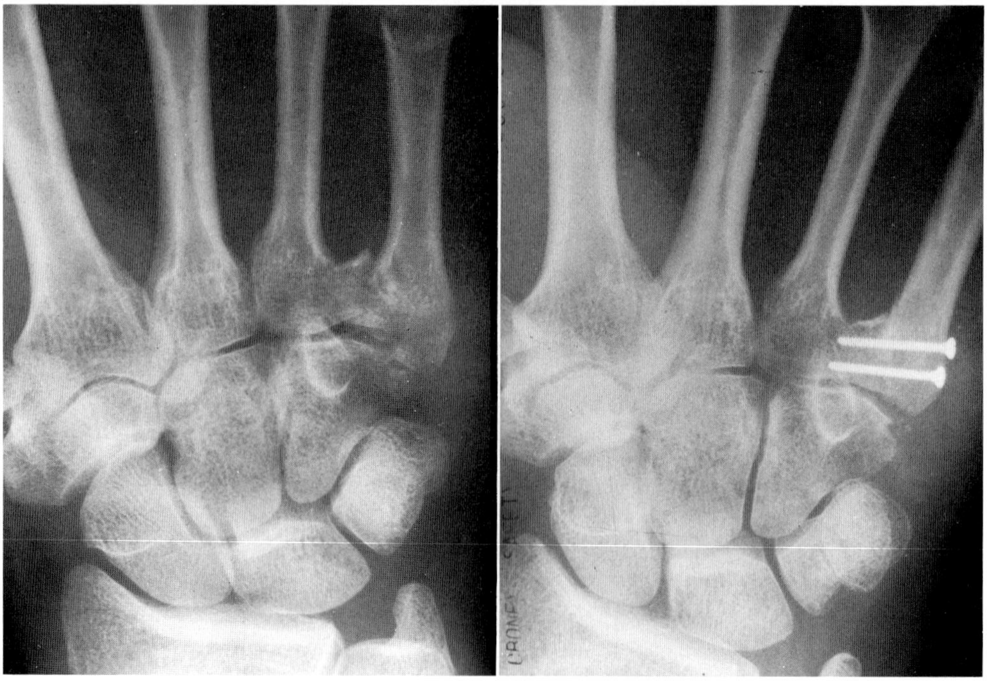

Fig. 15-12. A, Fracture-dislocation of the little-finger carpometacarpal joint irreducible by closed manipulation. **B,** Open reduction and internal fixation with 2 mm screws restores articular congruity and stability.

ligament, lateral mobility of this ulnar ray, unlike the thumb metacarpal, is limited. Thus it is often impossible to approximate by closed manipulation the displaced shaft fragment to the base fragment, which remains affixed to the hamate. Through a dorsoulnar approach, the fracture is accurately reduced and fixation achieved by either Kirschner wires or small screws.

SUMMARY

Prompt recognition of the magnitude of articular damage is essential to optimal treatment of complex joint injuries of the hand. Restoration of articular congruity and stability by a method of repair that facilitates early joint motion coupled with a supervised therapy program consistently leads to a satisfactory recovery. In contrast, one needs to read only the sports section of the daily newspaper to appreciate the frequency and degree of impairment resulting from neglected injuries: the pitcher or quarterback who cannot control the ball, the wide receiver with "no hands," the high-scoring guard who loses his touch, the hockey player who can't stick-handle, and the boxer without a knockout punch. Professional and enthusiastic amateur athletes require skillful care. The several-month period of disability necessary for rehabilitation of these complex injuries is a "minor penalty" compared to the "flagrant violation" of inadequate treatment.

REFERENCES

1. Baldwin, L.W., Miller, D.L, Lockhart, L.D., and Evans, E.B.: Metacarpophalangeal joint dislocation of the fingers: a comparison of the pathological analysis of index and little finger dislocations, J. Bone Joint Surg. (Am.) **49:**1587-1590, Dec. 1967.
2. Beasley, R.W.: Hand injuries, Philadelphia, 1981, W.B. Saunders Co.
3. Becton, J.L., Christian, J.D., Goodwin, H.N., and Jackson, J.G.: A simplified technique for treating the complex dislocation of the index metacarpophalangeal joint, J. Bone Joint Surg. (Am.) **57:**698-700, July 1975.
4. Bowers, W.H., and Hurst, L.C.: Gamekeeper's thumb: evaluation by arthrography and stress roentgenography, J. Bone Joint Surg (Am.) **59:**519-524, June 1977.
5. Dray, G., Millender, L.H., and Nalebuff, E.A.: Rupture of the radial collateral ligament of a metacarpophalangeal joint to one of the ulnar three fingers, J. Bone Joint Surg. **4:**346-350, July 1979.
6. Eaton, R.G., and Malerick, M.H.: Volar plate arthroplasty of the proximal interphalangeal joint: a review of ten year's experience, J. Hand Surg. **5:**260-268, May 1980.
7. Green, D.P., and Terry, G.C.: Complex dislocation of the metacarpophalangeal joint, J. Bone Joint Surg. (Am.) **55:**1480-1486, Oct. 1973.
8. Hammas, R.S., Horrel, E.D., and Pierret, G.P.: Treatment of mallet finger due to intra-articular fracture of the distal phalanx, J. Hand Surg. **3:**361-363, July 1978.
9. Kaplan, E.M.: Dorsal dislocation of the metacarpophalangeal joint of the index finger, J. Bone Joint Surg. (Am.) **39:**1081-1086, Oct. 1957.
10. Lister, G.: Intraosseous wiring of the digital skeleton, J. Hand Surg. **3:**427-434, Sept. 1978.
11. McCue, F.C., et al.: Ulnar collateral ligament injuries of the thumb in athletes, Sport Med. **2:**70-80, March-April 1974.
12. McCue, F.C., et al.: Athletic injuries of the proximal interphalangeal joint requiring surgical treatment, J. Bone Joint Surg. (Am.) **52:**937-955, July 1970.
13. McElfresh, E.C., and Dobyns, J.H.: Management of fracture-dislocations of the proximal interphalangeal joints by extension-block splinting, J. Bone Joint Surg. (Am.) **54:**1705-1711, Dec. 1972.
14. Neviaser, R.J., and Wilson, J.N.: Interposition of the extensor tendon resulting in persistent subluxation of the proximal interphalangeal joint of the finger, Clin. Orthop. (83):118-120, March-April 1972.
15. Palmer, A., and Louis, D.: Assessing ulnar instability of the metacarpophalangeal joint of the thumb, J. Hand Surg. **3:**542-546, Nov. 1978.
16. Peimer, C.A., Sullivan, D.J., and Wild, D.R.: Palmar dislocation of the proximal interphalangeal joint, J. Hand Surg. **9A:**39-48, Jan. 1984.
17. Redler, I., and Williams, J.T.: Rupture of a collateral ligament of the proximal interphalangeal joint of the fingers, J. Bone Joint Surg. (Am.) **49:**322-326, March 1967.
18. Smith, R.J.: Post-traumatic instability of the metacarpophalangeal joint of the thumb, J. Bone Joint Surg. (Am.) **59:**14-21, Jan. 1977.
19. Spinner, M., and Choi, B.Y.: Anterior dislocation of the proximal interphalangeal joint: a cause of rupture of the central slip of the extensor mechanism, J. Bone Joint Surg. (Am.) **52:**1329-1336, Oct. 1970.
20. Stark, H.H.: Troublesome fractures and dislocation of the hand. In American Academy of Orthopaedic Surgeons: Instructional Course Lectures **19:**130-149, St. Louis, 1970, The C.V. Mosby Co.
21. Stener, B.: Displacement of the ruptured ulnar collateral ligament of the metacarpophalangeal joint of the thumb: a clinical and anatomical study, J. Bone Joint Surg. (Br.) **44:**869-879, Nov. 1962.
22. Wilson, J.N., and Rowland, S.A.: Fracture-dislocation of the proximal interphalangeal joint of the finger: treatment by open reduction and internal fixation, J. Bone Joint Surg. (Am.) **48:**493-502, April 1966.
23. Zemel, N.P., et al.: Chronic fracture dislocatioin of the proximal interphalangeal joint: treatment by osteotomy and bone graft, J. Hand Surg. **6:**447-455, Sept. 1981.

16. Short-shrift problems: a grab bag of athletic injuries

James H. Dobyns

Anyone with a topic like this is in trouble. The first thing to do is to define "short shrift," which is the 'short space of time given to a condemned man for confession before execution.' "Short" is 'not having enough length'; "shrift" means 'an absolution of sins,' an area of such importance that many sinners feel that it should not be short! Many sinners feel the same way about the problems to be mentioned here—they don't get enough respect! There are so many such problems that many will not be mentioned here. There simply isn't time enough to give all the topics that might be appropriate, and so categories are provided along with a few specific examples. Anatomic areas, all of which have their problems, are perhaps more closely packed in the wrist than anywhere else in the musculoskeletal field. Let's review a few problem categories.

Skin problems are often overlooked but are addressed in Chapter 10. Muscle and tendon overuse problems are common at the elbow and forearm and also at the wrist. Muscle-tendon anomalies are seldom discussed, yet they are the underlying cause of many troublesome problems. Nerve-abuse problems were mentioned, but they are so important that they deserve more time;[1] likewise with vascular abuse problems. Bone and joint problems are usually discussed, but many still get overlooked. Ganglia are indeed a problem, though often minimized. Impingement syndromes other than at the shoulder are hardly mentioned in most discussions of athletic problems, but they are common at the wrist. Still other joint problems that receive short shrift are joint instability, joint shear, and compression injuries and even undisplaced fractures, which are often overlooked, particularly when in the scaphoid or the distal end of the radius. I treated my wife for 3 months for a distal radius fracture and never got a positive report from the radiologist, though it was quite clear as time went on that she had a fracture and that it was healing. This is also a common experience in fractures that become ischemic such as Kienböck's disease of the lunate (Fig. 16-1) and Preisser's disease of the scaphoid. It occurred to me one day that I was seeing many wrist problems that I could map by drawing an oval around the radial aspect of the wrist. Within that small area is a great multiplicity of diagnoses. The categories include

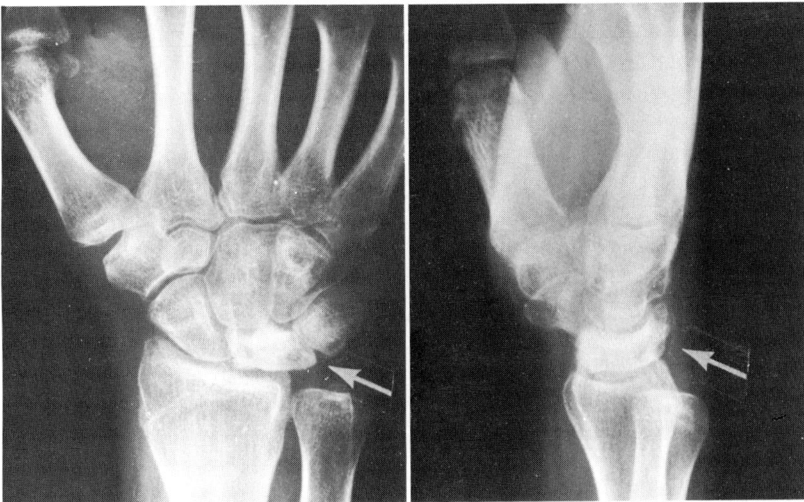

Fig. 16-1. Kienböck's disease. Anteroposterior and lateral roentgenograms of the wrist showing increased density of the lunate bone.

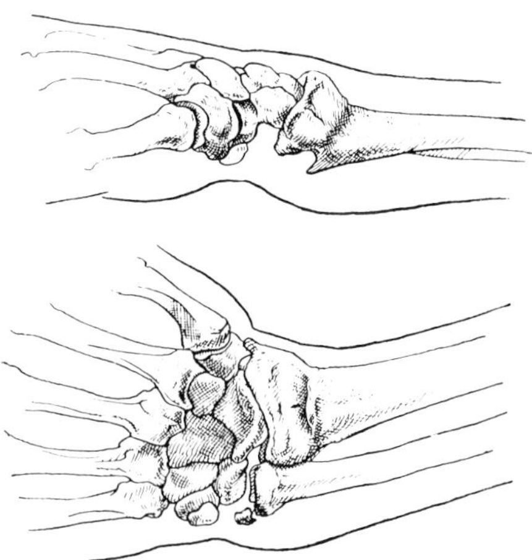

Fig. 16-2. Malunited fracture of the lower end of the radius (malunited Colles' fracture). Notice dorsal displacement of the distal fragment, posterior tilting of the articular surface of the radius, radial deviation of the hand, prominence of the distal end of the ulna, and ununited fracture of the ulnar styloid process.

sprains and dislocations, fractures that may become malunions (Fig. 16-2), synovitis that may become arthritis, tenosynovitis, tendinitis, ganglia, bone cysts (which may be tumors or may be ganglia), neuropathy or neuralgia problems, vascular problems, tendon rupture problems, articular and periarticular calcifications, and tumors.[2] Tumors are infrequent in this area, but they do occur. They may present with pain or

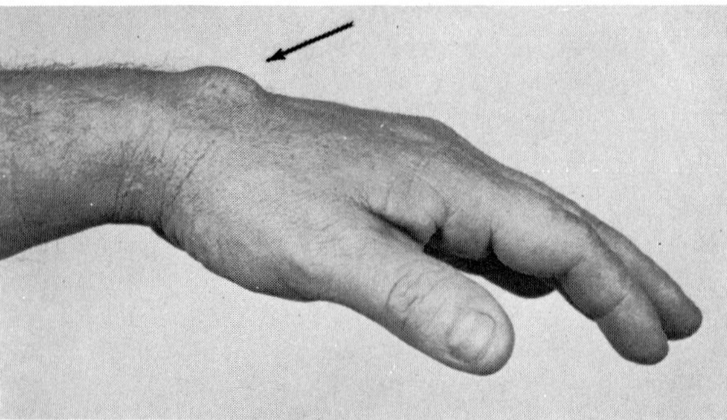

Fig. 16-3. Ganglion of the wrist, with rounded, well-demarcated swelling on the dorsum of the wrist.

simply as a mass. The more common ganglion also presents with pain or as a mass (Fig. 16-3). The literature tells us about conditions that resemble ganglia. This list reads much like the entities of the radial oval syndrome. It includes muscle anomaly, lipoma, neuroma of the posterior interosseous nerve, hamartoma, aneurysm, dorsal exostosis of the carpus or the radius, dorsal prominence of the scaphoid, dorsal prominence of the lunate, tendon injury, tenosynovitis, periarticular calcareous deposits, and tumors of the soft tissue or bone. We recently reviewed a few cases of recent years that resembled wrist ganglia[3] but instead were found to be a synovial carcinoma, two cases of clear cell sarcoma, a giant cell tumor of the tendon sheath, and a plexiform neuroma. Even a bony lesion may be similarly deceptive. A patient was seen with a history of night pain for 2 years, relieved by taking aspirin at night. A radiopaque lesion of bone with aspirin relief should be an osteoid osteoma. The scan was positive and tomography emphasized radiopaque lesion. At surgery, it was a ganglion, and so both types of deception are very possible. A ganglion may mimic another lesion; another lesion may mimic a ganglion. Either way the problem usually receives "short shrift"!

Another short-shrift group are the nerve-abuse problems, whether from one-time trauma or repetitive trauma. They are common and disabling. A simple example is the effect of wrist-encircling devices such as watches and manacles, which easily aggravate the sensitive radial sensory nerves. Many nerve-abuse syndromes are almost unique to special activities such as bowling, which may produce bowler's thumb.[1] This is a sports-stress syndrome because a bowling ball produces it. It almost exclusively involves the ulnar digital nerve of the thumb, which becomes greatly enlarged. Such nerves tethered in one spot by scar adapt by lengthening as well as thickening. At this stage the damaged nerve, once lysed, must be rerouted or reanastomosed. Since every tissue in the area can be abused, the lesion may be both an arterial and a nerve problem and is preceded by skin callus and soft-tissue fibrosis. The best treatment is to identify the problem early and stop the abuse. In bowling this may be done by redrilling the bowling ball but, of course, may require that the activity be stopped.

Muscle-tendon overuse problems are exceedingly common, and one that gets very little respect is the extensor intersection syndrome.[2,4] The signs are enlargement at the intersection where the abductor pollicis longus and extensor pollicis brevis cross the two radial wrist extensors. The unique, dramatic characteristic of this syndrome in the acute stage is the pronounced crepitus, so noteworthy that workers call this condition a "squeaker." The problem occurs near but not at the de Quervain stenosing tenosynovitis area. The cause has been said to be bursitis, peritendinitis crepitans, a muscle compartment syndrome, a tendon compartment syndrome. Athletic activities known to produce the syndrome include rowing, gymnastics, and weight lifting. The treatment is rest, protection, and stopping the causative activity. Surgery is best avoided but occasionally needed and in principally decompression.

The most important data to remember to avoid overlooking the short-shrift syndromes are the facts of anatomy. Knowledge of anatomy, variations in that anatomy, and knowledge that stress can cause any tissue to break down will lead to proper diagnoses, even if the problems are unique or seemingly trivial. With the proper diagnosis adequate treatment is selected, and the problem will then receive "long shrift"!

REFERENCES

1. Dobyns, J.H., O'Brien, E.T., Linscheid, R.L., and Farrow, G.M.: Bowler's thumb, diagnosis, and treatment: a review of seventeen cases, J. Bone. Joint Surg. **54A**(4):751-755, June 1972.
2. Dobyns, J.H., Sim, F.H., and Linscheid, R.L.: Sports stress syndromes of the hand and wrist, Am. J. Sports Med. **6**(5):236-254, 1978.
3. Fogel, G.R., Younge, D.A., and Dobyns, J.H.: Pitfalls in the diagnosis of the simple dorsal wrist ganglion, Orthopedics **6**(8):990-992, Aug. 1983.
4. Wood, M.B., and Linscheid, R.L.: Abductor pollicis longus bursitis, Clin. Orthop. (93):293-296, June 1973.

17. Peripheral nerve injuries and entrapments of the forearm and wrist

John F. Mosher

Peripheral nerve problems about the forearm and wrist are surprisingly rare when one considers the tremendous pounding and stresses to which this area is subjected. Add to this the exercise programs that lead to such exaggerated muscle development and I would believe that nerve compression syndromes would be frequent, but such is not the case.

NERVE INJURIES
Bowler's thumb (Fig. 17-1)

Bowler's thumb is a perineural fibrosis of the ulner digital nerve of the thumb at the metacarpophalangeal crease. It is a traumatic neuroma characterized by proliferation of the fibrous tissues around and within the digital nerve. The cause seems to be repetitive friction against the corner of the thumb hole. The patient notices a tender nodule at the base of the thumb (ulnar metacarpophalangeal crease). Tinel's sign can usually be elicited.

Early recognition and protective measures are the key. Change the position of the thumb hole, wear a splint, or stop bowling. Surgery is very rarely indicated. Belsky and Millander[2] reported a bowler's thumb in a baseball player. Because of unrelieved symptoms, they transposed the nerve posterior to the adductor pollicis tendon. This solution seems a very practical approach to this repetitive pressure problem.

Entrapment or nerve compression syndrome in athletes is a significant if not common problem.

Carpal tunnel syndrome

The carpal tunnel syndrome, a median nerve compression syndrome, though not widely recognized until the 1950s with the writings of Dr. George Phalen,[20] is now perhaps the most common diagnosis in a hand surgical practice and its incidence seems to be increasing. The incidence of carpal tunnel syndrome as a sports-related problem however is surprisingly low. Any condition increasing the volume of the contents of the rigidly confined carpal canal can be the initiating factor. Nonspecific

174

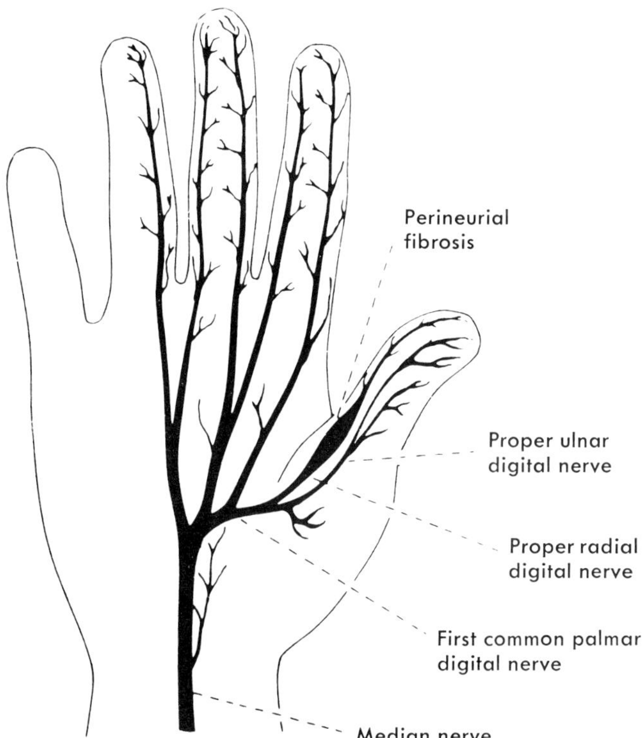

Fig. 17-1. Bowler's thumb. Distal sensory branches of median nerve in hand and location of perineural fibrosis of proper ulnar digital nerve of thumb. (From Minkow, F.V., and Bassett, F.H., III: Clin. Orthop. (83):115, 1972.)

synovitis is by far the most common cause. Hypertrophied or abnormal flexor superficialis[22] or lumbrical muscles[5,13] and thrombosis of the persistent artery[14] of the median nerve (5% occurrence) have been implicated. Each of these conditions would seem to have an increased potential in vigorous athletes, but somehow they seem to be almost immune to the problem.

Since carpal tunnel syndrome is so rare in the athlete when the diagnosis is entertained, unusual causes must be suspected. In addition to the above causes, fracture of the hamate hook[18] has been reported. Special roentgenograms may be indicated: carpal tunnel view, tomograms, and computerized tomography, which best shows soft-tissue masses in the carpal tunnel. Systemic diseases such as diabetes mellitus may present as a carpal tunnel syndrome.

Symptoms. The usual carpal tunnel syndrome is reported as night-time numbness[20] relieved by motion. Abnormal muscles in the carpal tunnel are more likely to produce the median nerve paresthesias with activity. Thrombosis of the persistent median artery is likely to cause the sudden onset of a "numbing pain" that is unremitting and will need more urgent surgical relief.

Signs. Tinel's tap sign and Phalen's test may be positive in the usual manner. Prior exercise with the abnormal muscle conditions has not proved to effect any change in the incidence of positive signs.

Tests. Nerve conduction study is recommended for all unusual nerve compression syndromes, and I consider the carpal tunnel syndrome in the athlete such a case. Prior exercise again has not been productive in clarifying the diagnosis.

I routinely order an arthritis panel and a fasting blood glucose test in younger patients.

Treatment. Orally administered anti-inflammatory agents and night splinting have been ineffective for our athletes. Cortisone injection[10,26] into the canal may be an effective temporary measure.

Surgery. Carpal tunnel surgery is generally quite simple, but the release of the flexor retinaculum may be a major event in the hand function of an athlete who vigorously uses the hand. Release of the flexor retinaculum "bowstring" has been shown to increase the distance between the pillars of the canal 2 to 3 mm but has been as great as 6 mm.[3] The resultant adjustment of the transverse carpal curve after the transection of the retinacular bowstring may be a cause of persistent wrist pain.

Subluxation of the flexor sublimis of the ring finger over the hook of the hamate has been reported after release of the flexor retinaculum. For this reason various retinaculum incisions have been advocated to avoid this problem.[9] I have not utilized anything but a straight retinaculum incision around 5 mm radial to the ulnar border of the canal. Postoperatively the wrist is splinted in extension for 2 to 3 weeks. Vigorous weight lifting (elbow flexion in supination) is curtailed for 8 to 10 weeks.

PROXIMAL ENTRAPMENT NEUROPATHIES OF MEDIAN NERVE

The proximal sites of entrapment of the median nerve are as follows:[15]

1. Supracondylar process and ligament of Struthers
2. Lacertus fibrosus
3. Within the pronator teres muscle
4. Arch of superficial head of flexor digitorum sublimis

With the designed muscle hypertrophy of today's athletes this problem of proximal entrapment would seem a likely repetitive type of injury. But once again the vigorous young athletes seem almost immune to the problem.

The problem with diagnosis of these problems is the vagueness of the complaint, the physical signs, and the electrodiagnostic studies. Only in the AINS (anterior interosseous nerve syndrome)[23] can the diagnosis be easily made.

The median nerve entrapments around the elbow generally present with a vague aching pain in the proximal end of the forearm and increase with activity and decrease with rest. There may be some complaint of median distribution numbness in the hand, but these patients are not awakened at night as those with the carpal tunnel syndrome. It is most helpful if the patient can localize the most symptomatic area with a fingertip and the examiner can palpate an area of point tenderness and produce a

Tinel's tap sign, but this rarely seems to be the case. Phalen's wrist flexion test may be positive, and that finding may further cloud the diagnosis.[15]

Various physical tests are described to localize the area of compression,[12,24] but they are often not specific.

The electrodiagnostic studies are not diagnostic in many cases (except AINS with defibrillation in the flexor pollicis longus, ulnar half of the flexor digitorum profundus, and pronator quadratus).

I routinely test for diabetes in suspected nerve entrapments in locations other than the cubital or carpal tunnel.

Except with AINS where there are obvious functional deficits a long course (4 to 6 months) of conservative therapy (anti-inflammatories, rest) may be justified. In the AINS with progressive or complete paralysis of the FPL and with or without the FDP index and middle finger, observation for 6 to 12 weeks is reasonable, since spontaneous recovery may occur.

The approaches for exploring the proximal median nerve have been well described.[8] The exploration is formidable and must extend from around 5 cm proximal to the elbow to beyond the flexor superficialis arch.

Ulnar nerve

Compression of the ulnar nerve occurs at the elbow (cubital tunnel) and the wrist (Guyon's canal). This nerve is easily palpated in the ulnar groove in its subcutaneous setting. It is frequently the recipient of minor stings, but it rarely is severely injured by direct trauma. It is however a frequent sight of compression problems but rarely associated with sports activity.

Cubital tunnel

Compression of the ulnar nerve occurs as the nerve slides forward with elbow flexion. It is trapped in the wedge-shaped space between the humeral origin of the flexor carpi ulnaris and epicondyle. Anterior subluxation of the nerve may magnify this problem. Rarely abnormal musculature such as the anconeus epitrochlearis may be implicated in the compression.

Symptoms
1. Uncomfortable sensations or tingling with or without numbness in the ulnar nerve distribution of the hand
2. Weakness and clumsiness of the hand may be noted early or gradually

Signs
1. Tinel's tap sign present over the ulnar nerve at some point along the cubital tunnel.
2. Elbow flexion test[25]: Maximal active elbow flexion may increase the ulnar nerve sensory symptoms.
3. Subluxation of the ulnar nerve over the medial epicondyle with flexion and extension of the elbow.

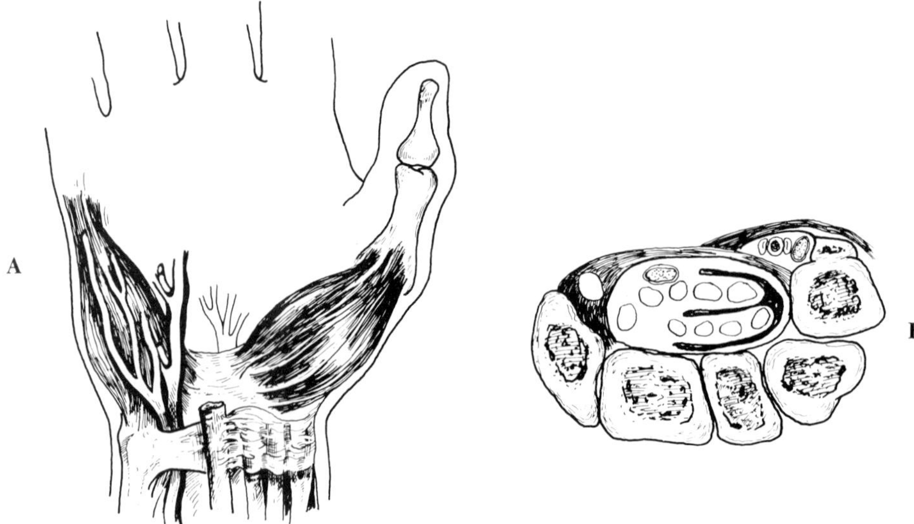

Fig. 17-2. Anatomic relations of structures within ulnar tunnel. **A,** Palmar view lies medial to ulnar artery. **B,** Cross section of both carpal and ulnar tunnels. Ulnar tunnel at top right is bounded anteriorly by superficial transverse carpal ligament, posteriorly by deep transverse carpal ligament, and medially by pisiform bone and pisohamate ligament. Structures within this tunnel from left to right are vein, artery, vein, and nerve. (From Milford, L.: The hand, ed. 2, St. Louis, 1982, The C.V. Mosby Co.)

4. Intrinsic weakness or atrophy in the hand.
5. A sensory deficit within ulnar distribution

Test. Nerve conduction study is definitive in this condition.

Treatment

1. Conservative trial—night splints to prevent elbow flexion
2. Intrinsic atrophy probably dictates rather urgent surgical intervention. It also is an indication of a possible poor final result.[1]

Surgery. If the nerve is hypermobile I prefer an anterior submuscular transposition.[4] Rarely, I have just released the flexor carpi ulnaris sling with or without epineurolysis.

Ulnar tunnel syndrome (Loge de Guyon) (Fig. 17-2)

Although this area is termed a tunnel,[16] there is not a substantial roof and there are few compression syndromes other than with tumors such as a ganglion or lipoma. Constant pressure such as bicycle handlebars may cause sensory and motor symptoms. Recurrent trauma may produce an ulnar artery thrombosis[16] or aneurysm and thus compromise the distal ulnar nerve function but usually with a more vascular (Raynaud's) type of presentation. A fall on the outstretched hand may injure the sensory branch of the nerve as it passes superficially to the hook of the hamate.

At the point where the motor branch exits deeply from this canal, there is a real compression area. The fibrous origin of the abductor and flexor of the fifth finger, which arches over the motor branch and the pisohamate ligament lying deep, create a fibrous ring encircling the motor branch against the hook of the hamate. Compression syndromes in this area often develop spontaneously and quickly with little complaint of discomfort or numbness but rapid development of weakness and motor wasting. In this instance hypothenar motor function is intact. More distal compression of the nerve has been reported at the fibrous arch of the adductor, and so a good physical exam is most important to elucidate the locale of the compression.

Radial tunnel syndrome

The diagnosis "tennis elbow" has appeared in the literature for more than 50 years. Lateral epicondylitis is a term frequently equated with "tennis elbow". But as we have come to know, of these four words only the lateral and elbow have been correct. The patient rarely is a tennis player and inflammation of the epicondyle is not the disorder. This entity has been well defined as a tear in the origin of the extensor carpi radialis brevis (ECRB).[19] and the area of pain can be covered by one fingertip over the lateral epicondyle.

Since the 1972 article by Roles and Maudsley[21] we have been aware of the "radial tunnel syndrome." The incidence of diagnosis of this entrapment is on the rise.

Anatomy. The radial nerve is almost totally (except for the brachioradialis, BR) a nerve of extension, and it seems to have wandered astray to appear in front of the elbow. To find its way back to the dorsal surface of the forearm, the motor branch (posterior interosseous nerve) passes through the "radial tunnel," under the mobile wad of Henry" (BR, ECRL, ECRB) and between the two heads of the supinator muscle. This "tunnel" is only about three fingerbreadths in length. There are four described anatomic compressive factors:[17]

1. Fibrous bands tethering the nerve to the radiohumeral joint
2. Fibrous border of extensor carpi radialis brevis
3. Radial recurrent "fan" of vessels
4. Arcade of Fröhse

The "radial tunnel syndrome" depicts a compression of the posterior interosseous nerve in the area of the head of the radius that manifests as an aching pain associated with activity. The posterior interosseous nerve is described as a purely motor nerve, but it is now recognized[7,17] that the so-called motor nerves such as the posterior interosseous or the deep motor branch of the ulnar nerve carry a significant number of sensory fibers from the joint, muscles, and even some skin receptors. This explains the aching pain resulting from compression of the "motor" nerve.

Symptoms. The following are symptoms of this radial tunnel syndrome or "resistant tennis elbow":

1. Aching pain in the extensor mass that may radiate to the dorsal side of the wrist. The pain increases with activity, particularly wrist flexion and pronation. This pain is commonly the only complaint.

2. Weakness of wrist, finger, or thumb extension is rare.
3. Numbness is rare.

Signs

1. *No* lateral epicondylar point localization.
2. Tenderness on deep palpation over the radial neck, just over or posterior to the "mobile wad."
3. Resisted extension of the middle finger. Increased pain with this manuever is said to indicate a radial tunnel entrapment, but this same action causes increased pain with "tennis elbow" and has not been an effective differential test in my experience.
4. Resisted supination of the extended elbow causes an increase in the aching pain.

Nerve conduction studies are not reliable in this condition. A delay in conduction from the spiral groove to the extensor digitorum communis is indicative of a pathologic condition in the tunnel area, but most patients do not show any conduction deficit. It has been suggested that this is attributable to the intermittent nature of the compression.

True posterior interosseous nerve syndrome (PINS) with paresis below the extensor carpi radialis longus is rare and to my knowledge has not been reported except with trauma, inflammation, rheumatoid arthritis, or tumor (ganglion, lipoma).

Therefore with the radial tunnel syndrome, like the proximal median nerve compression syndromes, the decision regarding surgical exploration is made almost entirely on clinical grounds.

Conservative care, such as changing activities to decrease the muscle stress about the radial tunnel and anti-inflammatories, may be effective.

Surgical approaches to this tunnel have been well described.[8,17] Most recently I traveled the path described by Hall et al.[11] The posterior interosseous nerve is approached between the brachioradialis and the extensor carpi radialis longus. The exposure was excellent and mobilization of surrounding muscles was only minimally necessary.

Although the diagnosis is not very exact in this condition, because of the lack of specific tests the relief of this chronic aching pain may be dramatic. The posterior interosseous nerve must be well exposed throughout the length of the tunnel (although the fibrous proximal border of the superficial head of the supinator, the arcade of Frohse) seems to be the most frequent area of constriction. Everyone seems to report good results with this surgery; the diagnosis however remains to be a problem.

SUMMARY

Peripheral nerve problems of the forearm and wrist are not common. We still must be alert regarding this entity. The specific diagnosis in many of the entrapment problems may be uncertain at best. Surgical decompression can give excellent relief but should never be considered a "minor" procedure even in a condition so common and "simple" as the carpal tunnel syndrome.

REFERENCES

1. Adelaar, R.S., et al.: The treatment of the cubital tunnel syndrome, J. Hand Surg. **9A:**90, Jan. 1984.
2. Belsky, M.R., and Millender, L.H.: Bowler's thumb in a baseball player: a case report, Orthopedics **3:**122, Feb. 1980.
3. Blablock, H.S.: ASSH Newsletter, p. 34, 1981.
4. Broody, A.S., et al.: Technical problems with ulnar nerve transposition at the elbow: findings and results of reoperation, J. Hand Surg. **3:**85, Jan. 1978.
5. Butler, B., and Bigley, E.: Aberrant index (first) lumbrical tendinous origin associated with carpal tunnel syndrome: a case report, J. Bone Joint Surg. **53A:**160, Jan. 1971.
6. Dobyns, J.H., et al.: Bowler's thumb: diagnosis and treatment, J. Bone Joint Surg. **54A:**751, June 1972.
7. Dykes, R.W., and Terzis, J.K.: Functional anatomy of the deep motor branch of the ulnar nerve, Clin. Orthop. (128):P167, Oct. 1977.
8. Eversmann, W.W.: In Green, D.P., editor: Operative hand surgery, New York, 1982, Churchill Livingstone, p. 958.
9. Fischer, E.: ASSH Newsletter, p. 13, 1982.
10. Green, D.P.: Diagnostic and therapeutic valve of carpal tunnel injection, Presented at meeting of American Society for Surgery of the Hand, Atlanta, Ga., Feb. 1984.
11. Hall, H.C., et al.: An approach to the posterior interosseous nerve, Plast. Reconstr. Surg. **74:**435, Sept. 1984.
12. Hartz, C.R., et al.: The pronator teres syndrome: compressive neuropathy of the median nerve, J. Bone Joint Surg. **63A:**885, July 1981.
13. Jabaley, M.: Personal observations on the role of the lumbrical muscles in carpal tunnel syndrome, J. Hand Surg. **3:**88, Jan. 1978.
14. Jackson, I.T., and Campbell, J.C.: An unusual cause of carpal tunnel syndrome: a case of thrombosis of the median artery, J. Bone Joint Surg. **52B:**330, May 1970.
15. Johnson, R.K., et al.: Median nerve entrapment syndrome in the proximal forearm, J. Hand Surg. **4:**48, Jan. 1979.
16. Kleinert, H.E., and Hayes, J.E.: The ulnar tunnel syndrome, Plast. Reconstr. Surg. **47:**21, Jan. 1971.
17. Lister, G.D., et al.: The radial tunnel syndrome, J. Hand Surg. **4:**52, Jan. 1979.
18. Manske, P.R.: Fracture of the hook of the hamate presenting as a carpal tunnel syndrome, The Hand **10:**181, 1978.
19. Nirschl, R.P.: The etiology and treatment of tennis elbow, J. Sports Med. **2:**308, 1974.
20. Phalen, G.S., et al.: Neuropathy of the median nerve due to compression beneath transverse carpal ligament, J. Bone Joint Surg. **32A:**109, 1950.
21. Roles, N.C., and Maudsley, R.H.: Radial tunnel syndrome, resistant tennis elbow as a nerve entrapment, J. Bone Joint Surg. **54B:**499, 1972.
22. Smith, R.J.: Anomalous muscle belly of the flexor digitorum superficialis causing carpal tunnel syndrome, J. Bone Joint Surg. **53A:**1215, Sept. 1971.
23. Spinner, M.: The anterior interosseous nerve syndrome, J. Bone Joint Surg. **52A:**84, Jan. 1970.
24. Spinner, M.: Injuries to the major branches of peripheral nerves in the forearm, ed. 2, Philadelphia, 1978, W.B. Saunders Co.
25. Wadsworth, T.G.: The external compression syndrome of the ulnar nerve at the cubital tunnel, Clin. Orthop. (124):189, May 1977.
26. Wood, M.R.: Hydrocortisone injections for carpal tunnel syndrome, The Hand **12:**62, 1980.

18. Upper extremity splinting and bracing (hand)

Frank C. McCue III
Vi A. Mayer
Joe H. Gieck

We have seen some of the protective devices that are available to prevent injury to athletes in various sports. However, when injury does occur, we like to get the athletes back to their activities as soon as possible without placing them in jeopardy by increasing their injuries or reinjuring structures that are in the healing phase.

It is reported that protective splints were first used in the Middle Ages by knights to protect their hands from lances and various other weapons used at the time. Although the concept of using splints for protection during sporting events is not new, today we have new materials to work with as well as a better understanding of hand function and the healing process.

STATIC VERSUS DYNAMIC SPLINTS

There are two basic types of splints, static and dynamic. Static splints prevent motion from occurring. Dynamic splints allow and may often create motion. Immobilization is required during the acute or healing phase of an injury. Static splints will protect an athlete's hands, thereby allowing him to participate in activities earlier. It should be noted that dynamic splints may be used to substitute for paralyzed muscles. In the rehabilitation phase of recovery, dynamic splints are generally used to overcome soft tissue as well as joint contractures. Static splints may also be used to overcome deformity.

Successful splint fabrication requires that one be familiar with the planes and contours of the normal hand, as well as the deformities each joint is prone to develop. In fabricating protective devices for athletes, one must be familiar with the kinematic differences of the hand at rest versus the hand at work. It is helpful to have the appropriate sports equipment available while one is molding the splints.

Some principles of splint design may be altered when one is working with athletes. A general rule of splinting is to leave as much of the palmar surface free as possible. However, it may be more important to provide greater stability than to

182

allow for sensibility input on the volar surface of the hand depending on the functional need of an individual athlete.

SPLINTING PRINCIPLES

Hand splints may be molded in either a functional position or in an intrinsic-plus or antideformity position. Whenever possible after trauma, the wrist should be positioned in dorsiflexion because the wrist is the key joint in maintaining mechanically balanced hand function. When immobilized in a functional position, the wrist is usually placed in 30 degrees of dorsiflexion. The metacarpophalangeal (MCP) joints are flexed approximately 45 degrees. The proximal interphalangeal (PIP) joints are in 10 to 20 degrees of flexion. It is necessary to maintain all three skeletal arches of the hand (proximal and distal transverse as well as longitudinal) when one is fabricating splints.

When immobilized in an intrinsic-plus or "clam-digger" position, the wrist is positioned in from 30 to 60 degrees of dorsiflexion, the MCP joints are placed in close to maximal flexion whereas the PIP joints are placed in slight flexion, approximately 10 degrees. MCP and PIP joints are especially vulnerable to contracture.

By positioning the MCP joints in flexion, the length of the collateral ligaments is maintained. This position discourages MCP extension contractures from occurring. Early mobilization is always advocated because positioning of the MCP joints in acute flexion for long periods of time may result in intrinsic contracture. One may prevent intrinsic tightness by providing an exercise program to position MCP joints in extension while passively flexing the PIP and DIP joints. Placing the PIP joints in extension will maintain ligamentous length and thereby prevent flexion contractures. The PIP joints are the most important joints in the hand, and so maintaining motion through an early exercise program is of utmost importance. Position of the thumb in both the intrinsic-plus or functional position may vary from near opposition to various degrees of abduction. Thumb position is dependent on diagnosis, its extent of involvement, and the functional needs of the player.

Bony prominences must always be accommodated when splinting is undertaken. These prominences should either be avoided or have the pressure decreased by dispersal of the area of contact or by use of padding. Neglecting to do so may result in pressure areas or even skin breakdown.

Low-temperature materials available today have been a boon to those involved in splinting. Orthoplast, Kay Splint, Polyform, Polyflex, Aquaplast, and Manorthos are just a few. Most may be heated by a dry or wet method and are legal for use in competition. You should choose the type of material that is durable and one with which your therapist or trainer is most familiar. In most cases, solid materials are preferable to those that are commercially perforated. In our experience, perforated materials are not so durable. Because of the degree of stress placed on perforated materials by athletes, breakage may occur between the perforations in areas where a great deal of force is exerted.

Several other principles may be utilized to improve the strength of materials used in splinting. The principle of strength through contour definitely applies to splint fabrication. Rounded internal corners will disperse forces, thereby making the splint more durable. Imperfections along the edge of a splint may increase the chances for breakage.

FINGER SPLINTS

The following are splints that may be used for various injuries.

There are five pathologic causes of mallet finger. In most young persons, if they are treated early and protected adequately with a splint, they will heal. Molded Polythene (polyethylene) splints first discussed by Stack are effective in treating mallet fingers. Care must be taken to ensure that the splint fits properly. The DIP joint should be placed in slight hyperextension. The splint should be taped, not closed with Velcro. When the tape is changed, care should be taken that the distal phalanx not be allowed to drop into flexion.

Dorsal metal splints without padding may also be molded to protect mallet fingers as well as boutonnière and swan-neck deformities. These splints are useful in that they may be molded to the dorsal surface of the hand and do not interfere with stereognosis in ball handling. Unfortunately, any metal splint, no matter how small in size, is illegal to use during either high-school or college competition.

Hollis has devised two splints that are helpful in controlling swan-neck and boutonnière deformities[1] (Fig. 18-1, *A*). The swan-neck control splint prevents hyperextension from occurring at the PIP joints but allows complete flexion. The boutonnière control splint encourages complete PIP extension but allows the DIP joint freedom for flexion. (Fig. 18-1, *B*). Both splints are excellent for treating early injuries. When one is to engage in athletic activities, other stronger means of protection are necessary.

Various other commercial splints are available for treatment of boutonnière deformities. All may play an important role in deformity prevention, but none are appropriate for use on the athletic field. Commercial Polythene splints are not appropriate if PIP flexion contracture has already occurred.

A dynamic extension type of splint originally described by Capener is appropriate in cases when a PIP contracture has occurred. (Fig. 18-2). A Bunnell safety pin splint and joint jack are two additional types of splints. (Fig. 18-3). In use of the safety pin splint, it is necessary to apply the splint with less tension for a longer period of time. Maximal tension that is tolerable only for short periods of time is the downfall of many dynamic splinting programs. Use of the joint jack requires careful supervision. Improper positioning of the splint may result in hyperextension of the DIP joint. If the splint is positioned properly but excessive pressure is applied to the strap tissue, breakdown may occur. Successful splinting requires three equal points of fixation. If one of the forces is unequal, the result may be detrimental to rehabilitation.

Commercial wrist splints available at your local drugstore do not provide adequate stability for the competitive athlete. They often allow older or noncompetitive athletes to resume athletic activities earlier than they could without support.

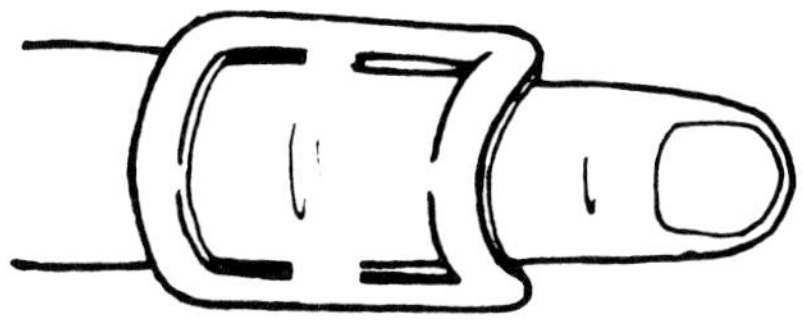

A

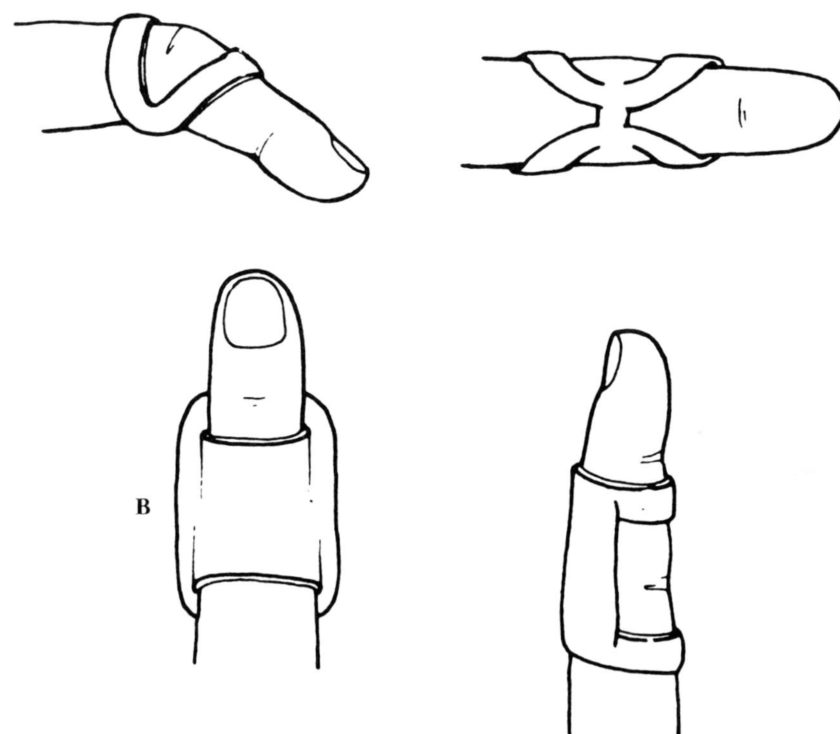

B

Fig. 18-1. **A,** Hollis's swan neck splint allows complete flexion but prevents hyperextension of the proximal interphalangeal (PIP) joint. **B,** Hollis's boutonnière splint supports the PIP joint in extension but allows the distal interphalangeal joint freedom to flex.

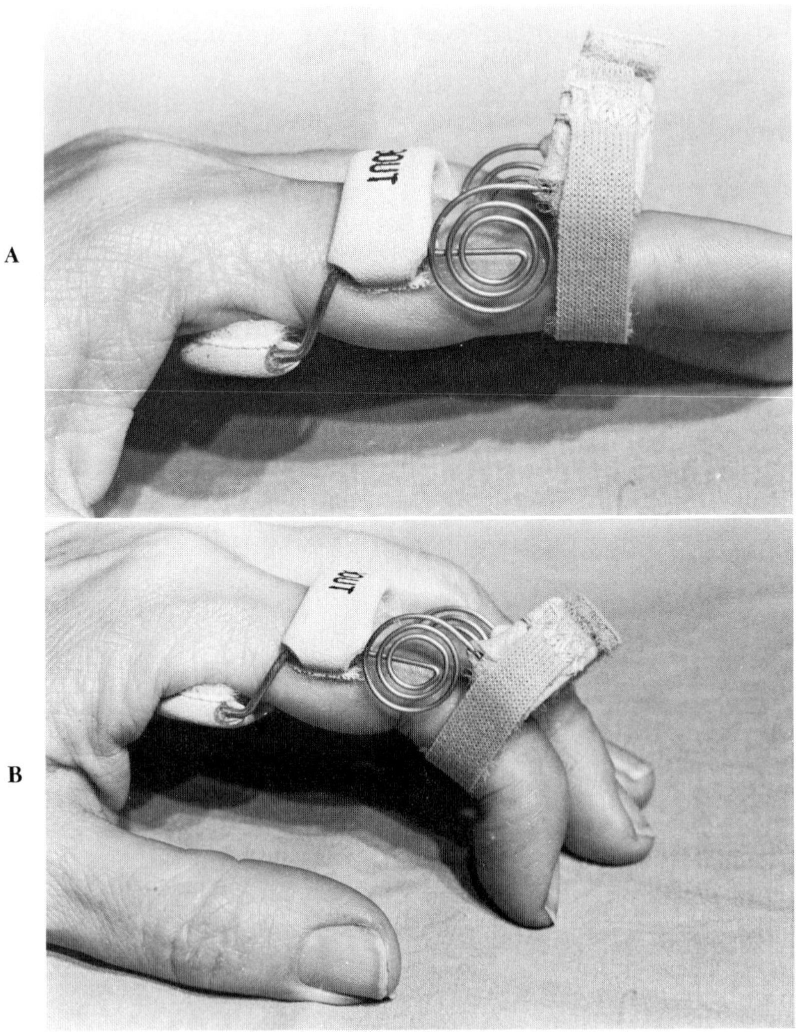

Fig. 18-2. **A,** Capener splint with proximal interphalangeal joint (PIP) held in extension. **B,** Capener splint allows flexion of the PIP joint.

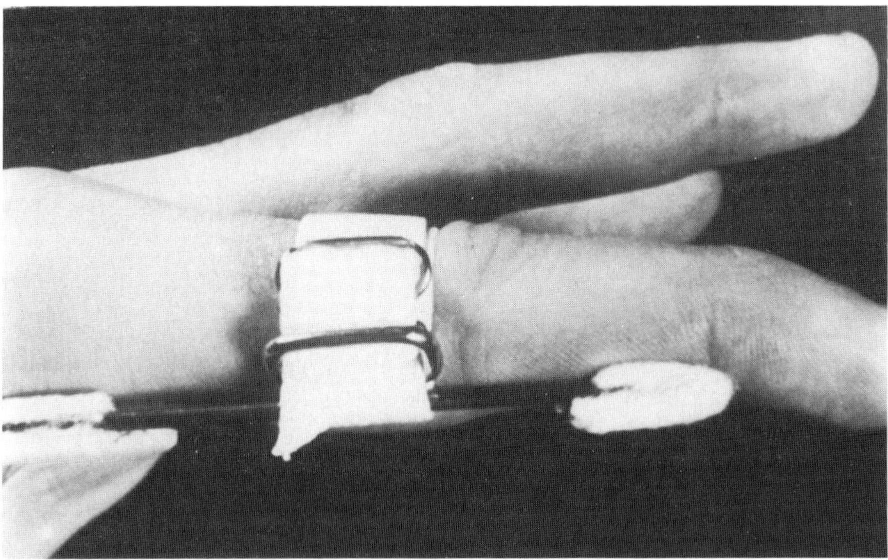

Fig. 18-3. Safety-pin splint requires less tension for longer periods of time.

EXERCISE AIDS

Web strap, buddy tapes, and flexor gloves are examples of exercise aids that are useful in the upper extremity. Web strap is one-half inch webbing with a buckle attached to one end. The strap is applied as a figure of eight and can be used to draw the proximal and distal finger joints into flexion. Buddy splints may be made from Velcro. (Fig. 18-4). Just as fingers may be taped together, the double Velcro may be used to stabilize one finger to an adjoining digit. This provides stability but may also be used to encourage active assistive exercises to an involved digit. A flexor glove is a means of tractioning fingers into flexion. In utilizing the glove, one must follow two basic principles. The tension exerted on the fingers should be reasonably comfortable for longer periods of time. The direction of the pull should be constructed so that the force of traction is oblique to the fingertips and directed toward the scaphoid. (Fig. 18-5). This device is most helpful in overcoming limitations of MCP flexion.

SILICONE CASTS

Silicone casts can be very useful in providing adequate mobilization while allowing the athlete to participate much earlier than he would with other means of protection. They are excellent for mobilizing carpal and metacarpal fractures.

The following is information regarding purchasing of materials and application of silicone casts:

GE RTV-11
Available in 1-pound can or 12-pound bucket; should be kept in the
   freezer to prevent deterioration

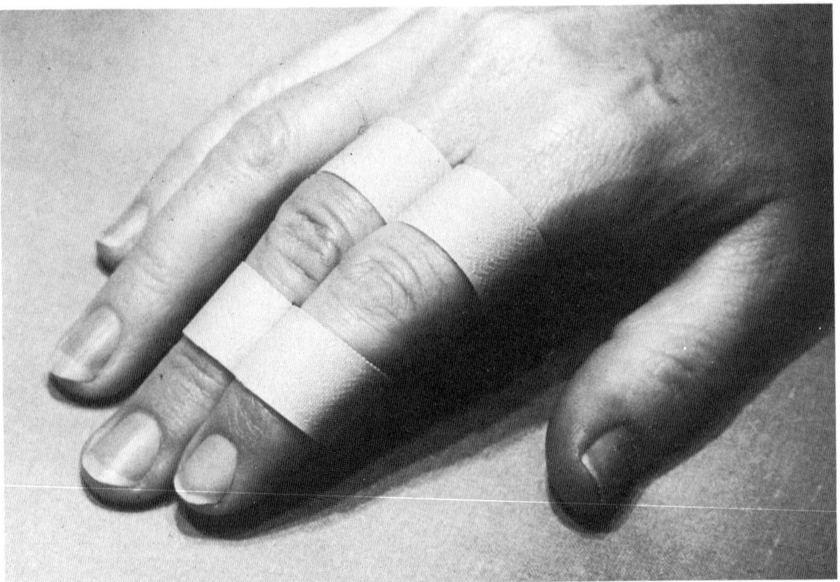

Fig. 18-4. Buddy tapes provide stability and active assistive exercise to the involved digit.

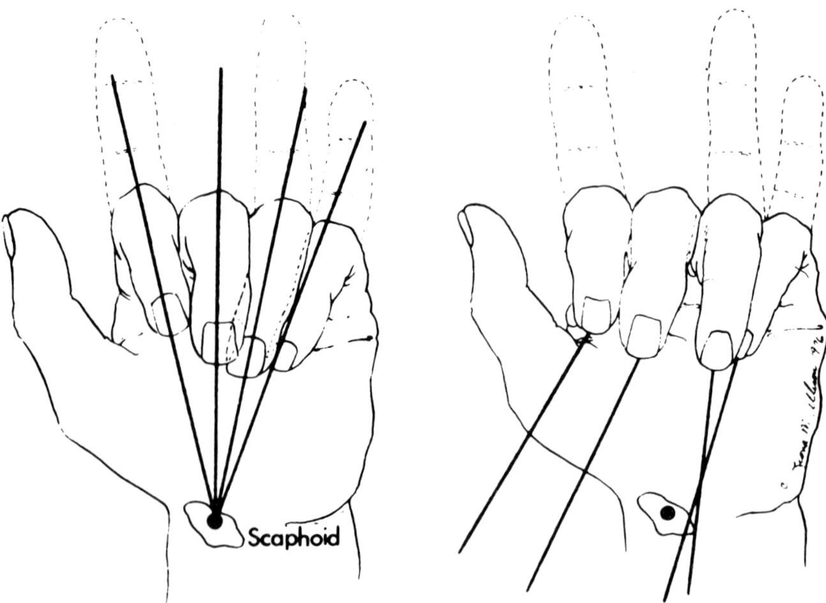

Fig. 18-5. When one is fabricating the flexion glove, forces on the fingers should be directed toward the scaphoid.

Vendor: S.E. Radio Supply
          Industrial Department
          414 Hillsborough Street   (800)-334-7742
          Raleigh, NC 27611   (919)-828-2311

Directions for applying silicone arm and hand cast:

1. Tape and pad area as necessary.
2. Apply Vaseline over area to be covered.
3. Apply layer of silicone (15 drops of catalyst per ounce of silicone) to area.
4. Apply a half roll of Kling to area.
5. Repeat steps 3 and 4 until three rolls of Kling are used.
6. To strengthen cast (e.g., to prevent wrist motion) soak 4 × 4 inch gauze pads in silicone mixture and incorporate in layers of Kling.
7. When finished, encase cast and area in plastic bag and secure with 2-inch elastic wrap.
8. When dry after 2 or 3 hours, cut off along ulnar side of arm.
9. Wear bivalved plaster cast during the day but silicone cast for practice and games.
10. Apply additional layers to strengthen cast as needed.

REFERENCES

1. Hollis, L.I.: Innovative splinting ideas. In Hunter, J.M., et al., editor: Rehabilitation of the hand, St. Louis, 1978, The C.V. Mosby Co.

SUGGESTED READINGS

1. Barr, N.R.: The hand: principles and techniques of simple splintmaking in rehabilitation, London, 1975, Butterworth & Co., Ltd.
2. Boyes, J.H.: Surgery of the hand, ed. 5, Philadelphia, 1970, J.B. Lippincott Co.
3. Crawford, G.P.: The molded Polythene splint for mallet finger deformities, J. Hand Surg. **9A:**231-237, 1984.
4. Fess, E., Gettle, K., and Strickland, J.: Hand splinting principles and methods, St. Louis, 1981, The C.V. Mosby Co.
5. Flynn, J.: Hand surgery, ed. 2, Baltimore, 1975, The Williams & Wilkins Co.
6. Hunter, J.M., et al.: Rehabilitation of the hand, St. Louis, 1978, The C.V. Mosby Co.
7. Hunter, J.M., et al.: Rehabilitation of the hand, ed. 2, St. Louis, 1984, The C.V. Mosby Co.
8. Kulund, D.N.: The injured athlete, Philadelphia, 1982, J.B. Lippincott Co.
9. Parry, C.B.W.: Rehabilitation of the hand, ed. 3, London, 1973, Butterworth & Co., Ltd.

PART THREE

Elbow and shoulder

19. Functional anatomy of the shoulder and elbow

George P. Bogumill

SHOULDER
Skeleton

The clavicle is a short S-shaped bone that functions as a "tie rod" of the upper limb to the axial skeleton and by its rotation allows for adaptive changes in the functional activity. It has rounded prominences on each end but does not have a true hinge joint. There is a normal secondary ossification center medially but none laterally. However, there is a lateral epiphysis, which can be dislocated traumatically. Thus diagnosis of a slipped epiphysis versus acromioclavicular dislocation must be made clinically rather than roentgenographically. The clavicle is one of the most frequently fractured bones in the body.

The scapula is ensheathed in muscle and more or less "floats" on the chest wall, depending on where the muscles are going to take it. It is a flat blade with multiple projections for muscle attachments.

The humerus is the proximal lever arm of the upper limb. It is a large long bone with a number of growth centers that can be injured in the adolescent. The rounded proximal end articulates with the glenoid surface of the scapula, though they do not fit well. The distal end is fairly complex and has a number of growth centers that can cause confusion on a roentgenogram. Fortunately one has a normal control of the other side in the adolescent athlete. The shaft of the humerus is occasionally fractured by torsional muscle pulls.

Joints

The sternoclavicular joint is the only one that attaches the upper extremity directly to the axial skeleton. The joint surfaces of the manubrium and clavicle are flat with a limited, mainly adaptive, range of motion (Fig. 19-1). There is an articular disk that allows increased freedom of motion while functioning as an intra-articular ligament. Its function is to resist upward displacement of the medial end of the clavicle when a weight is carried in the hand as well as to cushion compressive forces through the clavicle. Other ligaments are the anterior and posterior sternoclavicular and the cos-

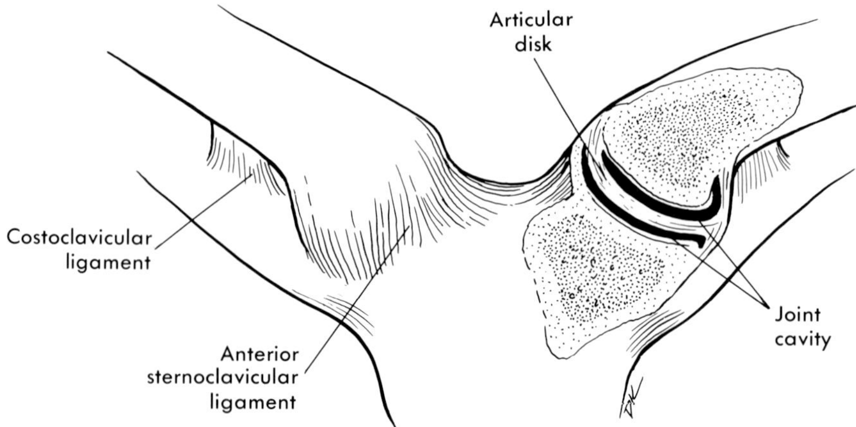

Fig. 19-1. Anatomy of sternoclavicular joint. Intra-articular disk attaches to cranial portion of medial clavicle and helps resist upward displacement when weight is borne in hand and in cushioning impacts directed medially along clavicle.

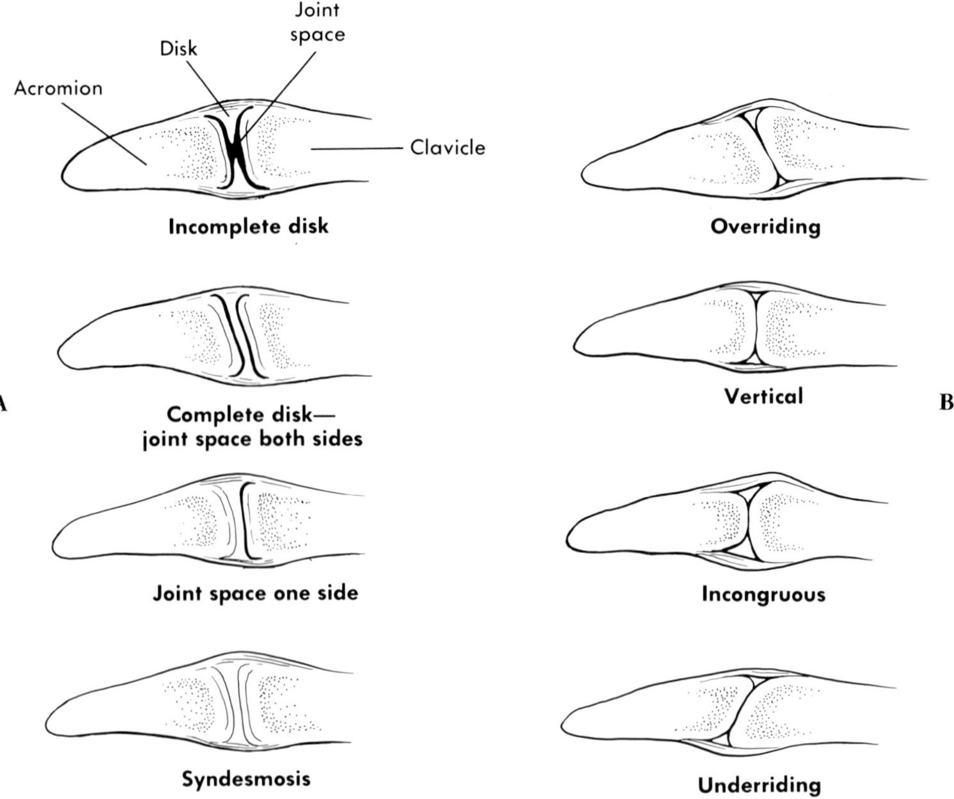

Fig. 19-2. Variations in acromioclavicular and sternoclavicular joints. **A,** Articular disk often incomplete, especially in older persons.

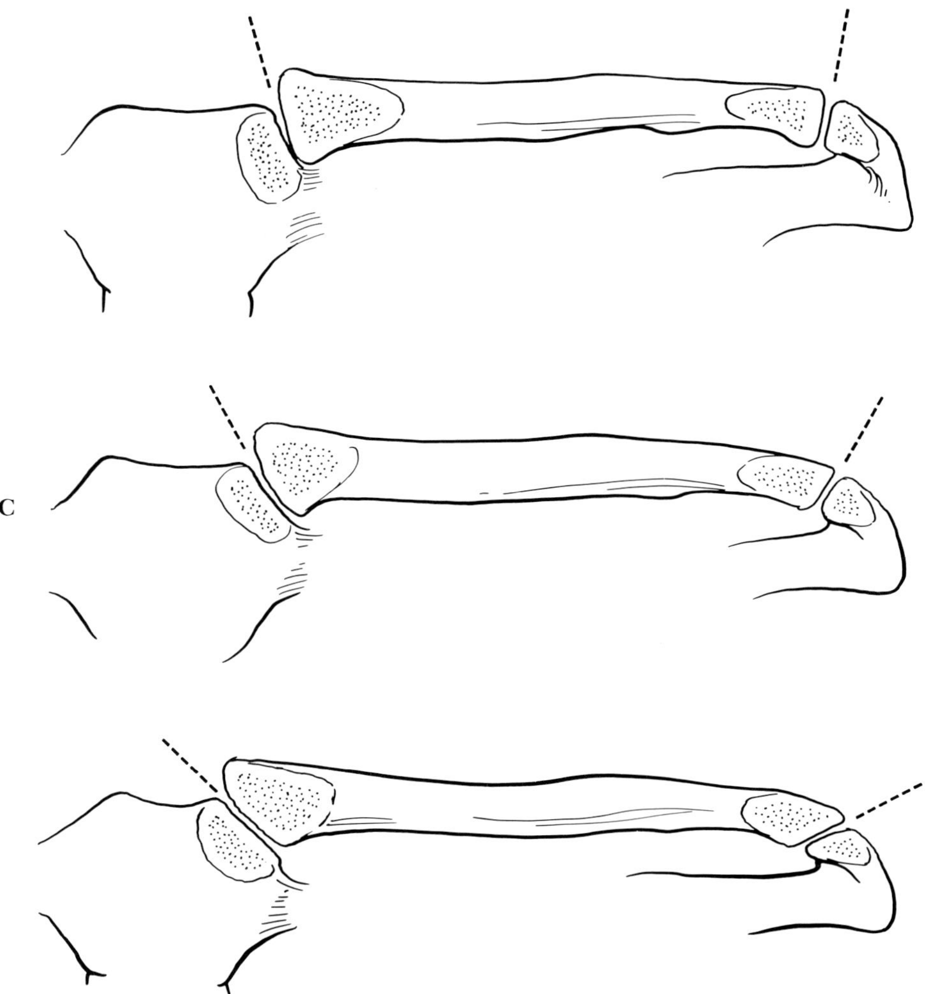

Fig. 19-2, cont'd. **B,** Varied shapes of clavicular end. **C,** Varied angles of ends of clavicle provide varying degrees of stability.

toclavicular ligament, a strong ligamentous attachment to the first rib. The posterior sternoclavicular ligament is the strongest support of the joint and maintains the elevation of the outer end of the clavicle at rest. It also helps to resist upward or backward displacement of the medial end of the clavicle.

The acromioclavicular joint is frequently injured in athletics. It has a relatively weak, easily disrupted capsular ligament. The main support of the joint comes from the coracoclavicular ligaments divided into conoid and trapezoid portions. The shape of the joint is quite variable (Fig. 19-2), but usually the slope of the distal end of the clavicle fosters slipping of the acromion beneath the clavicle when an impact is placed on the outer aspect of the shoulder. There is an interarticular disk, which may be partial or may completely divide the acromioclavicular joint into two. Occasionally there is no synovial cavity but merely a syndesmosis. Like the sternoclavicular joint, the acromioclavicular joint is not a true hinge joint but is mainly a sliding planar joint providing for adaptive motions.

The shoulder joint has a small glenoid surface of the scapula. The humeral surface is approximately two to three times larger than the true glenoid surface. The glenoid labrum acts to broaden the articular surface but doesn't deepen it. There are capsular ligaments and some reinforcements of these, but they are not truly very effective. The capsule itself is large, lax, and easily distensible. There is often a defect anteriorly that connects the joint cavity with the subscapularis bursa. Most of the support of the shoulder comes from the musculature around it rather than from the capsule and ligaments. This joint has the greatest range of motion of any joint in the body, and it does so at the sacrifice of stability. There is some deepening of the joint socket by the coracoacromial ligament, which caps the shoulder. The scapula must be rotated to tilt the glenoid upward in order to prevent the coracoacromial ligament from impeding overhead activities in throwing or racket sports. The long head of the biceps is contained within the joint capsule; however, it is covered by synovium and thus is separated from the joint fluid (Fig. 19-3, *B* to *D*). Its attachment to the supraglenoid tubercle helps it to resist upward displacement of the humeral head. With its long intra-articular course, it obviously has to obtain its blood supply from its bony attachment or the musculotendinous junction, or both. There are frequently deterioration and pain syndromes from this tenuous blood supply.

The same situation is present with the supraspinatus tendon, which is surrounded on both sides by the synovium of the glenohumeral joint inferiorly and the subcromial (subdeltoid) bursa superiorly (Fig. 19-3, *A*, *C*, and *D*). Thus the supraspinatus tendon must get its blood supply from the bony attachment or musculature junction, and since it is also subject to compression between the humeral head and the acromion, the watershed area of this tendon probably is related to its frequent deterioration and subsequent rupture. The infraspinatus and subscapularis do not have the same problem, since they are not between the acromion and the humeral head.

The subacromial bursa tends to be quite large. It separates the acromion and deltoid from the supraspinatus tendon. It facilitates motion of the shoulder and rotator cuff beneath the acromion and the coracoacromial ligament. It is more anterior than one would expect, and thus most of the painful impingements occur during anterior elevation rather than during pure abduction.

Muscles

The large muscles attaching to the upper limb can be divided conveniently into an extrinsic group, which attach the axial skeleton to the limb girdle or to the limb itself, and an intrinsic group, which go from the limb girdle to the limb.

Extrinsics. Muscles attaching from the thorax to the limb girdle are the subclavius, pectoralis minor, serratus anterior, and, in a sense, the omohyoid. The large muscle attaching from the thorax to the humerus is the pectoralis major. Muscles attaching from the vertebrae to the limb girdle are trapezius, levator scapulae, rhom-

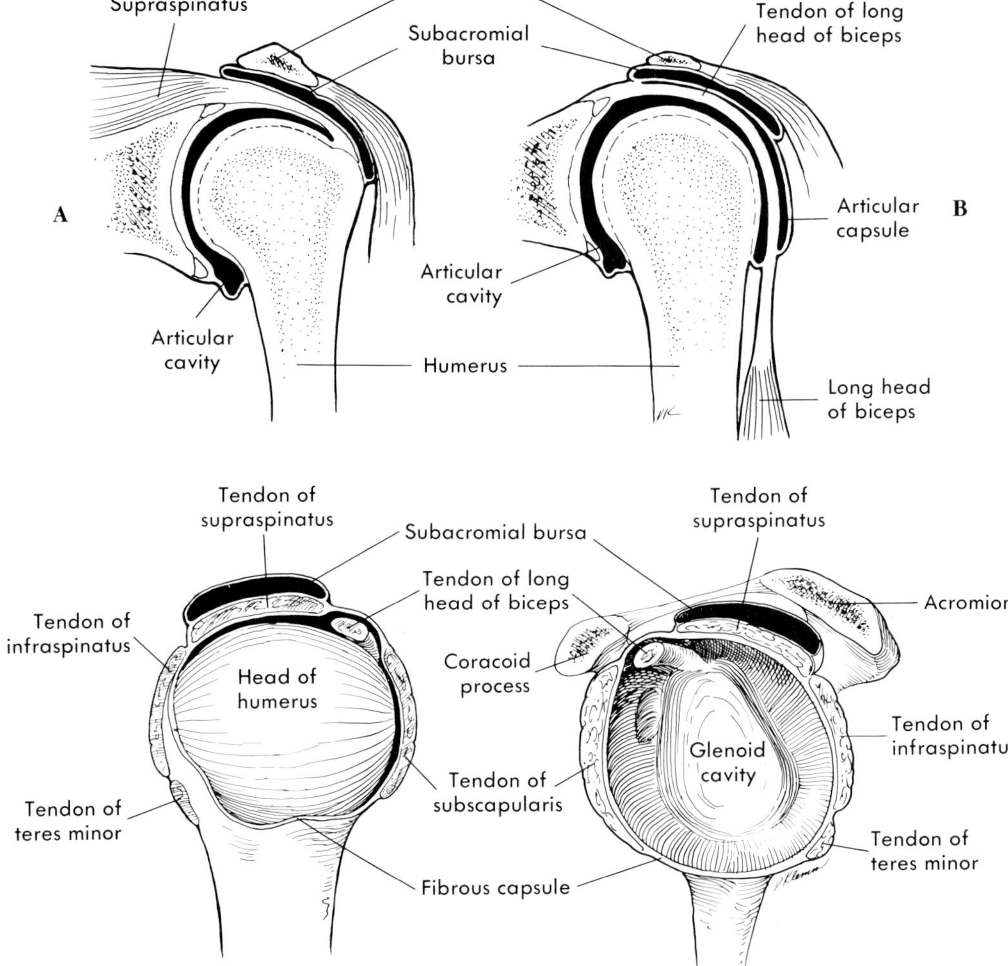

Fig. 19-3. Relationships of glenohumeral joint cavity, rotator cuff, and subacromial bursa. **A, C,** and **D,** Supraspinatus tendon covered by synovial cavity on both surfaces. **B, C,** and **D,** Long head of biceps has long intra-articular course and is separated from joint fluid by synovial covering.

boideus major, and rhomboideus minor. The single muscle attaching from the vertebral column to the humerus is the latissimus dorsi.

Intrinsics. The deltoid is the only muscle running from clavicle to humerus, and it joins with numerous muscles going from scapula to humerus. These muscles are deltoid, subscapularis, supraspinatus, infraspinatus, teres major, teres minor, and coracobrachialis. The long and short heads of the biceps go from scapula to radius, and the long head of the triceps attaches from scapula to ulna.

Functions of the shoulder

Limb girdle. The sternoclavicular joint is the point of fixation of the upper limb to the axial skeleton. Since the length of the clavicle is finite, and its medial end is spatially tied to the sternoclavicular joint, the clavicle functions as a spoke or radius of limb-girdle motion on this medially fixed point. We can change its position, but we can't change its length. The scapulothoracic joint is not a true synovial joint, of course, but is provided for rotation of the scapula "floating" on the chest wall. The radius of curvature of the chest wall is different from the functional radius of motion provided by the length of the clavicle. Thus the acromioclavicular joint, which has no prime movers, that is, no muscles crossing the joint to move it solely, has purely adaptive motions between the clavicle and scapula.

Movements of the scapular girdle are added to the glenohumeral range to place the proximal limb segment in a functional position. Protraction, that is, hunching the shoulder forward as seen when boxers try to protect their chin, is done by the large strong serratus anterior and pectoral muscles (Fig. 19-4, *A*). The muscles that retract the shoulder, that is, bring it posteriorly, are also large and strong and include the latissimus dorsi, trapezius, and rhomboids (Fig. 19-4, *B*). The elevators of the scapula are the levator scapulae, rhomboideus major, and rhomboideus minor, attaching to the medial border and the upper portion of the trapezius, which is the only muscle attaching to the outer end of the shoulder girdle (Fig. 19-5). With accessory nerve paralysis, drooping of the outer aspect of the scapula is only partially compensated for by the rhomboids and levator scapulae medially. The serratus anterior, pectoralis minor, lower fibers of the pectoralis major, latissimus dorsi, and lower trapezius are depressors of the scapula (Fig. 19-6) and are very important in lifting body weight from a chair or the floor when one presses up with the hands. The latissimus dorsi particularly is necessary for using crutches.

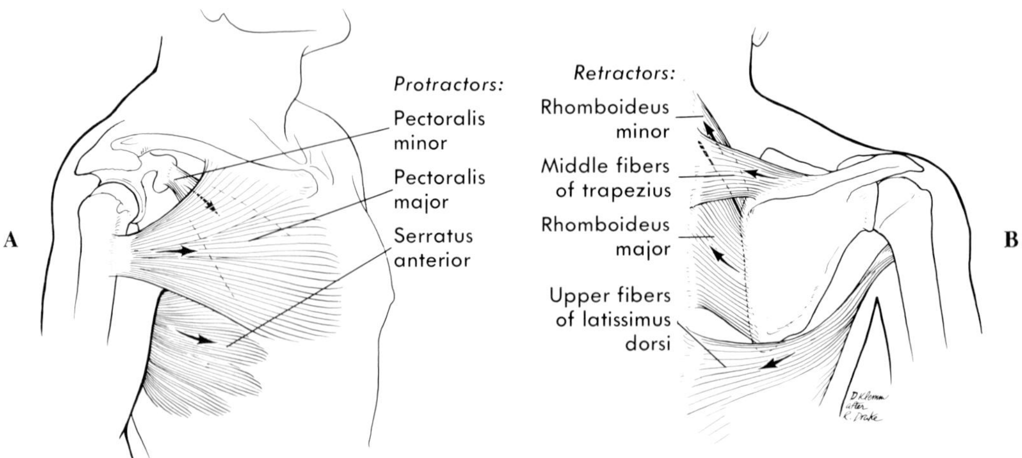

Fig. 19-4. Protractors, **A,** and retractors, **B,** of scapula.

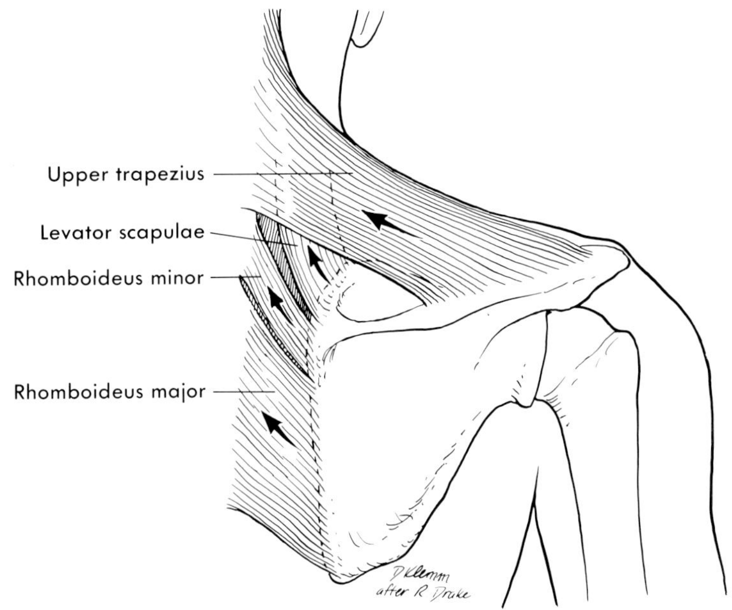

Fig. 19-5. Elevators of scapula.

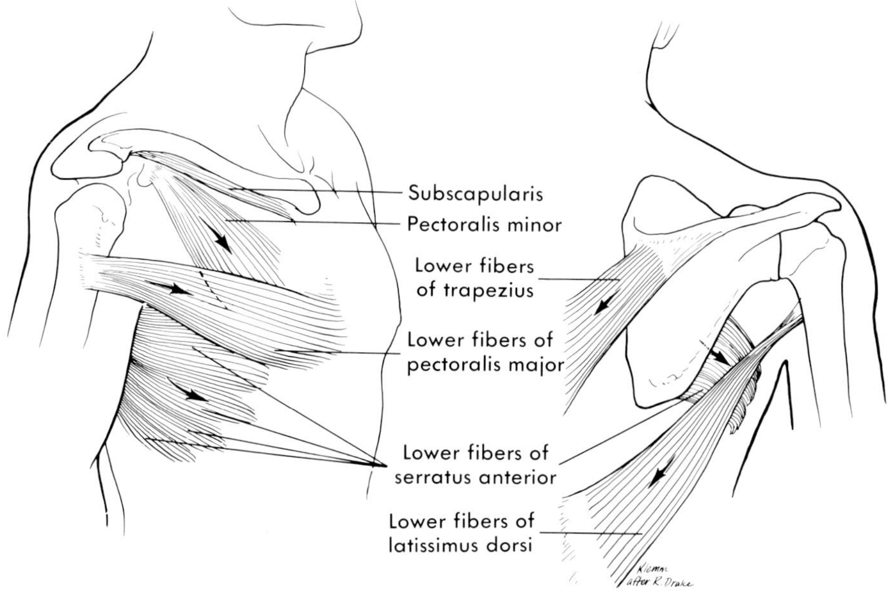

Fig. 19-6. Depressors of scapula.

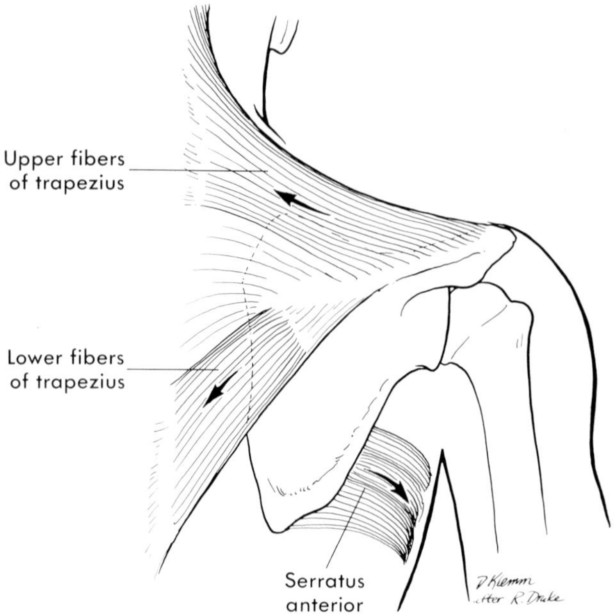

Fig. 19-7. Upward rotators of scapula.

Rotation of the scapula is used to augment the range of motion of the glenohumeral joint. Upward rotation of the glenoid face is done by upper and lower fibers of the trapezius and by the serratus anterior (Fig. 19-7). It has long been a truism that these two muscles are essential for successful use of the limb with a shoulder arthrodesis because rotation of the scapula then brings about elevation of the upper limb. Downward rotation of the glenoid surface of the scapula is done by gravity and by the levator scapulae, rhomboids, latissimus dorsi, pectoralis minor, and the lower fibers of the pectoralis major (Fig. 19-8).

Shoulder joint. The glenohumeral joint allows the greatest motion of any joint in the body at the expense of stability. It is difficult to define this motion because the glenoid faces forward 30 to 40 degrees; thus the motions in the planes of the body are not true motions in the planes of the joint. However, the motions are usually described in relation to the planes of the body. Thus there are motions in the sagittal and coronal planes as well as rotation about an axis down the shaft of the humerus regardless of the position of the humerus in space. In general, glenohumeral range of motion brings the arm slightly above horizontal, and adding scapulothoracic range of motion brings it vertical. Each person has a distinct "scapulohumeral rhythm," which is approximately two thirds glenohumeral and one third scapulothoracic.

Flexion of the humerus is accomplished by the clavicular head of the pectoralis major, the anterior portion of the deltoid, the coracobrachialis, and the biceps brachii (Fig. 19-9, *A*). Extension is accomplished by the triceps, teres major, latissimus dorsi,

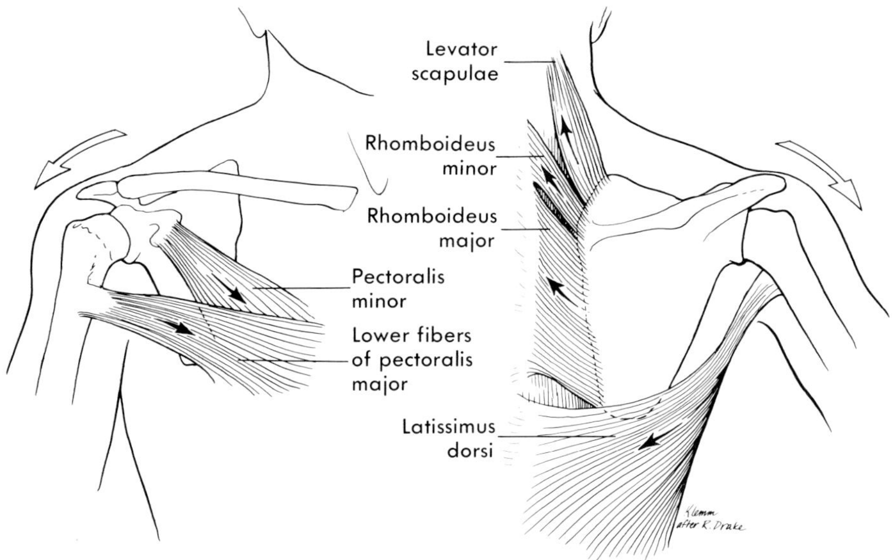

Fig. 19-8. Downward rotators of scapula.

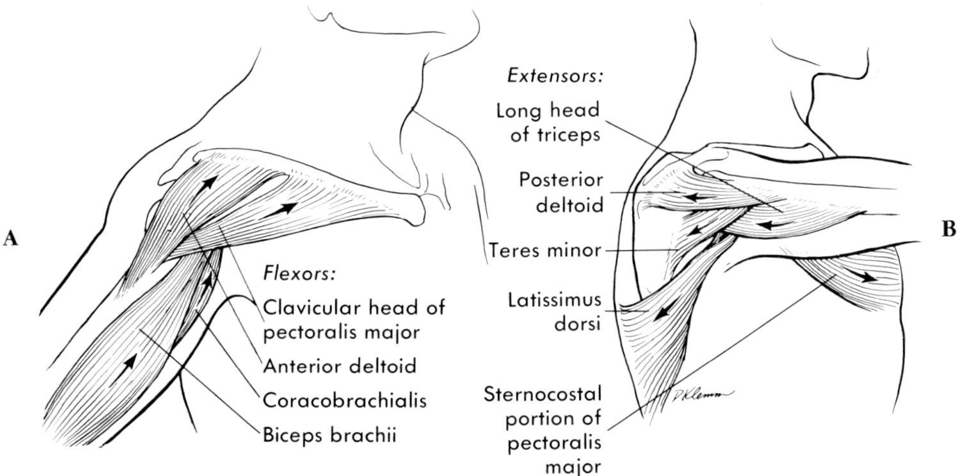

Fig. 19-9. Flexors and extensors of arm.

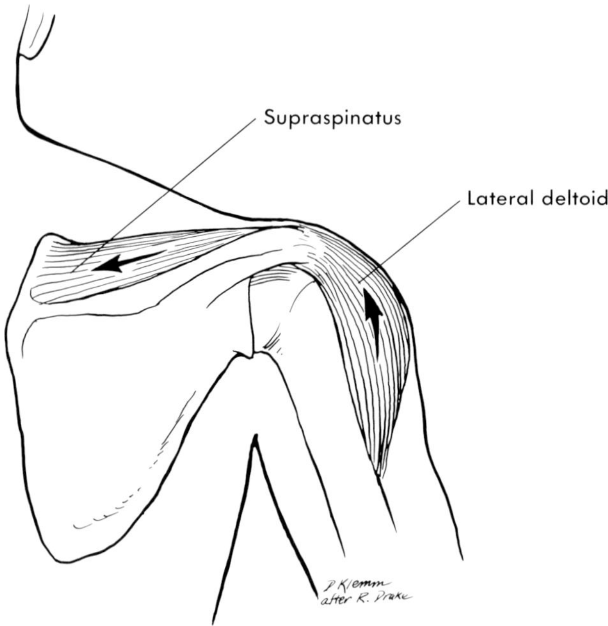

Fig. 19-10. Abductors of arm.

and the posterior portion of the deltoid (Fig. 19-9, *B*). The sternocostal portion of the pectoralis major is also an extensor as one can observe by placing the hand on the edge of a table and pushing down while palpating the muscle; the sternocostal portion of the pectoralis major will contract. Conversely, the action of placing the hand beneath the edge of the table and lifting up causes contraction in the clavicular portion. The abductors of the arm are primarily the supraspinatus and the central portion of the deltoid (Fig. 19-10). The adductors of the arm are large and numerous; they include the pectoralis major, the anterior and posterior portion of the deltoid, the coracobrachialis, teres major, and latissimus dorsi (Fig. 19-11). The relative strength of adductors over abductors helps explain why one cannot hold much weight with the arm extended horizontally but can press downward with enough power to do the "iron cross" in gymnastics with the powerful adductor muscles.

A similar situation pertains with the rotators of the arm. The internal rotators are larger, stronger, and more numerous than external rotators (Fig. 19-12). Although the latissimus dorsi and teres major originate dorsally from the trunk, they attach to the front of the humerus and are added to the pectoralis major, subscapularis, and anterior portion of the deltoid (Fig. 19-13). The external rotators are much smaller and weaker and include the infraspinatus, teres minor, and posterior portion of the deltoid (Fig. 19-14). The discrepancy between internal rotator-adductor power versus external rotator-abductor strength is considered to have survival value; it helps the infant to hang on to its mother when she flees from a tiger.

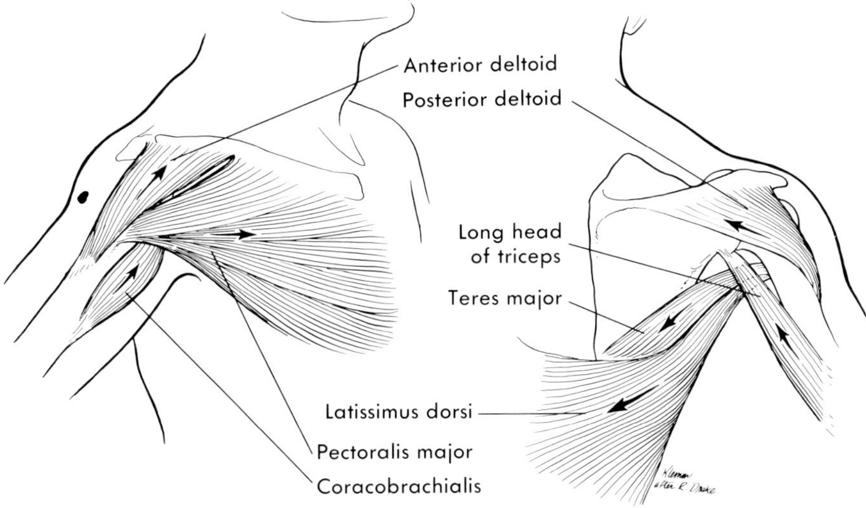

Fig. 19-11. Adductors of arm.

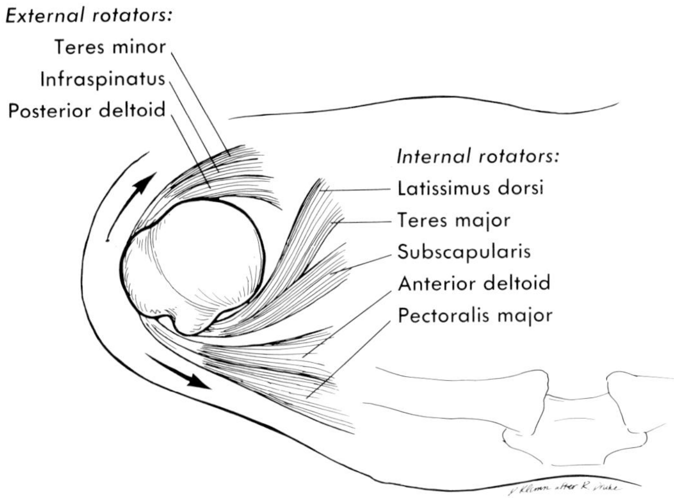

Fig. 19-12. Rotators of arm from above.

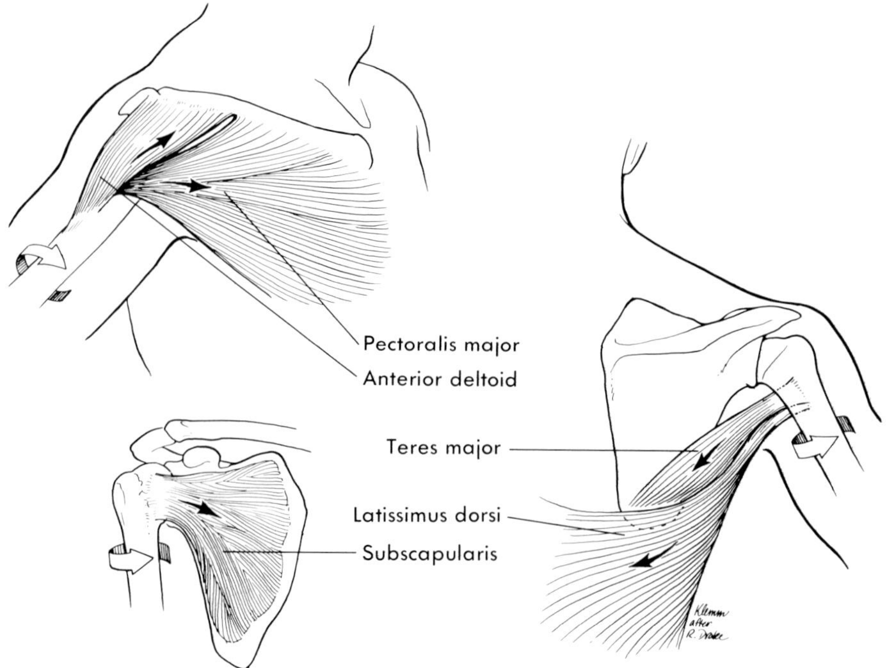

Fig. 19-13. Internal rotators of arm.

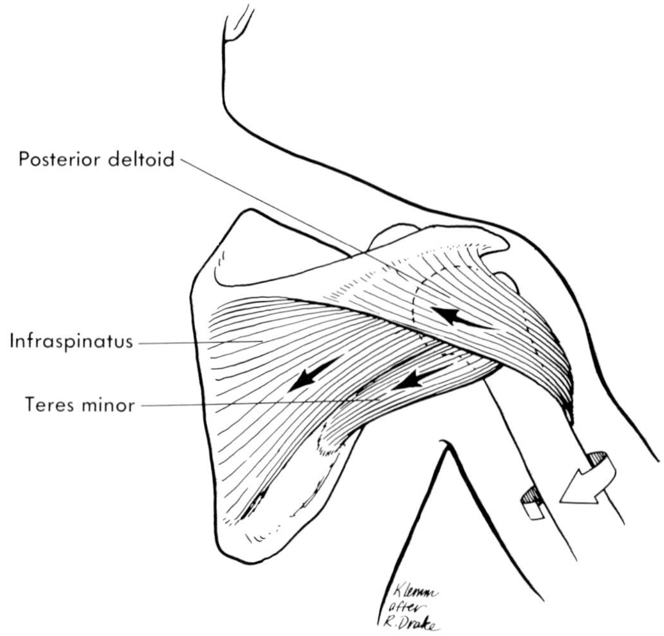

Fig. 19-14. External rotators of arm.

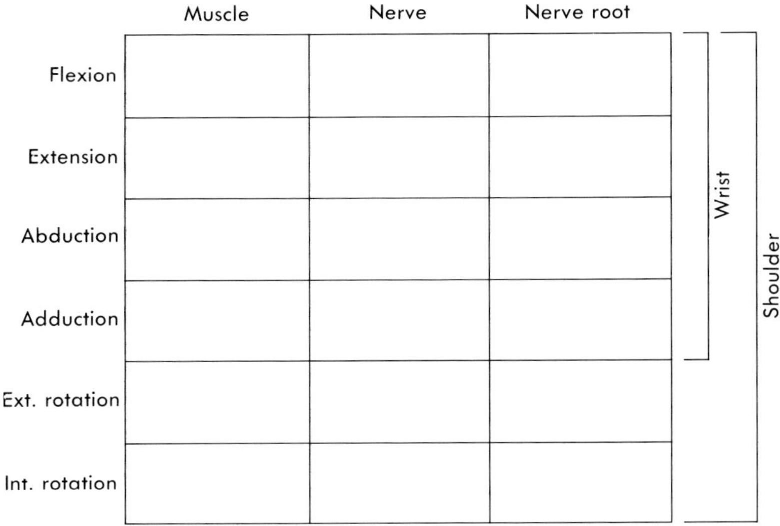

Fig. 19-15. Table of factors involved in motor function of shoulder and wrist. Filling in the blank spaces is an excellent functional exercise for the student of limb function and has clinical value in diagnosis of dysfunction.

Muscular dysfunctions may be attributable to problems of the muscles, problems of the nerves to these muscles, or problems with the nerve roots supplying those nerves. Many times diagnosis of the specific site of injury is difficult. Filling the blanks in a chart such as illustrated in Fig. 19-15 is a practical learning exercise to determine which muscles, nerves, or nerve roots are involved in the specific motions of the shoulder area (or wrist, elbow, and so on).

ELBOW
Skeleton

The distal humerus articulates with the proximal radius and ulna, which in turn articulate with each other. The ulna glides as an almost pure hinge joint in the trochlear groove of the humerus. There is slight side-to-side wobble, but it is insignificant in the normal elbow, though it is enough to loosen a prosthesis over a period of time. The radial articulation with the humerus is a gliding joint with a concavity on the proximal end of the radius. Since this gliding motion must be available in all positions of elbow flexion and extension as well as forearm rotation, the concavity of radial head moves on a large rounded prominence on the distal humerus called the "capitellum." Another major portion of the elbow articulation is between the proximal radius and ulna, which allows for rotation of the forearm. These three joints, radiohumeral, humeroulnar, and radioulnar, are encased in one capsule. With injury there will be an effusion into the entire cavity. There are anterior and posterior fat pads that lie inside the joint capsule but outside the synovium; thus, when the joint is distended with fluid or blood, the fat pads are lifted out of the coronoid and olecranon fossas and become visible on the lateral roentgenogram ("fat-pad sign"). The capsule is lax anteriorly and posteriorly until the extreme of extension or flexion is reached; the capsule then becomes quite tight and acts as a tether to further motion. The stronger ligaments are on the medial aspect extending from the humeral condyle to the ulna; they attach to bone on each end and have a fixed length. Radially the ligament is also strong but attaches to bone only on its humeral end. Distally it attaches to the annular ligament and thus indirectly to the ulna but not directly to the radius. Thus the radial collateral ligament is not a true hinge type of collateral ligament. There is also the very long and strong interosseous membrane that holds the radius and ulna together throughout their length. The fibers of this membrane are shortest in full pronation. The annular ligament holds the radial head against the proximal ulna while allowing rotation. Distally the triangular fibrocartilage complex serves a similar purpose of allowing the distal radius to rotate around the distal ulna.

Movements

Elbow motions are primarily flexion and extension in the ulnohumeral joint about a slightly oblique axis through the humeral epicondyles. A consequence of the obliquity of this axis is the "carrying angle." Elbow motions also include pronation and supination of the forearm; this is done about an axis through two fixed points. The head of the radius does not move in space, but the distal end of the radius does. However, the distal end of the ulna does not move in space; so the axis for pronation and supination is an oblique one, connecting points in the head of the radius proximally and the head of the ulna distally. The distal end of the radius rides around that relatively fixed distal point. Pronation is accomplished by several large muscles (Fig. 19-16, *A*): the pronator teres and pronator quadratus, flexor carpi radialis, and palmaris longus. The brachioradialis can pronate from a fully supinated position to the midposition, and it can also supinate from the fully pronated position to the midposition but not beyond. The brachioradialis does not have any function on the wrist joint, since it attaches to the distal radius. Other supinators are the biceps brachii and the supinator itself with weak help from the extensor carpi radialis longus (Fig. 19-16, *B*).

The flexors of the elbow are strong and include the biceps, brachioradialis, and brachialis. The pronator teres and finger flexors are also quite strong muscles, but they don't have a very good moment arm at the elbow joint; thus they don't function very well as elbow flexors. Elbow extension is done most often by gravity but powerfully by the large triceps muscle. Again a chart listing elbow movements can be completed as a learning exercise. (Fig. 19-17).

Nerves

Nerves to the upper limb appear very early in fetal development. As soon as a limb bud is formed and the central axis begins to condense to form the musculoskeletal element, nerve fibers grow from the primitive spinal cord and extend into the

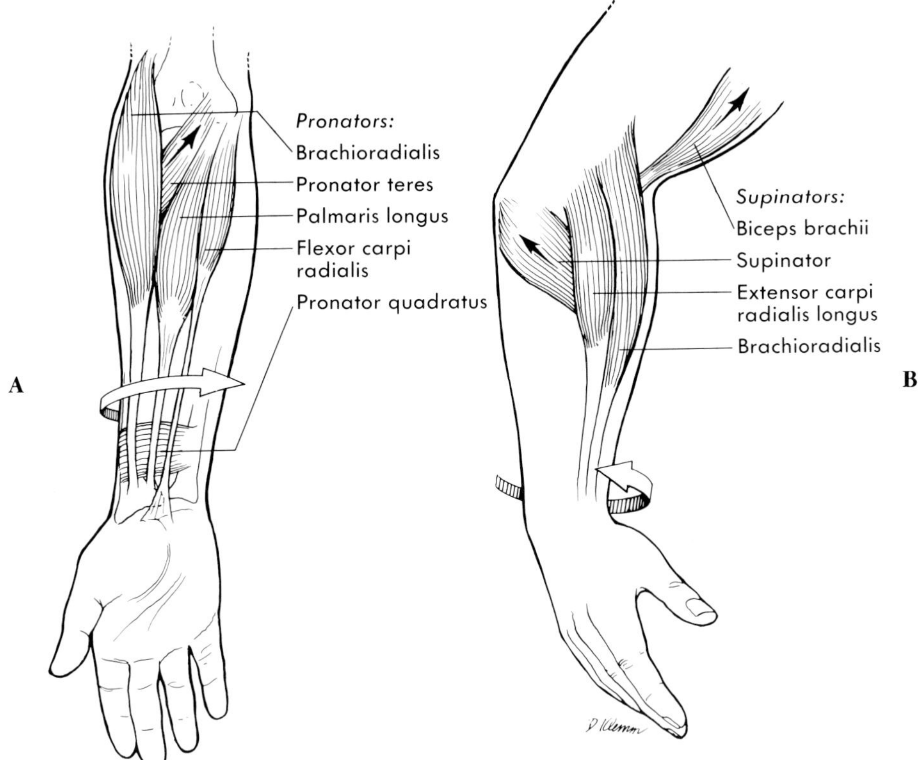

Fig. 19-16. Pronators and supinators of forearm.

Elbow

	Muscle(s)	Nerve(s)	Nerve root(s)
Flexion			
Extension			
Pronation			
Supination			

Fig. 19-17. Table of factors involved in motor function of elbow.

limb. These nerves soon divide into anterior and posterior primary divisions as well as several smaller branches. The posterior primary divisions extend into the segmental musculature in the back of the neck and thorax and do not form plexuses. On the other hand, the anterior primary divisions do form plexuses as they enter the limb bud with portions located anterior or posterior to the skeletal axis. Since the fifth cervical through first thoracic roots pass almost entirely into the upper limb, there is a gap in the sensory dermatome anteriorly between the C4 and T2 nerve roots. One has to keep this in mind when checking for sensory loss of a brachial plexus injury.

The dermatome distribution in the extremity is somewhat variable but has a reasonable constancy. The C6 nerve root supplies the thumb; C8 the ring and little fingers; and C7 the long and middle fingers. C5 and T1 end on the radial or ulnar aspect of the forearm respectively. The brachial plexus is fairly well compressed around the axillary artery in the axillary sheath from which the various branches extend to their point of distribution, frequently passing through a gap between muscle origins or between muscle and bone.

The brachial plexus is formed in the base of the neck by the anterior primary rami of the C5 to T1 nerve roots. The roots pass through the gap between the anterior and middle scalene muscles; at this point they cross the first rib and then pass beneath the clavicle and coracoid process anterior to the shoulder joint. The roots of the plexus itself can be compressed in the neural foramina of the vertebral column, in the interscalene notch, against the first rib, or against the coracoid or clavicle. Occasionally, protective equipment worn to protect bony prominences can become a source of compression of the nerves. Traction injuries often occur to the upper roots or the lower roots of the plexus by traction on the arm. Lower-root injuries are fairly common in thoracic surgery when the chest wall is opened by a median sternotomy incision. A large callus from a fractured clavicle can also cause compression in this region.

The named nerves then depart from the brachial plexus by various roots, and where they cross bony prominences, they may be subject to injury. Anteriorly the nerves penetrating the costoclavicular membrane into the pectorales major and minor are seldom injured. Posteriorly the suprascapular nerve passes through the suprascapular notch beneath the transverse scapular ligament. A syndrome of paralysis of the supraspinatus and infraspinatus muscles has been described because of compression in this region, occasionally by pressure in this area from equipment or straps.

The axillary nerve passes through the quadrilateral space posteriorly around the neck of the humerus, where it may be compressed causing isolated deltoid muscle palsy. The radial nerve is relatively protected until it gets to the lateral intermuscular septum, where it passes from the posterior compartment to the anterior compartment of the arm. It is tethered to the bone in this area and is subject to injury by fractures or by compression. Slightly more distally, it divides into sensory and motor portions; the latter passes through the arcade of Fröhse into the supinator muscle from which it exits as the posterior interosseous nerve. Each of the major nerves entering the forearm passes between two heads of a muscle. The radial nerve passes through the supinator as we have just described.

The musculocutaneous nerve splits the coracobrachialis before it continues distally between the biceps and brachialis muscles. Compression syndromes have not been described affecting the motor branch, but rupture of the biceps muscles in paratroopers from the ripcord passing across the biceps occasionally injures the musculocutaneous nerve. A compression syndrome has been described for the sensory portion of the nerve, where it penetrates the deep fascia just lateral to the biceps tendon in the cubital fossa. This would interfere with sensation down the radial side of the forearm from the elbow to the wrist. I have seen this nerve compressed after weight lifting.

The ulnar nerve has to pass from anterior to posterior through the medial intermuscular septum. It goes through a fibrous canal called the "arcade of Struthers" and then lies behind the intermuscular septum to the elbow where it is occasionally compressed at the elbow joint or just distal to it. As the elbow is flexed, the distance between the two heads of the flexor carpi ulnaris increases. Occasionally, a transverse fibrous band between these two heads of origin becomes taut and can compress the nerve in the cubital fossa.

The median nerve is free in the arm itself but can be compressed by the lacertus fibrosus (bicipital aponeurosis), or by a supracondylar process with its ligament of Struthers passing from the process to the medial epicondyle. The nerve is more commonly injured where it traverses a gap between the two heads of origin of the pronator teres or at the proximal leash of the flexor superficialis muscle origin.

The long thoracic nerve is subject to spontaneous paralysis with loss of function in the serratus anterior and winging of the scapula.

The cutaneous nerves of the forearm are first the medial antebrachial cutaneous nerve from the medial cord, supplying sensation from the region of the elbow to the level of the wrist on the ulnar aspect. One must keep in mind when examining for ulnar nerve injury that the sensation provided by the ulnar nerve does not begin proximal to the wrist. Then come the lateral antebrachial cutaneous nerve, which supplies the radial aspect of the forearm from elbow to wrist, and the posterior antebrachial cutaneous from the radial nerve, which supplies the variable region over the olecranon and proximal ulna.

VESSELS
Arteries

The subclavian artery supplies the muscles about the scapula. It becomes the axillary artery at the level of the first rib. The axillary supplies the humeral head and anastomoses about the scapula and then becomes the brachial artery, which supplies muscles of the arm and nutrient vessel to the humerus. The brachial ends by dividing into radial and ulnar arteries at the elbow level. The radial passes down the radial aspect of the forearm into the hand, supplying forearm muscles and the deep vascular arch of the hand. The ulnar artery traverses the ulnar side of the forearm into the hand, supplying muscles of the forearm, providing the anterior and posterior interosseous vessels, and ending in the superficial arch of the hand from which the digital arteries arise.

Veins

The basilic vein begins on the dorsum of the hand and passes up the ulnar aspect of the forearm to end in the brachial vein. The cephalic vein begins on the dorsum of the hand and passes up the radial and volar aspect of the forearm and arm to end in the subclavian vein. Both of these have numerous valves.

Lymphatics

Lymphatics are vessels that travel with the veins and empty into numerous nodes in the axilla. The drainage region of the axillary nodes is the upper limb, the body wall above the umbilicus, and the back above the level of the waist.

20. The adolescent elbow

Frank A. Pettrone

The recent explosion of interest in sports, fitness, and health is apparent to all. What may be less apparent is that this interest has also been demonstrated in children, with a parallel increase in the frequency of sports-related childhood injuries. These injuries fall into two main categories: trauma and overuse syndromes. Although we tend to think of the latter as occurring only in the adult recreational athlete, the phenomenon of overuse syndromes is being seen with ever-increasing frequency in the childhood athlete. Little Leaguer's elbow was the first to receive public notoriety, but numerous other sites are now well known. Problems such as tendinitis of the shoulder, elbow, wrist, and knee; stress fractures; heat stress syndromes; and runner's knee problems are seen with increasing frequency in children. As opposed to the adult, causes of this overuse syndrome are not primarily "training errors" but include significant other predisposing factors such as (1) growth imbalance, which produces muscle–bone length imbalance, loss of flexibility, and relative incoordination; (2) skeletal malalignment, such as leg-length inequality, genu valgum, and anteversion, which predispose to knee symptoms; (3) flatfoot, noticed frequently with shin splints or chondromalacia, which benefits from orthotics; (4) improper footwear (worn-out shoes); (5) training errors that are attributed to inadequate conditioning exercises, or too rapid increase in duration of play; (6) recurrent microtrauma to articular cartilage, which may predispose to osteochondritis dissecans of the elbow (capitellum), knee, and talus; (7) osteochondrosis or traction apophysitis, that is, Osgood-Schlatter's or Sever's disease, which are caused by tight muscle groups leading to avulsion minifractures.[4]

THE IMMATURE SKELETON

Before discussing specific injury patterns, a review of the developing skeletal system is needed. An awareness of epiphyseal plate appearance, closure, and roentgenologic clues as to normal development versus a pathologic condition is necessary.[3]

The specific timing of appearance of growth centers about the elbow is of particular importance. The sequence of growth-center appearance in the elbow is as fol-

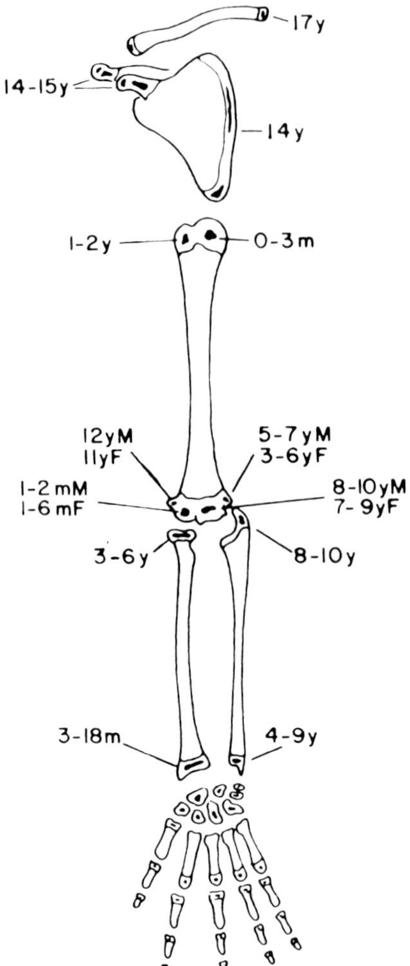

Fig. 20-1. Sequence of growth center appearance in the upper extremity.

lows: capitellum (5-month-old male, 4-month-old female); medial epicondyle (7-year-old male, 5-year-old female); trochlea (9-year-old male, 8-year-old female); lateral epicondyle (12-year-old male, 11-year-old female) (Fig. 20-1). In addition, the radial head appears at 5 years in males and 4 years in females, and the olecranon at 10 years in males and 8 years in females.[11]

Closure just occurs at the distal humerus, with the capitellum, lateral epicondyle, and trochlea fusing together at puberty (17-year-old male, 14-year-old female), and then fusing to the shaft. The medial epicondyle fuses later at 18 years in males and 15

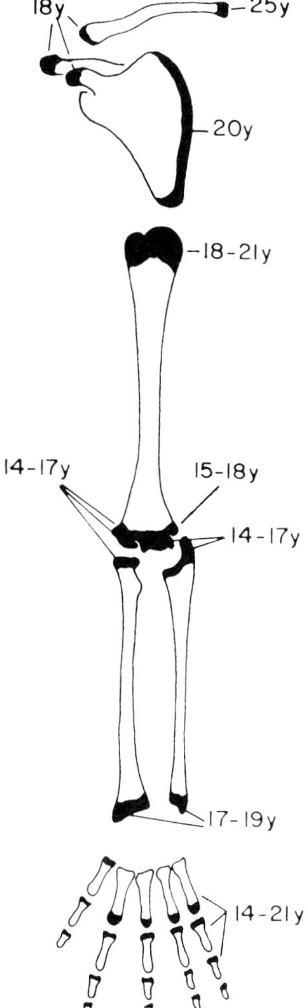

Fig. 20-2. Sequence of physeal closure in the upper extremity.

years in females. The radial head and the olecranon both close at 15 years in males and 14 years in females (Fig. 20-2).

ROENTGENOLOGIC EVALUATION OF THE ELBOW

Standard evaluation includes anteroposterior and lateral views; however, oblique views may be useful, particularly in trauma or specific lesions. The olecranon view is useful for evaluation of posterior spurs and loose bodies and is taken in 30 or more degrees. Stress films are helpful in the evaluation of medial instability (Fig. 20-3).

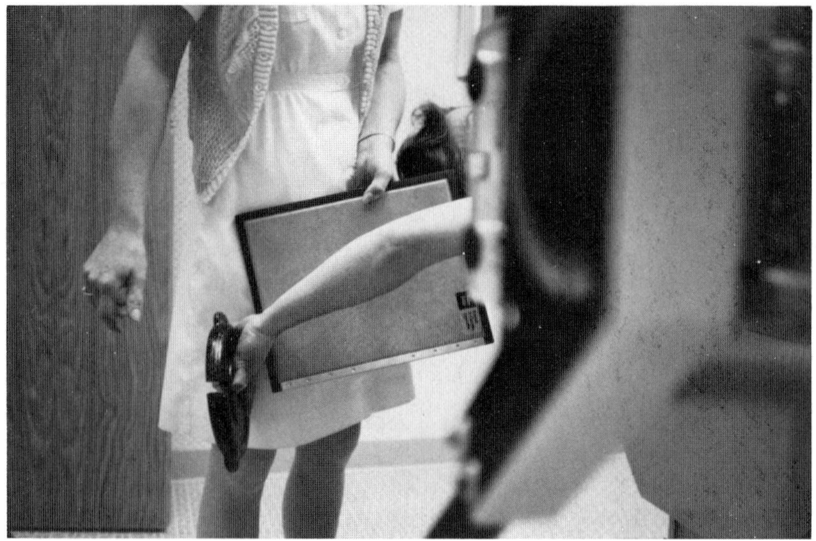

Fig. 20-3. Technique for valgus stress roentgenogram of elbow.

One can also infrequently see a supracondylar process that may be associated with medial symptoms or neurovascular compromise. The supratrochlear foramen may occasionally contain an ossicle and should not be misread as a loose body.

VAGARIES OF THE ELBOW

In evaluating the child with elbow pain, one needs an awareness of normal variation versus a pathologic condition.

Olecranon

The physis normally enters the joint surface and is wider posteriorly than anteriorly. This is sometimes mistaken for a fracture; however, a fracture is wider anteriorly. The physis always closes from the joint side outward[9] (Fig. 20-4).

Radial head

The radial head aligns in all projections with the capitellum. With maturation, it becomes curved or saucerized and may demonstrate two distinct surfaces. (A notch may be found on the lateral aspect of the proximal radial metaphysis, which is a normal variant and not a fracture.) A displaced fracture of the radial head is rarely difficult to diagnose, and the presence of a fat-pad sign is diagnostic. However, a cortical infraction or radial neck fracture may show no fat pad. A vertical fracture of the radial head will produce a joint effusion. A roentgenologic pitfall may occur with the biceps tubercle, which may mimic a lytic lesion when seen straight on.

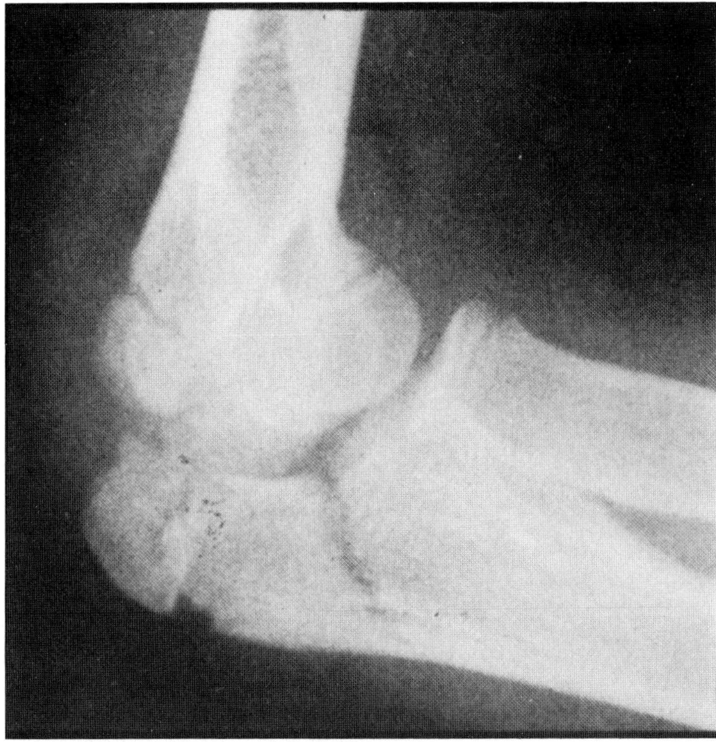

Fig. 20-4. Differentiation of olecranon epiphysis from a fracture (wider anteriorly). (From Silberstein, M.J., Brodeur, A.E., and Graviss, E.R.: J. Bone Joint Surg. **63A**(5):722-725, 1981.)

Capitellum

The capitellar ossification center is the first to appear and lies between the anterior shaft of the humerus and a line up from the coronoid (Fig. 20-5). The center is tilted downward early, and the epiphyseal plate is wider posteriorly and remains so as the child grows. The capitellum fuses with the trochlea first and then the lateral epicondyle, before uniting with the humerus.[10]

Lateral epicondyle

The distal part of the epiphysis first fuses to the capitellum before uniting with the humerus, and the remaining proximal part of the physis should not be misread as a fracture. The lateral epicondyle begins to ossify distally and proceed to a smooth-curved sliver shape and then to a triangular shape[6] (Fig. 20-6).

Medial epicondyle

The ossific center may be multicentric, lies posteromedially to the distal humerus, and is better seen on a lateral roentgenogram. It is readily differentiated from an

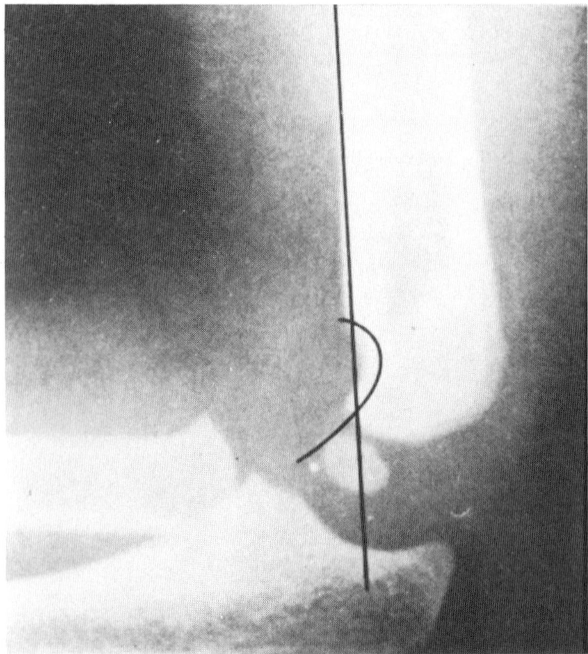

Fig. 20-5. The coronoid line and the humeral-shaft line describe an angle within which normally lies most of the ossified portion of the capitellum. (From Silberstein, M.J., Brodeur, A.E., and Graviss, E.R.: J. Bone Joint Surg. **61A**(2):244-247, 1979.)

A   B   C

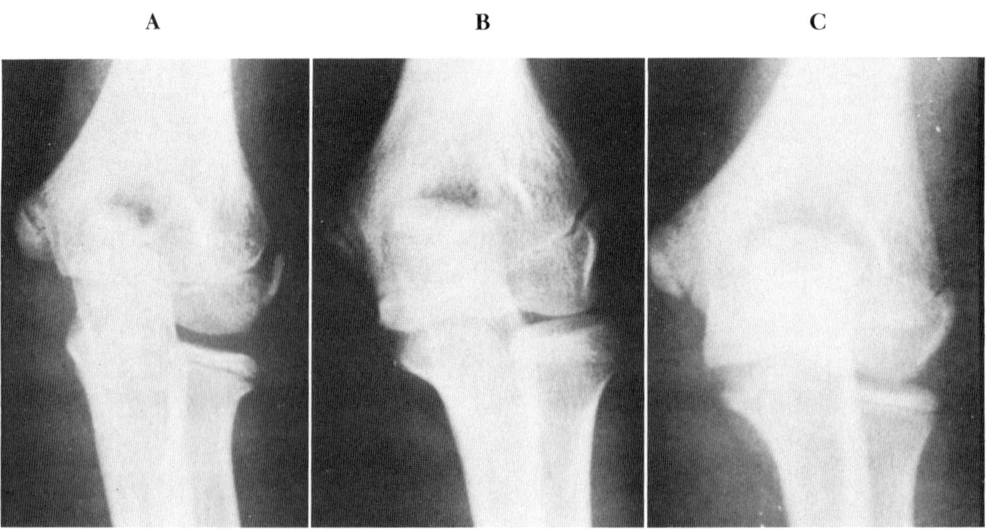

Fig. 20-6. A, Lateral epicondyle ossifies to a smooth curved sliver of bone. **B,** Distal part of epiphysis of lateral epicondyle fused to capitellum. **C,** Distal portion of lateral epicondyle fuses, and the proximal portion resembles a fracture. (From Silberstein, M.J., Brodeur, A.E., and Graviss, E.R.: J. Bone Joint Surg. **64A**(3):444-448, 1982.)

avulsion fracture in which the fragment is inferiorly and medially displaced with loss of parallelism. Fractures of the medial epicondyle may not be associated with joint effusion or metaphyseal avulsion fragments.[8]

LITTLE LEAGUER'S ELBOW (Fig. 20-7)

The problems of the professional baseball pitcher are well documented—ulnar traction spurs, ulnar neuropathy, loose bodies, and degenerative osteoarthritis. Soft-tissue lesions include muscle rupture and medial collateral ligament sprains or rupture. The single most important cause is valgus elbow stress with the throwing motion.

According to Little League Baseball, Inc., there are now over 2 million active

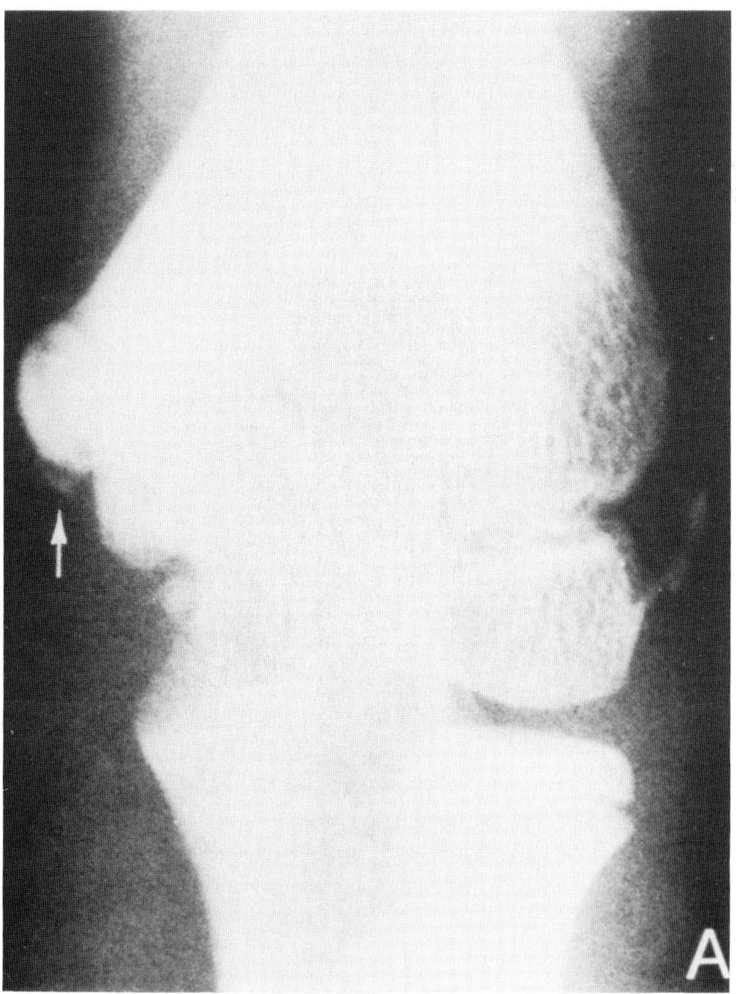

Fig. 20-7. Little Leaguers' elbow.

Little League Baseball players. One percent of those participating sustained injuries from throwing. Twenty percent of the epiphyseal injuries to the elbow were sustained by players other than pitchers.[2]

In the skeletally immature child, the valgus strain in the throwing motion affects the weakest area, which is the cartilaginous apophyseal growth area. This area is disrupted in the throwing motion. Little Leaguer's elbow is truly a misnomer, used to describe several different problems involving the growth plate of the distal end of the humerus. The epicondyle is the site of origin of the flexor and pronator muscles of the forearm. Complete avulsion is the most dramatic injury and is easily diagnosed. More important, however, are other subtle roentgenographic findings that result from valgus strain to the elbow. The biomechanical forces are tensile strain applied to the medial side and compression forces on the lateral side. These findings include (1) delayed closure of the medial epicondylar growth plate; (2) traction apophysitis producing fragmentation and widening of the medial epicondylar apophysis; (3) further progression leading to frank medial epicondylar avulsion; (4) osteochondrosis of the capitellum and radial head; (5) osteochondritis dissecans.

Delayed closure of the medial epicondylar growth plate is seen in an arm subjected to excessive pitching. The pitcher in Little League Baseball makes 15 to 20 pitches per inning and is allowed to pitch six innings per week. If three innings are pitched in 1 day, the child must rest 3 days before pitching again. Thus it is clear that practice and play outside Little League must be contributing to this injury. The symptoms are minimal, and rest until the pain is gone is sufficient. If the stress has been going on for a long period of time, there may be hypertrophy of the distal end of the humerus with acceleration of bone growth.

Traction apophysitis is also secondary to repetitive abuse. The elbow is frequently more tender and swollen, and diminution of motion is present. Rest until pain free with restoration of full motion is recommended.

Avulsion of the medial epicondyle is seen with both a violent forceful throw or trauma. If the fragment is displaced less than 5 mm, cast immobilization for 3 weeks is recommended. If the fragment is separated more than 5 mm and rotated, open reduction and pin fixation are recommended. Another important surgical indication (often missed) is acute valgus instability, which, if present, should be repaired.

Osteochondrosis of the radial head and capitellum is fortunately rare. Clinically, pain, tenderness, and limitation of motion are seen. Roentgenologically, sclerosis, fragmentation, and bony deformity with articular incongruity are seen. Rest not only until pain free but also until the lesion has roentgenologically healed is recommended. The healing process may take 12 to 18 months to complete.

Osteochondritis dissecans is seen as a consequence of the osteochondrosis, whereby a fragment may become dislodged and become a loose body. Surgical removal (arthroscopically) is recommended.

Incidence

Adams, in a classic article, reported on the frequency of roentgenographic changes in Little League pitchers' elbows.[1] Among the 80 pitchers studied, he observed fragmentation of the medial epicondylar apophysis in 39 and osteochondrosis of the humeral capitellum or radial head in six. Torg, in another study, similarly followed 44 pitchers and found only two cases of traction apophysitis.[12] The difference is explained by the decreased competitiveness of practice and play in Torg's study. This emphasizes the consequence of excessive play outside the structured bounds of Little League Baseball and agrees with the data I initially presented from Little League Baseball.

SOCIAL AND PSYCHOLOGICAL ASPECTS OF SPORTS IN CHILDHOOD

One important factor in a child's emotional health is free play. Relaxation, play, and interaction with peers are essential to a sense of well-being. Intrusive, domineering parents or an overly rigid play structure all work to the detriment of the child. Participation of children in sports is almost universal between 6 and 12 years of age and then gradually declines. At the onset of pubescence, the decline accelerates dramatically in girls. What causes this dramatic loss of motivation? It can be lost because of our failure to appreciate the child's self-esteem needs. Private or public ridicule and derogation of the child who is acquiring motor skills is extremely detrimental. The inevitable loss of self-esteem through participation in activities that produce anxiety and self-doubt can produce a lifelong adverse reaction to sports participation. We must provide every child with the opportunity to develop a strong sense of personal worth through the process of motor learning and skills acquisition.

The stereotype "tennis mother" or "Little League dad" may be overgeneralizations, but such parent-child interactions extinguish the child's desire to participate in sports. Consider the following examples: (1) The parent may be unwilling to allow the activity to remain child oriented (a full football uniform on a 12-year-old does not make a man out of the child). (2) The parent may also be unable to maintain an appropriate emotional distance from the child's activity. The child then feels he is being exploited by the parent and rebellion can occur. (3) The parent may inflict guilt upon the child producing a form of emotional bondage. The parent may say, "Look at all I've done for you." The child is then unable to feel good about himself or the activity. (4) The parent may lose sight of the true meaning of sports and see the child's ability as a passport to status and economic freedom—"my child, the champion." However, the probability of a gifted childhood athlete becoming a successful professional athlete is near infinity.[5]

In summary, the value of participation in sports during childhood is inestimable. Lifelong traits, behavior patterns, and social as well as athletic skills are developed through sports. We, as parents, must be conscious of the child's need for play as an essential component of psychologic growth. We indeed must enhance, not impede, this need.

SELECTED READINGS

1. Adams, J.: Injuries to the throwing arm: a study of traumatic changes in the elbow joints of boy baseball players, Cal. Med. **102**:127, 1965.
2. Hale, C.: Little League Baseball, Presented at United States Olympic Committee meeting: Upper Extremity Injuries, Atlanta, Georgia, February 1983.
3. Kohler, A.: Borderlands of the normal and early pathology in skeletal roentgenology, ed. 3, New York, 1968, Grune & Stratton, Inc.
4. Micheli, L.: Overuse injuries in children's sports: the growth factor, Orthop. Clin. North Am. **14**(2):337-360, April 1983.
5. Ogilvie, B.: The orthopedist's role in children's sports, Orthop. Clin. North Am. **14**(2):361-372, April 1983.
6. Silberstein, et al.: Some vagaries of the lateral epicondyle, J. Bone Joint Surg. **64A**:444, 1982.
7. Silberstein, et al.: Some vagaries of the radial head and neck, J. Bone Joint Surg. **64A**:1153, 1982.
8. Silberstein, et al.: Some vagaries of the medial epicondyle, J. Bone Joint Surg. **63A**:524, 1981.
9. Silberstein, et al.: Some vagaries of the olecranon, J. Bone Joint Surg. **64A**:722, 1981.
10. Silberstein, et al.: Some vagaries of the capitellum, J. Bone Joint Surg. **61A**:244, 1979.
11. Tachdjian, M.O.: Pediatric orthopedics, Philadelphia, 1972, W.B. Saunders Co.
12. Torg, J.: Little League: the theft of a carefree youth, Physician Sportsmed. **1**:72-78, June 1973.

21. Bony injuries about the elbow in the throwing athlete

James R. Andrews

Pure bony injuries do occur in the elbow of the throwing arm, but most often they have some associated soft-tissue counterpart. This is a discussion of the more common problems including their pathophysiology, diagnosis, and treatment.

Pain in the elbow of the throwing arm is a common problem best exemplified by the baseball pitcher. Tullos and King[14] reported that 50% of professional pitchers experienced elbow or shoulder joint symptoms that caused them to be unable to pitch at various times in their careers. Much has been written about baseball player's elbows since the initial works of George Bennett.[3,4] Slocum[11] was one of the first to classify throwing injuries into medial tension and valgus compression overload injuries. Barnes and Tullos[2] and Tullos and King[14] have subclassified these categories into various bony and muscular lesions. It is well known that the throwing arm undergoes both general bony and muscular hypertrophy.[7] The bony hypertrophy must surely account for some of the lesions seen in the throwing arm. King et al.[8] explained that 50% of all pitchers have flexion contractures, and about 30% of these players have a concomitant cubitus valgus deformity. They observed that the combination of hypertrophy of the olecranon fossa and the humerus, with cubitus valgus, causes impingement on the medial aspect of the olecranon fossa. Indelicato et al.[6] recognized this area of bony impingement and believed that it was attributable to the stress imposed during the acceleration phase of pitching. Some authors have been negative about the chances for players to return to competitive pitching when these lesions occur.[5] We have recently emphasized the importance of the posteromedial osteophyte on the olecranon and the corresponding contact area of chondromalacia on the medial wall of the olecranon fossa and reported a surgical technique to correct this problem.[15]

BIOMECHANICS

Baseball pitchers, as well as other throwing athletes, suffer similar injuries to the elbow. To best understand the pathophysiology of these injuries, one must under-

This work was supported in part by the Hughston Sports Medicine Foundation, Inc., Columbus, Georgia.

stand the pitching mechanism. Analysis of the pitching mechanism is well documented.[1,9,13,16] It consists of several phases: windup, cocking and acceleration, release point, deceleration and follow-through.

Windup

The windup starts from a two-legged stance to a position with the ipsilateral leg planted and the ball just being removed from the glove. The body is now ready to commence forward motion. The contralateral leg is cocked, and the ball is being removed from the glove. There are no violent moves during this phase, and no excessive strain is placed on the pitcher. This is a very smooth preparation phase.

Cocking

This phase has been aptly named. It is characterized by planting the contralateral leg in front and internally rotating the pelvis to an anteroposterior direction. This causes the ipsilateral abdominal oblique muscles to be stressed. During this time, the ball is elevated and positioned such that the humerus is approximately horizontal, the elbow flexed at approximately 90 degrees (depending on the pitch and the pitcher), and the humerus externally rotated to about 160 degrees. There is very little, if any, forward motion of the ball during this phase, so that at the end of the cocking phase the shoulder has advanced to prestress (or to extrinsically load) both the humeral adductors, such as the pectoralis major and the subscapularis, and internal rotators, such as the latissimus dorsi and the teres major muscles. The development of the extrinsic loading is a smooth, well-controlled process.

Acceleration

The acceleration phase refers to the portion of the pitching mechanism that occurs at the end of the cocking phase when the forward velocity of the ball is still essentially zero to the point of ball release. The ball must be accelerated from zero to a speed in excess of 80 miles per hour in about 50 milliseconds. This acceleration is affected in two ways. The anterior motion of the shoulder is stopped to allow a transfer of anterior momentum from the trunk to the arm. At the same time the anterior muscles (pectoralis and subscapularis) are contracted adding an intrinsic acceleration loading to the extrinsic load set up during cocking. The humerus is accelerated anteriorly for the first half of this acceleration phase. The internal rotator muscles, latissimus dorsi and teres major, are also contracted extrinsically to start the internal rotation of the humerus. This process is well controlled, but as the rate of humeral adduction increases, the torque on the elbow joint necessary to accelerate the forearm is relatively high. It is, however, smoothly applied.

At the halfway point of this phase, the rate of adduction on the humerus is decreased by imposition of a deceleration from the teres minor, infraspinatus, and supraspinatus muscles. This deceleration allows a transfer of momentum to the forearm and adds to the rate of internal rotation, further accelerating the ball. During this phase, the centrifugal force imposed on the ball and the forearm extends the elbow joint. The rate of extension is dependent on the pitching style but is controlled by the elbow flexors. It appears as extrinsic loading primarily on the biceps and the brachialis. The acceleration torque on the elbow joint, when coupled with a high rate of extension of this joint, can cause relatively high shear forces to be imposed on the articular cartilage. The greater the extension velocity, the greater will be the shear stress with its consequent articular surface degeneration.

The end of acceleration occurs before ball release. The wrist is slightly extended and the arm is at 0 degrees of adduction. The external rotators, such as the posterior deltoid and teres minor, are starting to contract to stop the arm. The transfer of momentum is to the hand and the ball. The wrist flexes to about 0 degrees, and the ball is released. This phase between the stopping of the acceleration of the arm to complete extension of the wrist and subsequent ball release is called the "release point." It occurs in about 6 milliseconds and is also the start of the deceleration phase.

Deceleration

The deceleration phase is the most violent phase in the mechanism. The phase lasts from the start of deceleration at ball release to the end of humeral internal rotation, which is evidenced by the point of maximum pronation of the forearm. All the shoulder muscles are contracting violently at this point. There is a force outwards on the arm of approximately 300 pounds that must be opposed to maintain some appositional stability of the glenohumeral joint. The muscles opposing this force are also decelerating the rotary motions of the arm. The deceleration torques are more than twice as great as the acceleration torques. In general, the deceleration forces are much higher but of shorter duration than the acceleration forces. This is true with the pitching mechanism because the ball is accelerated over 50 milliseconds and the arm is decelerated in less than 20. If the elbow-extension velocity is not decelerated entirely, the overextension injuries common to the elbow can occur. Additionally, if the elbow extension is decelerated too rapidly, the extremely high flexion forces required can overstress the biceps tendon.

Follow-through

In the follow-through phase the body moves forward with the arm to reduce shoulder distraction force and to allow the pitcher to regain his balance. The planted contralateral leg position is the controlling factor during this phase.

CLASSIFICATION

Valgus stress with forced extension is the major pathologic mechanism of the elbow. Tension stress is produced on the medial side of the elbow and compression on the lateral side with a shear force because of the angular velocity of the elbow joint. Forced extension also contributes to chronic injuries and leads to injury of the olecranon process and olecranon fossa.

Injuries to the elbow can be classified as (1) medial stress, (2) lateral compression,

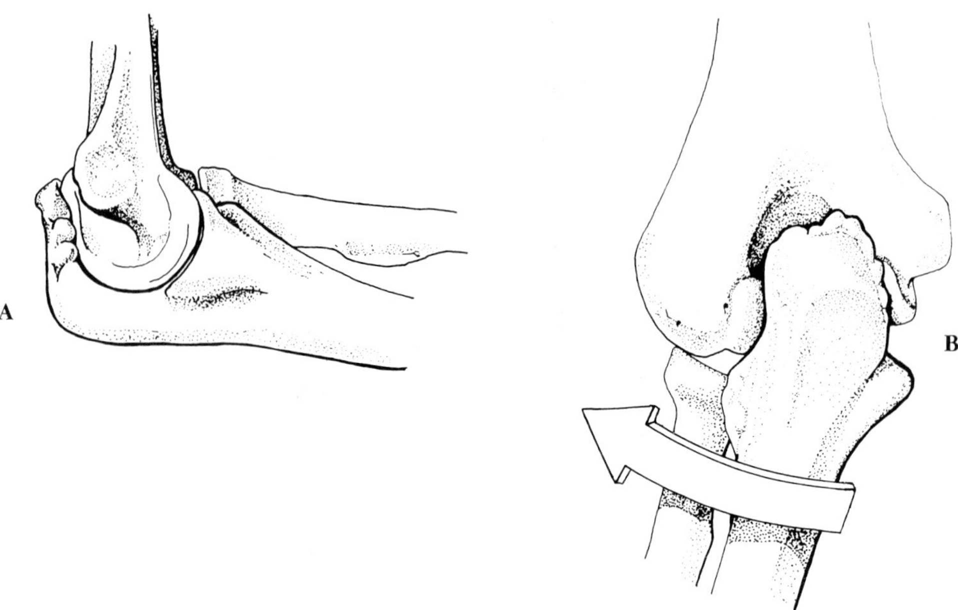

Fig. 21-1. Side view, **A,** of elbow showing medial extent of osteophytes around the olecranon. **B,** Posterior aspect of olecranon showing extent of posterior and posteromedial osteophytes as elbow impinges into olecranon fossa. *Arrow,* Direction of dynamic stress and resultant impingement of olecranon process in olecranon fossa. (From Wilson, F.D., Andrews, J.R., Blackburn, T.A., and McCluskey, G.: Am. J. Sports Med. 11(2):83-87, 1983.)

or (3) forced extension injuries. Medial stress injuries include strain and tears of the flexor muscles, avulsion of the medial epicondyle, tears or attenuation of the medial collateral ligament or traction on the ulnar nerve. Lateral compression injuries include osteochondral fractures of the humeral capitellum or the radial head, avascular necrosis of the capitellum, or hypertrophy of the radial head and capitellum. Forced extension injuries include scarring and fibrous tissue deposition in the olecranon fossa, osteophyte formation of the tip of the olecranon process, primarily posteromedially, and loose body formation[1,5,11] (Fig. 21-1).

Secondary soft-tissue contractures associated with bony injuries about the throwing elbow are a result of radial head hypertrophy, extension block, or pain on forced extension. Considerable overlap in these classifications occurs with specific clinical cases.

STABILITY OF THE ELBOW

Because of biomechanical stresses opposed on the throwing elbow, it is constantly being overloaded with distraction medially and compression laterally and posteriorly. Stability is afforded the throwing elbow by its primary stabilizer, the medial collateral ligament, and its secondary stabilizers, the medial flexor musculotendinous mass, the bony articulation of the radial head and capitellum, and the olecranon-olecranon fossa bony complex. These primary and secondary stabilizers resist the valgus vector forces of the throwing act and thereby are also areas of concern in the injured throwing elbow.

DIAGNOSIS

Pain in or about the elbow is the number one complaint. A detailed history should include the precise location of the pain. Referred pain to the forearm may indicate soft-tissue inflammation or peripheral nerve irritation. Alterations in the distal sensory function of the ulnar nerve can also be found with a medial distraction instability pattern. Locking or catching may indicate loose body formation and can usually be localized to the anterior or posterior compartment of the elbow.

A history of loss of full range of motion is common and nonspecific and is usually a combination of both soft-tissue contracture and bony disturbance.

The physical examination should be carried out in a systematic fashion, usually with the patient sitting. The stability of the medial collateral ligament should be tested and compared to the opposite elbow. A detailed examination of the ulnar nerve includes evaluation of motor and sensory function, direct palpation for tenderness with or without Tinel's sign in the ulnar groove, and examination for ulnar nerve subluxation over the medial epicondyle. Deep palpation of the flexor-pronator medial muscle mass may pinpoint a muscle strain. Range of motion of the elbow in flexion-extension and pronation-supination of the forearm is recorded.

Examination of the lateral and posterior compartment of the elbow may elicit specific points of tenderness. Specific tenderness posteromedially along the tip of the olecranon may indicate valgus extension overload.

Occasionally the thrower can voluntarily demonstrate crepitation in the lateral compartment attributable to chondromalacia between the radial head and capitellum. This compressive maneuver uses the extensor muscle mass in a dynamic way to elicit the same symptoms the patient gets when he throws. Quite frequently the thrower can also demonstrate his posterior compartment symptoms by forcefully hyperextending his elbow and using his other hand to feel the exact origin and site of pain.

Roentgenograms taken include an anteroposterior, a lateral, and, in the thrower, an axial view (Fig. 21-2). Occasionally, oblique views will be of help in identification of a loose body or osteophyte.

Arthrograms and arthrotomograms are special roentgenographic tests that have been beneficial in special situations. In acute cases, the arthrogram may demonstrate capsular incompetency and arthrotomograms may demonstrate articular cartilage defects, osteophytes, and loose bodies. These specialized tests are certainly not needed in routine problems of the throwing elbow.

Arthroscopy of the elbow is rapidly becoming useful in the establishment of a definitive diagnosis in chronic conditions of the throwing elbow. It is useful in the diagnosis of loose bodies, definition of areas of chondromalacia, and visualization of direct areas of osteophyte formation, especially in the posterior compartment.

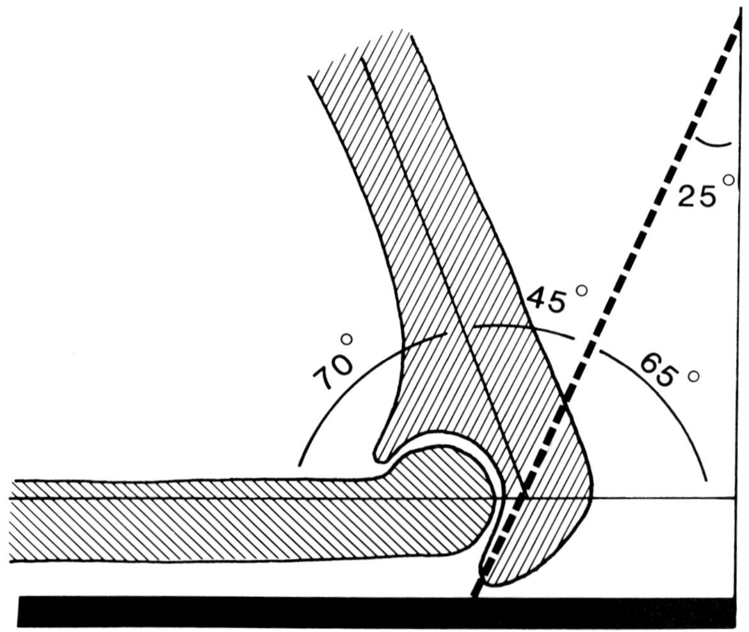

Fig. 21-2. Illustration showing technique of axial view that best demonstrates articulation of olecranon with trochlea and posteromedial osteophyte. (From Wilson, F.D., Andrews, J.R., Blackburn, T.A., and McCluskey, G.: Am. J. Sports Med. 11(2):83-87, 1983.)

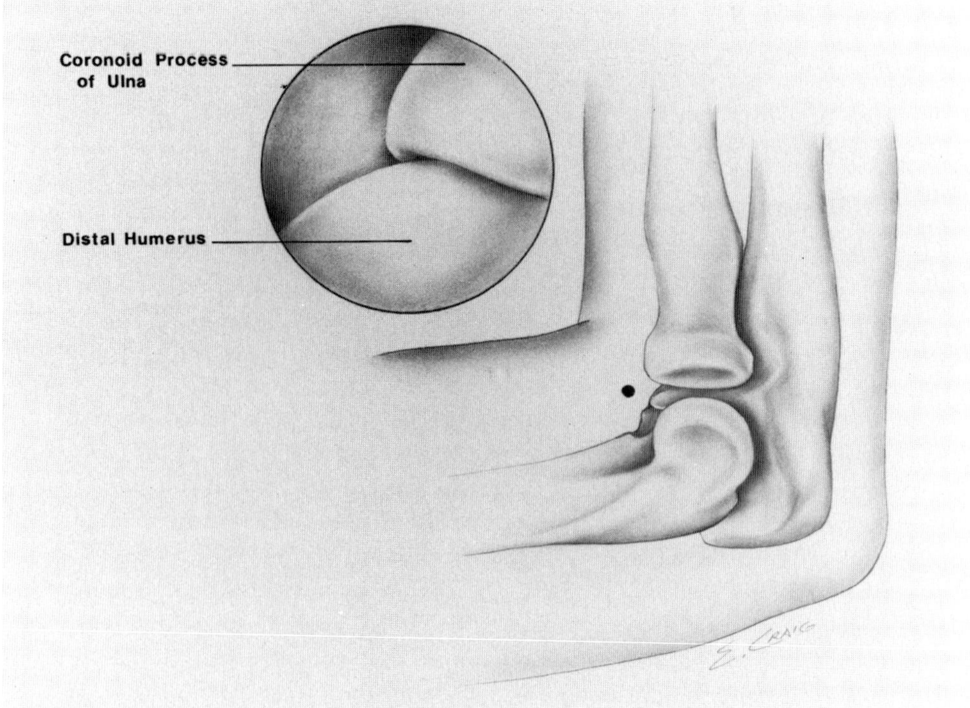

Fig. 21-3. Arthroscopic anatomy as seen through the anterolateral portal includes the distal humerus and coronoid process of the ulna.

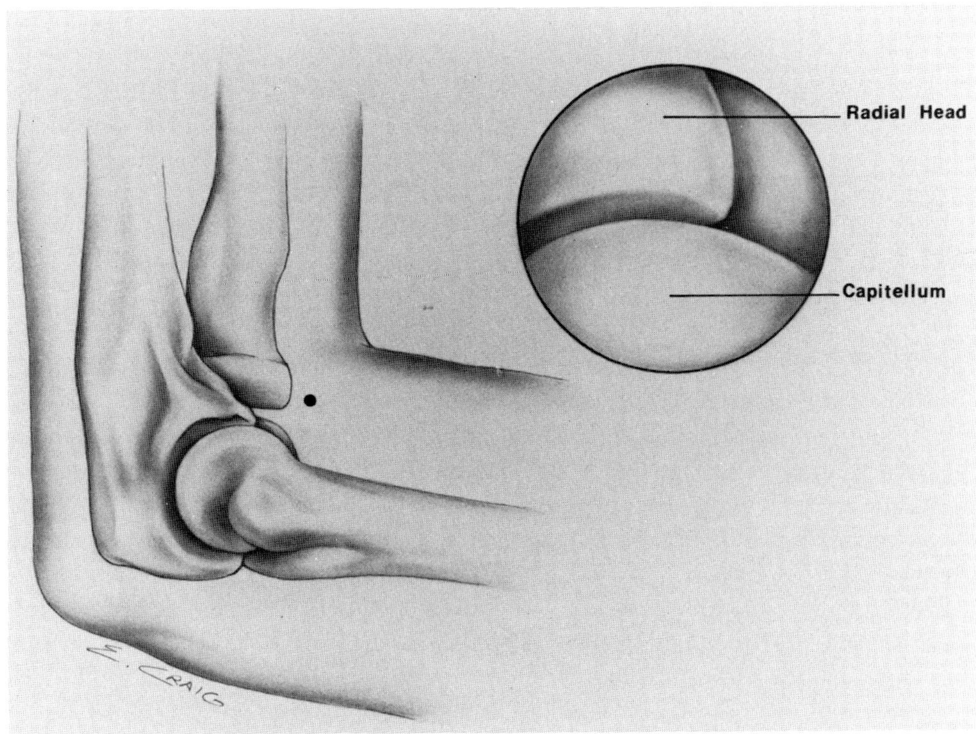

Fig. 21-4. Arthroscopic view through the anteromedial portal includes the capitellum and radial head.

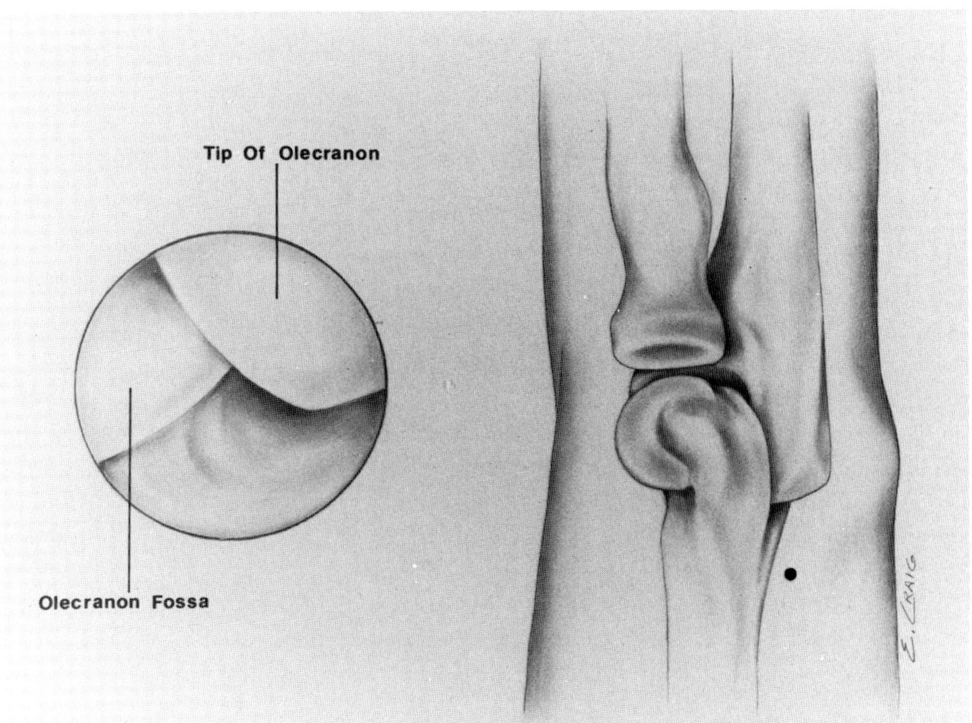

Fig. 21-5. The posterolateral portal is established with the arm extended for visualization of the tip of the olecranon and the olecranon fossa.

The general setup for arthroscopy of the elbow is carried out under general anesthesia with the patient supine with the arm suspended and the elbow in 90 degrees of flexion. A standard 4 mm 30-degree-angled arthroscope is used. Three standard portals are established in the following order: (1) anterolateral (Fig. 21-3), (2) anteromedial (Fig. 21-4), and (3) posterolateral (Fig. 21-5). Excellent visualization of the intra-articular structures of both the anterior and posterior compartment of the elbow is obtained with the use of these portals.

TREATMENT

Medial stress injuries of the throwing elbow occur because of repetitive distraction tensile loads applied to the bony and soft-tissue structures of the medial side. In the adolescent thrower the entire medial epicondyle may be avulsed. In these cases where the bone fragment is large, open reduction and internal fixation are appropriate, regardless of the displacement. Early motion after treatment is extremely advantageous in the adolescent. Occasionally the medial collateral ligament of the elbow will avulse only a small fragment of bone (less than 3 or 4 mm), and in general this does not have to be reduced. Occasionally the small fragment will create late symptoms of pain in the adult thrower but can be excised by a fiber-splitting, flexor muscle incision without jeopardizing the integrity of the medial collateral ligament.

Many medial stress injuries that involve the bone may also involve adjacent soft-tissue injuries as in the anterior capsule and the proximal-flexor muscle mass. These structures must also be considered in both nonoperative and operative treatment.

Associated ulnar nerve neuritis must also be considered and decompression or transposition is sometimes necessary.

Lateral compression injuries of the throwing elbow are best exemplified by the osteoneurosis of the lateral compartment in the "Little Leaguer's elbow." Osteochondritis dissecans[12] is the leading cause of permanent elbow disability in pitching athletes. Lateral compression injuries occur in the youngest, least experienced pitchers.

This group usually has the most severe flexion contractures and get the least benefit from surgery. Their return to pitching is also poor. The osteochondritis most often involves the capitellum.

Panner[10] first described this disease in the 1920s and believed that it was similar to Legg-Perthes disease. He believed it was self-limiting and did not require treatment. The exact cause of Panner's disease is unknown, but the most commonly accepted explanation is overuse of the elbow.[17] The disease displays a familial tendency and occurs more frequently in males than females at a ratio of 10 to 1. Hypertrophy of the radial head is a frequent finding. Hughston believes that the presence of radial head hypertrophy is an ominous finding regarding return of full extension and full function of the elbow (J.C. Hughston, personal communication).

Dramatic chondral defects can also be seen in the skeletally mature pitching elbow because of lateral compression. They can be found on both sides of the lateral compartment including the radial head articular cartilage and the capitellum. Exfoliated articular cartilaginous loose bodies can present a problem as well as pain. One must be very conservative in the skeletally immature throwing athlete with osteochondritis dissecans involving the lateral compartment of the elbow. Frequently these young throwers present with lateral compartment pain and loss of range of motion, both in extension and in flexion. It is very tempting to treat these elbows by either an open or arthroscopic surgical approach to remove the loose bodies and correct the areas of necrotic bone and promote a healing response. It has been my experience that an overly aggressive approach to the problems of these patients may very well lead to progressive loss of motion although they may experience some pain relief. It is my recommendation that they be treated conservatively until they are skeletally mature except in the very unusual case of an obvious loose body that is mechanically interferring with the elbow joint.

In the skeletally mature throwing elbow with osteochondritis dissecans and loose bodies, the loose bodies can be safely removed either through an open lateral approach or an arthroscopic approach. Quite frequently these loose bodies will be found dislodged and lying in the posterolateral compartment of the elbow. For this reason, the three previously described portals are quite frequently needed for complete evaluation and removal of loose bodies in the elbow joint. In the skeletally mature elbow, débridement of the articular defects can be done to promote a fibrocartilaginous healing response. I have not attempted to pin back osteocartilaginous loose fragments found in the lateral compartment of the elbow joint.

In the lateral compression category, early mobilization of the elbow is considered important if range of motion is to be reestablished or increased.

Valgus extension overload is a result of the valgus vector forces applied to the elbow joint during the normal pitching act. The extension block is a result of trauma to the posterior compartment of the elbow associated with extensive pitching activity. The degenerative changes are usually the result of two mechanisms: (1) extension overload resulting in osteophyte formation on the tip of the olecranon, fibrous tissue deposition of the olecranon fossa, and loose body formation and (2) valgus stress that results in abutment of the medial aspect of the olecranon process against the medial olecranon fossa. This causes local chondromalacia along with osteophyte formation on the posterior corner of the olecranon tip, which, in itself, can produce an extension block.

Treatment is by both a conservative and a surgical approach. In most cases of mild extension overload, patients will respond to rest from pitching gentle range-of-motion exercises and a flexibility and strengthening program. Some pitchers who have developed a valgus extension overload with osteophytes of the posterior compartment have continued to pitch successfully while being treated conservatively. These pitchers do develop a flexion deformity of their pitching elbow, but it does not appear to alter their pitching performance. Quite frequently they are able to overcome their painful pitching arc and resume their previous level of pitching.

In athletes with persistent pain, surgery is frequently recommended. Also requiring surgical intervention are those patients in whom loose body formation becomes a

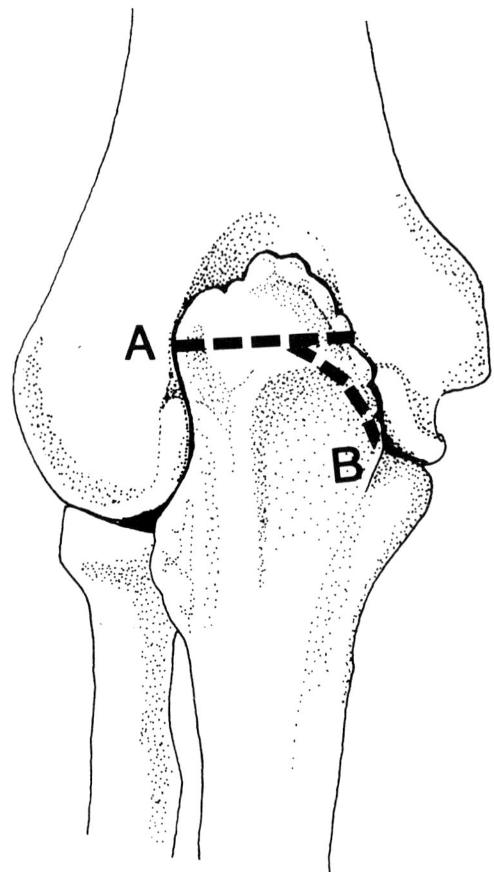

Fig. 21-6. A, posterior view of olecranon. First cut made straight across. **B,** Second cut made with curved osteotome. (From Wilson, F.D., Andrews, J.R., Blackburn, T.A., and McCluskey, G.: Am. J. Sports Med. 11(2):83-87, 1983.)

factor with mechanical blocking and locking in the elbow joint. I recommend a lateral approach to the posterior compartment of the elbow to debride the olecranon tip and to remove loose body formation. This lateral approach offers easy access to the radiocapitellar joint as well as olecranon and olecranon fossa. The skin flap can be adequately retracted to expose the medial aspect of the olecranon. Soft-tissue contractures can also be released with a skin incision. The offending tip of the olecranon with its posterior osteophyte as well as its posterior medial osteophyte can be debrided by either a rongeur or an osteotome (Fig. 21-6). I am now recommending that a minimal débridement of the posterior tip of the olecranon be done lest stabilization of the secondary stabilizer against the valgus vector forces of the elbow be disturbed.

In any of the conditions including valgus extension overload and lateral compression disorders the primary stabilizer, that is, the medial collateral ligament, may also be involved. If this is the case, primary stabilization of the medial collateral ligament of the elbow is important.

Recently we have begun treating valgus extension overload of the elbow by operative arthroscopy. First, we evaluate the anterior compartment of the elbow in a routine manner for diagnosis. Loose bodies exfoliated from the posterior compartment of the elbow frequently migrate into the anterior compartment and vice versa.

On completion of the diagnostic or operative arthroscopy of the anterior compartment of the elbow, a posterolateral portal to the posterior compartment of the elbow is established for evaluation with a 4 mm 40-degree arthroscope. Excellent visualization is achieved with this technique of the osteophyte formation on the posterior tip of the olecranon as well as the posteromedial tip of the olecranon. Loose bodies, frequently found in the posterior compartment, can readily be seen and removed arthroscopically. A second portal to the posterior compartment of the elbow is frequently needed. The selection of this portal depends on the exact site of the posterior disorder but is usually a trans–triceps tendon portal.

Operative instruments can be introduced through this trans–triceps tendon, fiber-splitting portal to approach the tip of the olecranon. Operative instruments including chisels, motorized synovial resectors, motorized cutting instruments, and motorized burrs can be used to debride the posterior compartment. Using a posteriorly placed instrument, one can more selectively debride the olecranon tip while protecting the bony secondary stabilizer.

Postoperative care of valgus extension overload treated by arthrotomy is by use of a posterior splint to immobilize the elbow for soft-tissue healing. Early range of motion activities are recommended along with a progressive exercise program to strengthen the muscles about the elbow. When operative arthroscopy is the treatment for this condition, the elbow is immobilized in a soft-tissue dressing with a posterior splint for a period of 2 to 3 days before one begins range-of-motion activities and rehabilitation. In general, pitchers are allowed to resume some pitching activity at approximately 6 to 8 weeks postoperatively.

SUMMARY

Tremendous valgus stress during the acceleration phase of pitching is the primary cause of elbow injury in the pitcher. Lateral compression injuries are usually found in pitchers in their early teens, and osteochondritis dissecans is the primary underlying cause. Severe flexion contractures and even partial ankylosis of the elbow may occur. Prognosis after surgery is generally poor. Medial tension injuries with either soft-tissue damage or bony damage usually require surgery. The medial collateral ligament should be considered the primary stabilizer against the valgus vector overload. The medial collateral ligament or bony avulsion from the medial compartment of the elbow should be primarily corrected. Results of early surgical correction to these lesions should produce excellent results.

Pitchers with extension block injuries are generally older, more experienced athletes. These pitchers have had symptoms for some time with progressive loss of full extension of the elbow and increasing pain. Valgus extension overload can be surgically corrected by an open surgical approach or an operative arthroscopic approach. Basically these approaches are palliative and progression of symptoms at a later date may be expected. Finally, the postoperative rehabilitation of any elbow problem is extremely important and should be pre-planned for the specific pathologic condition treated.

ACKNOWLEDGMENT

I wish to thank the *American Journal of Sports Medicine* for permission to reprint material that appeared in volume 11, pages 83 to 88, 1983.

REFERENCES

1. Andrews, J.R., McCluskey, G.M., and McLeod, W.D.: Musculotendinous injuries of the shoulder and elbow in athletes. Schering Symposium, Athletic Training **11**:68, 1976.
2. Barnes, D.A., and Tullos, H.S.: An analysis of 100 symptomatic baseball players, Am. J. Sports Med. **6**:62-67, 1978.
3. Bennett, G.E.: Shoulder and elbow lesions of the professional baseball pitcher, J.A.M.A. **117**:510-514, 1941.
4. Bennett, G.E.: Elbow and shoulder lesions of baseball players, Am. J. Surg. **98**:484-492, 1959.
5. DeHaven, K.E., and Evarts, C.M.: Throwing injuries of the elbow in athletes, Orthop. Clin. North Am. **4**:301, 1973.
6. Indelicato, P.A., Jobe, F.W., Kerlan, R.K., Carter, V.S., et al.: Correctable elbow lesions in professional baseball players: a review of 25 cases, Am. J. Sports Med. **7**:72, 1979.
7. Jones, H.H., Priest, J.D., Hayes, W.C., Tichenor, C.C., et al.: Humeral hypertrophy in response to exercise, J. Bone Joint Surg. **59A**:204, 1977.
8. King, J.W., Brelsford, H.J., and Tullos, H.S.: Analysis of the pitching arm of the professional baseball player, Clin. Orthop. **(67)**:116-123, 1969.
9. McLeod, W.D.: The pitching mechanism. In Andrews, J.R., Carson, W.G., and Zarins, B., editors: Clinics in sports medicine: injuries to the throwing arm, Philadelphia, 1985, W.B. Saunders Co.
10. Panner, H.J.: A peculiar affection of the capitellum humeri resembling Calvé-Perthes' disease of the hip, Acta Radiologica **10**:234, 1927.
11. Slocum, D.B.: Classification of the elbow injuries from baseball pitching, Am. J. Sports Med. **6**:62, 1978.
12. Tivnon, M.C., Anzel, S.H., and Waugh, T.R.: Surgical management of osteochondritis dissecans of the capitellum, Am. J. Sports Med. **4**:121-128, 1976.
13. Torg, J.S.: Little League: "The theft of a carefree youth," Phys. Sports Med. **1**:72-78, 1978.
14. Tullos, H.S., and King, J.W.: Throwing mechanism in sports, Orthop. Clin. North Am. **4**:709-721, 1973.
15. Wilson, F.D., Andrews, J.R., Blackburn, T.A., and McCluskey, G.: Valgus extension overload in the pitching elbow, Am. J. Sports Med. **11**:83-88, 1983.
16. Woods, G.W., Tullos, H.S., and King, J.W.: The throwing arm: elbow joint injuries, J. Sports Med. **1**:43-47, 1973.
17. Woodward, A.H., and Bianco, A.J.: Osteochondritis dissecans of the elbow, Clin. Orthop. **(110)**:35-41, 1975.

22. Tennis elbow (epicondylitis)

Epidemiology and conservative treatment

Russell F. Warren

Lateral epicondylitis is a common condition confronting the physician that has been termed "tennis elbow." A wide variety of activities and occupations have been associated with its onset.

Originally described by Runge in 1873,[14] Cyriax in 1936 noted 26 possible causes.[6] Bernhang noted that over half of his patients described tennis as the contributing factor.[1] Various large series by Coonrad,[5] Boyd,[3] Nirschl,[11] and Gruchow[8] have noted certain common points. The prevalence of lateral epicondylitis appears to be nearly equal for males and females. The patient's age is commonly in the fifth decade with a range from the second to the eighth. The dominant arm is more frequently involved, with Bernhang noting an 87.2% incidence and a bilaterality of 5.8%.[1] Several authors have noted the low prevalence of the condition in blacks, with Bernhang[1] showing 1 of 190 and Coonrad[5] none in 339. Medial epicondylitis, which appears to affect more experienced players, is considerably less common, representing 9.8% of Bernhang's patients.

INCIDENCE

Although studies vary, it appears that age and activity level are the critical factors. Most authors have noted an increasing incidence with age, peaking during the fifth decade. Gruchow and Pelletier,[8] in a study of recreational club players, overall noted an incidence of 39.7%, with 24% under 50 years of age describing their symptoms as severe in contrast to 42% of those over the age of 50.

Priest, in two separate studies, noted a 45% incidence in world-class players, whereas 47% of "average" players had symptoms at some time. Nirschl in 1977 reported on a random study of 200 club players, noting that 50% of those over 30 had symptoms of "tennis elbow" at some point in time with half having a duration of less than 6 months. The remaining 50% had symptoms averaging 2½ years.[11]

AGE AND SEX

Gruchow and Pelletier noted a significant increase in reported cases in players after 40 years of age with a fourfold increase in prevalence in men and a twofold increase in women. However, there was no significant difference in the prevalence rate between males and females. In addition, they noted that the recurrence rate for players with a prior history was also greater after 40 years of age.[5]

EFFECT OF ABILITY AND PLAYING TIME

Gruchow and Pelletier in evaluating playing time noted an association between playing time and incidence of new cases of tennis elbow. In particular this was apparent in players under 40 years of age. In players less than 40 years of age with a playing time greater than 2 hours per week, the risk of developing tennis elbow was 3.5 times more than those playing less than 2 hours per week. In players over 40 years of age this ratio was approximately 2.[5]

When experience and ability were studied, no relationship to the onset of symptoms was noted. However, with greater experience a greater proportion of players report a history of tennis elbow. In evaluating playing ability, they noted a higher incidence among class A and B players compared to class C and novice players. However, after evaluating these data as to playing time, one would find that the effect was mainly attributable to increased playing time rather than ability. This is somewhat in contrast to Bernhang[2] and Nirschl who have noted that inexperienced players often use poor stroke techniques that result in greater mechanical load on the elbow. This appears to be particularly the case in using a one-handed backhand stroke where the player leads with his elbow flexed, thus forcing the elbow and wrist extensors to take most of the stress rather than the shoulder. In addition, off-center hits have been noted to increase the torque forces at the handle thus creating greater load on the wrist extensors and flexors. Bernhang has noted the importance of grip size and indicates that a grip that is too small results in the need for higher loads in the muscle tendon unit at the elbow.[2]

Most authors believe that lateral epicondylitis in the tennis player is a result of repeated overloading of the muscle tendon unit resulting in small tears, and inflammation within these tendon origins. Overall it appears that the cause is multifactorial, with age and playing time being the most important variables.

Etiology of lateral epicondylitis
1. Repeated overload to extensor tendons
2. Age with tendon degeneration
3. Playing time (repeated activity)
4. Strength of tissue
5. Flexibility of tissues
6. Technique of sports (ability)
7. Type of equipment

Ability alone will not prevent tennis elbow, but poor mechanics of stroke production seem likely to predispose to overload resulting in early injury and chronic conditions. Certainly anyone treating tennis elbow knows the futility of treating this condition if poor stroke production persists.

PATHOLOGY

A wide variety of descriptions of the pathologic condition of "tennis elbow" or lateral epicondylitis are present, including bursitis, tendinitis and synovitis.[7] However, some uniformity of opinion appears to be forming, with many authors describing tears within the tendon origins including Cyriax,[6] Coonrad,[5] and Nirschl.[12] Coonrad[6] noted in 39 operative cases that a tear within the tendon origin was seen in 28. In 22 the tear was superficial, and in 6 it was deep, hidden beneath the superficial tendons. In 11 patients no tear was seen, but 9 of these had extensive scar formation. Nirschl and Pettrone, in reviewing the findings in 88 surgical cases, noted a consistent finding of immature fibroblastic and vascular infiltrate in the origin of the extensor carpi radialis brevis (ECRB) tendon.[12] They believe this is a result of microscopic tears with a subsequent healing response. They localized this area of injury to the origin of the ECRB tendon and noted that simply releasing the tendon from the epicondyle will not allow visualization of the site of injury. Our findings have been more variable than this with tears seen both superficially and more deeply within the ECRB tendon. Often the tendon may appear pale without an obvious tear being present, but a biopsy may demonstrate a healing response with inflammation.

It should be noted, however, that the findings at surgery are often at least partially related to the repeated steroid injections that have been used before surgery. Thus Coonrad noted that on average his patients had been injected six times with a range of 1 to 13 injections. Depending on the site and type of injection, injury to the tendon origin may be expected.[5]

PATIENT EVALUATION

We are all well familiar with the typical complaints of lateral epicondylitis; however in evaluating these patients one should consider some other conditions including cervical disk disease, thoracic outlet syndrome, radial tunnel syndrome, and conditions affecting the local tissue including the bone and joint directly.

Probably the most common condition is cervical spondylosis with referred distal pain. These patients may present with local pain and tenderness that to some degree can mimic the finding of tennis elbow. Certainly local tenderness over the epicondyle alone does not imply that the complaint does not have a more proximal origin. Similarly the thoracic outlet syndrome may present with elbow pain. In my experience this has been more commonly the medial humeral epicondyle with local tenderness and pain over the tendons of the flexor muscles. In addition, the surgeon needs to be aware of the double-crush syndrome whereby a nerve compressed proximally may be more sensitive to pressure distally. This should be considered in any type of entrapment, particularly in dealing with carpal tunnel syndrome, ulnar nerve entrapment, or radial tunnel syndrome.

The radial tunnel syndrome has been referred to by several authors as causing confusion and inappropriate treatment of tennis elbow. Roles and Maudsley in 1972 described performing a release of the posterior interosseous nerve to treat the entrapment that presented with symptoms similar to tennis elbow.[13] They noted that their patients had local tenderness directly over the radial nerve with pain at the lateral epicondyle and on passive stretching of the extensor muscles. In addition, they noted that resisted extension of the middle finger produced pain proximally.[13] In addition, Lister et al. have reported on some 20 patients with this condition. In each case reported there was a site of compression involving the radial nerve including the "radial recurrent fan" of vessels, the arcade of Fröhse, the tendinous margin of the extensor carpi radialis brevis, and fibrous bands anterior to the radial head. They reported that EMGs were positive in four of six patients in which they were obtained.[10] Although undoubtedly entrapment of the radial nerve does occur, it does not appear to be very common, nor does it routinely require the use of EMGs in evaluating patients with tennis elbow. There does appear to be considerable overlap in their symptoms and findings. Interestingly, Heyse-Moore has reported on the release of the radial tunnel in the treatment of resistant tennis elbow and noted that the results were similar to other treatments. He concluded that dividing the proximal origin of the supinator essentially released the extensor carpi radialis brevis, since their tendons of origin originated together from the lateral epicondyle. He concluded that the radial tunnel syndrome should not be considered as a common cause of resistant tennis elbow.[9] Certainly our experience would support Heyse-Moore's approach in that the radial tunnel syndrome is quite uncommon. EMG changes are infrequent in patients with tennis elbow, and surgery directed to the extensor tendon origins is highly successful.

MANAGEMENT OF LATERAL HUMERAL EPICONDYLITIS IN THE TENNIS PLAYER (Table 22-1)

Basically in the treatment of patients with epicondylitis there are three approaches:

1. Decrease inflammation by rest, anti-inflammatories, and ice
2. Improve strength and flexibility of the involved arm
3. Decrease the forces that the forearm muscles are subjected to

In managing patients that present with several months of pain over the lateral humeral epicondyle, relief of acute inflammation is the initial goal. Once the symptoms have quieted down a progressive exercise program emphasizing strength and flexibility throughout the forearm and shoulder is started. Finally, a variety of equipment and technique alterations may lower the loads generated on the extensor tendon origins. Rest is a variable in the prescription that is dictated by the duration and amount of discomfort. However, simply resting the arm will generally not allow the patient to return if his strength and flexibility have not improved.

Symptoms are graded I, II, and III, with the degree of rest corresponding to the severity of complaints.

Grading symptoms of lateral humeral epicondylitis

Grade I   Mild pain developing after activity not interfering with play
Grade II   Pain during and immediately after activity interfering with play
Grade III   Pain throughout daily activities precluding racket sports

Table 22-1. Tennis elbow treatment program

1. Rest (variable)	2 to 12 weeks
2. Anti-inflammatories given orally	Indocin (25 mg PO q.i.d. × 10 days)
3. Strength	At 7 to 10 days
	Wrist: Extensors/flexors
	Pronation/supination
	½ to 1 lb/week with 10 to 12 lbs maximum
	3 sets with 10 repetitions
	Shoulder: biceps, triceps
Flexibility	Stretch before and after exercise
	Slow: static for 20 seconds with 15 repetitions
Ice	After program for 15 minutes
4. Techniques	Lessons: backhand
	Surface: clay
	Racket: flexible; strung 52 lbs
	Opponent: low speed
5. Return to play	Painfree
	1. Prestretch
	2. 15 minutes: forehand/backhand, increase speed and duration slowly, alternate days
	3. After play use ice for 15 minutes
	4. Strength maintenance
	5. Brace

Mild complaints not limiting play and occurring only after activity (grade I) are treated by exercise combined with equipment alterations. In grade II, where the symptoms occur during play and interfere with activity, the rest period will range from 4 to 6 weeks. In grade III, where symptoms persist in all daily activity, racket sports are generally precluded for 8 to 12 weeks.

Initially patients are placed on anti-inflammatory agents given orally for 2 to 3 weeks. Generally I do not use steroid injections in the initial treatment of tennis elbow but rather reserve it for the resistant case not responding to the exercise program. Care to avoid the insertion of steroids into the tendon must be made because the tendon will be weakened by a direct injection. Instead the injection should be made close to the tendon near the bony insert to decrease inflammation without weakening the tendon. In addition, fat atrophy and loss of pigment may be noted if the injection is placed in the subcutaneous tissues. Thus we have reserved injections for more difficult conditions. However, injections of methyl prednisolone and hydrocortisone acetate often will only have a temporary affect unless an exercise program is performed. In Clarke and Woodland's study a significant recurrence rate of 43% with hydrocortisone and 66% for methyl prednisolone was noted.[4]

If injections are resorted to, a period of avoiding stress on the elbow for the next 2 to 4 weeks would appear to be warranted.

Icing after play or after exercise is valuable in decreasing local inflammation and allowing an exercise program to be continued. This is carried out by application of ice over a pad to the tender area for 15 to 20 minutes to gain any benefit. This is performed both after play and after weight lifting during the treatment phase.

STRENGTH AND FLEXIBILITY

The basic key to managing most patients with epicondylitis, either medial or lateral, is to improve the strength and flexibility of the involved muscles. Depending on the level of symptoms, the program will require 6 to 12 weeks and should be continued after the resumption of play.

One should perform strengthening on a daily basis attempting to stay below pain thresholds and exercising principally the wrist extensors and flexors. The exercises start with light weights, often 1 or 2 pounds, and progress to 10 to 12 pounds. Three sets of 15 repetitions are performed with the eccentric contraction phase twice as long as the concentric phase (Fig. 22-1). Before performing the strengthening routine, one should follow a stretching program for the extensors and flexors. Generally the extensors in lateral epicondylitis are contracted, and thus stretching with the elbow in extension and the wrist fully flexed is performed. This is alternated with stretching of the flexor muscles by extending the wrist passively. These are repeated 15 times, holding each set for 15 to 20 seconds at the point of maximum stretch on the extensors and flexors (Fig. 22-2). Stretching is performed both before and after lifting weights or playing tennis. Additional strengthening exercises include the development of forearm pronation and supination (Fig. 22-3) as well as elbow extension and flexion. Some work on the shoulder is also indicated. Often tennis players will have excessive development of the internal rotators at the shoulder with weak external rotators. This may result in tendinitis and limited motion at the shoulder with pain developing in the elbow as the forces are inappropriately placed on the elbow. In patients with any limitation of shoulder motion or shoulder complaints, attention to improving the balance between the rotators and restoring shoulder flexibility is important. To develop the rotator cuff, Theraband elastic or spring exercises are helpful.

FORCE TRANSMISSION

To decrease the forces that the elbow and the muscle tendon units are subjected to, several approaches are useful, as follows:
1. Patient education and improved technique
2. Equipment alteration: racket, surface, counterforce devices
3. Alteration in play: opponent

In dealing with tennis elbow the patient has to be made to understand his role in managing the condition. In addition, although the patient's level of play has not been proved as a causative factor, poor technique appears to result in creating an overload on the extensor or flexor muscle origins resulting in recurrent injury. Thus, if a player persists in leading with a flexed elbow, it is unlikely that any type of medication or surgery will have a long-lasting affect on his condition. In addition, their role in treating the symptoms with strengthening exercises and flexibility must be empha-

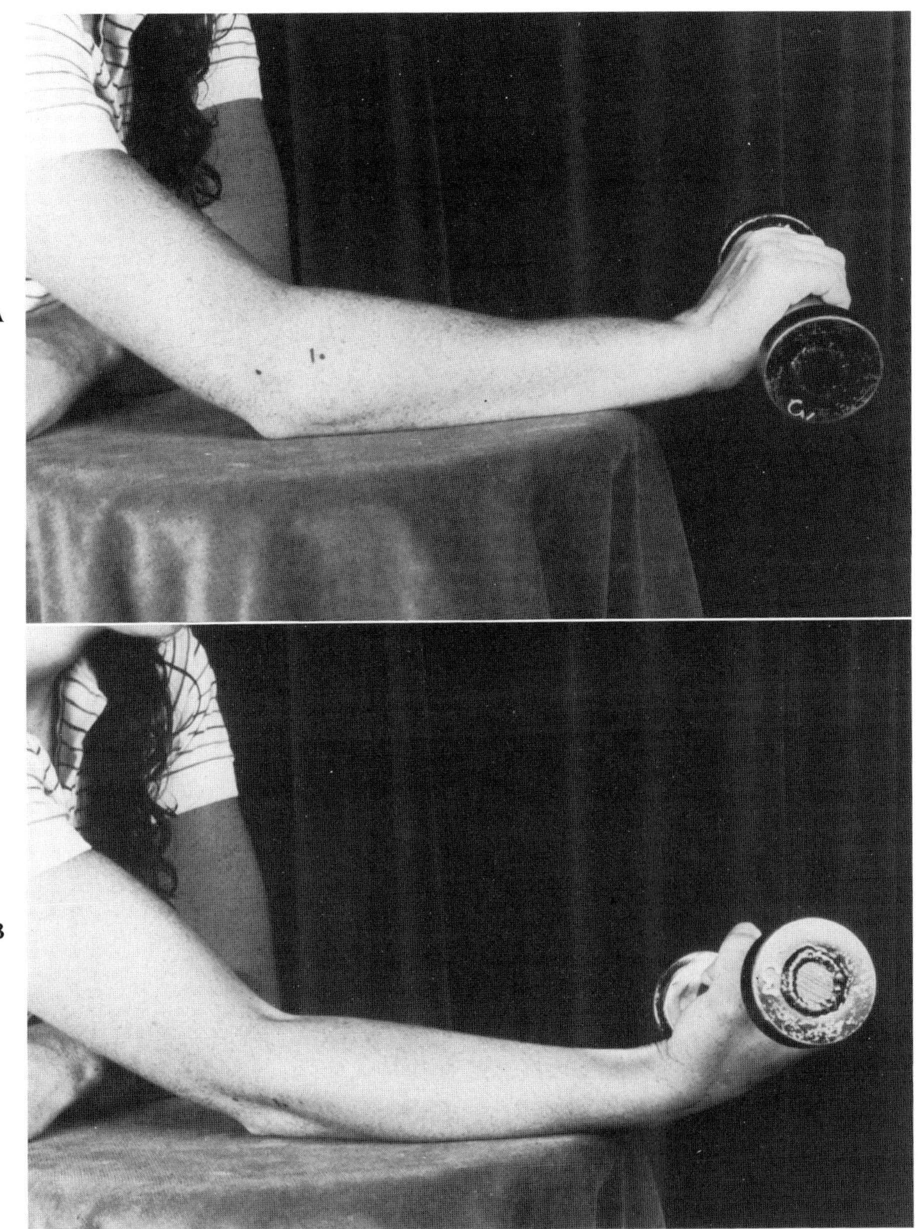

Fig. 22-1. Wrist extension-flexion weights.

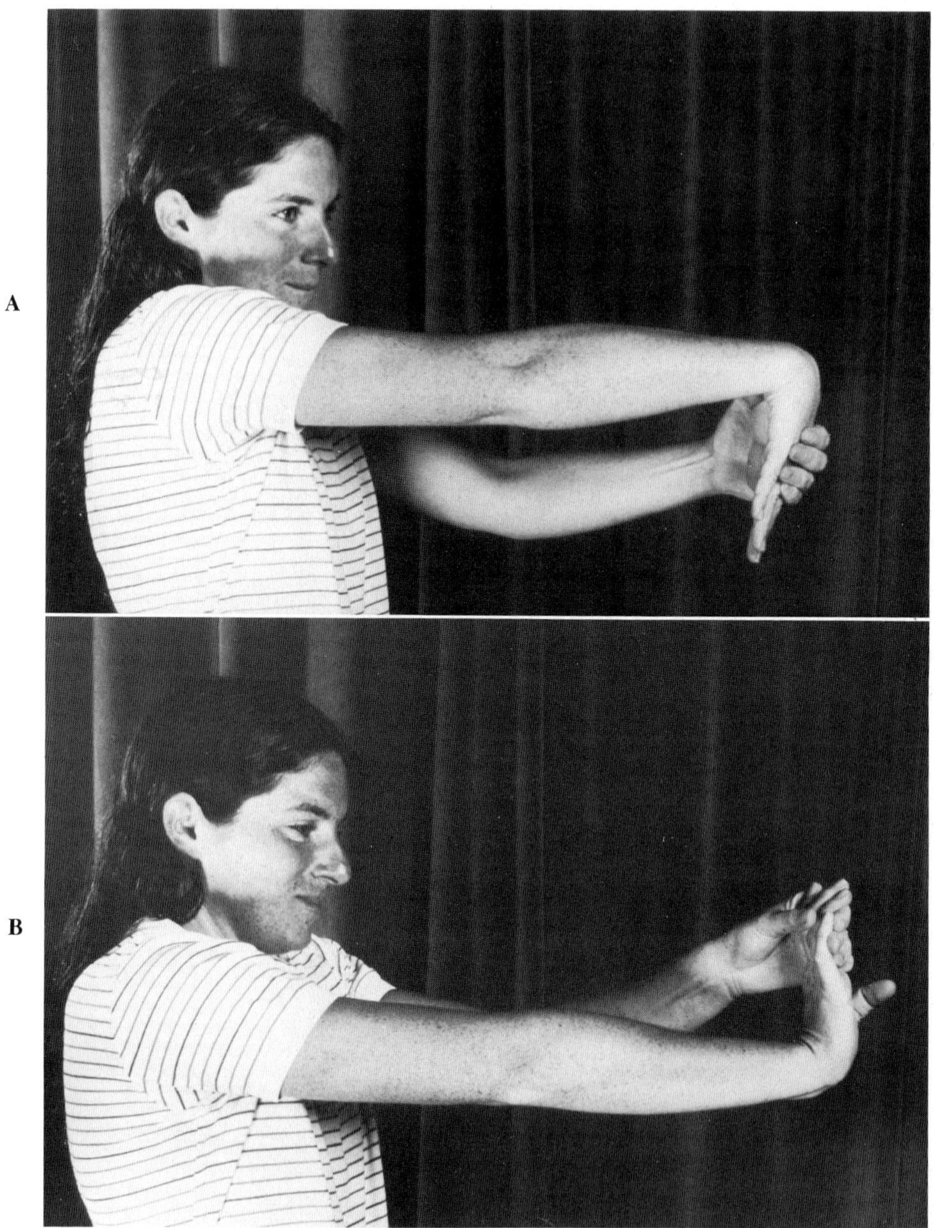

Fig. 22-2. Wrist stretch: flexion and extension.

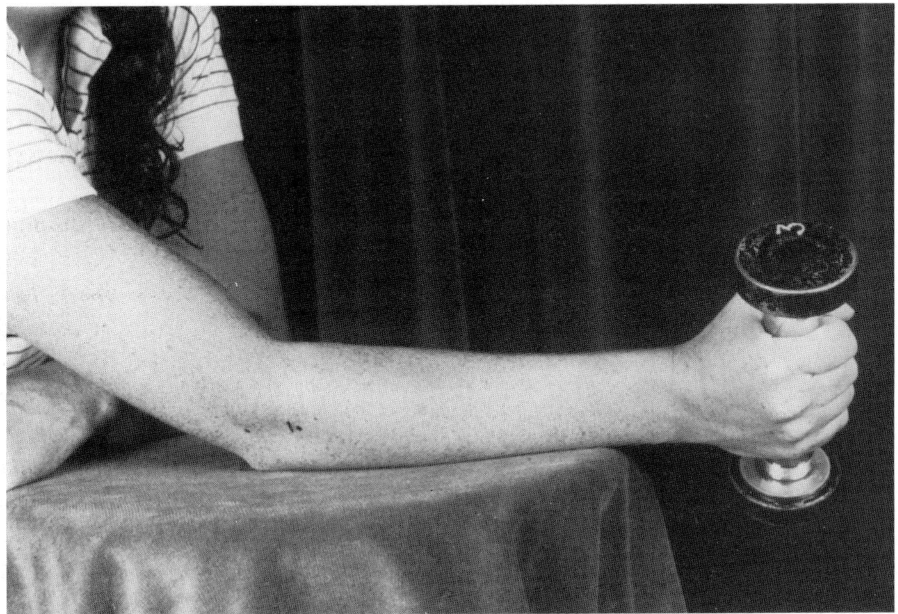

Fig. 22-3. Pronation and supination.

sized. Often we will ask patients to have several lessons on resuming play to see if their form is appropriate. At times resorting to a two-handed backhand technique will be helpful. In addition, teaching proper methods of developing top spin may decrease the patient's medial epicondylitis.

Equipment modification is a favorite area, with many statements both pro and con for various methods. In general it appears that racket alterations, as going to a lighter racket with improved flexibility, is helpful for some patients. In addition, stringing the racket at 50 to 55 pounds is helpful in contrast to a racket strung higher or lower. In an attempt to avoid off center hits, which increase the torque at the elbow, a racket with a larger sweet spot is often of value. Bernhang[2] has emphasized that a racket with a small handle makes it difficult to control the rotation of the racket and thus a larger grip may be better than a smaller one. Nirschl has noted that by placing a tape measure along the radial side of the ring finger and measuring from the proximal palmar crease to the tip of the finger will provide one with the appropriate size of the racket handle (Fig. 22-4). The utilization of counterforce bracing appears to be useful in some patients both in restoring them to activity and possibly decreasing the recurrence of the patient's pain (Fig. 22-5). The mechanism of how these braces work is not clear, but it would appear that they decrease the force transmission to the tendon's origin. Generally these braces are used only during activities that are known to cause the patient's problems.

In addition, a variety of methods may decrease the load transmission to the elbow

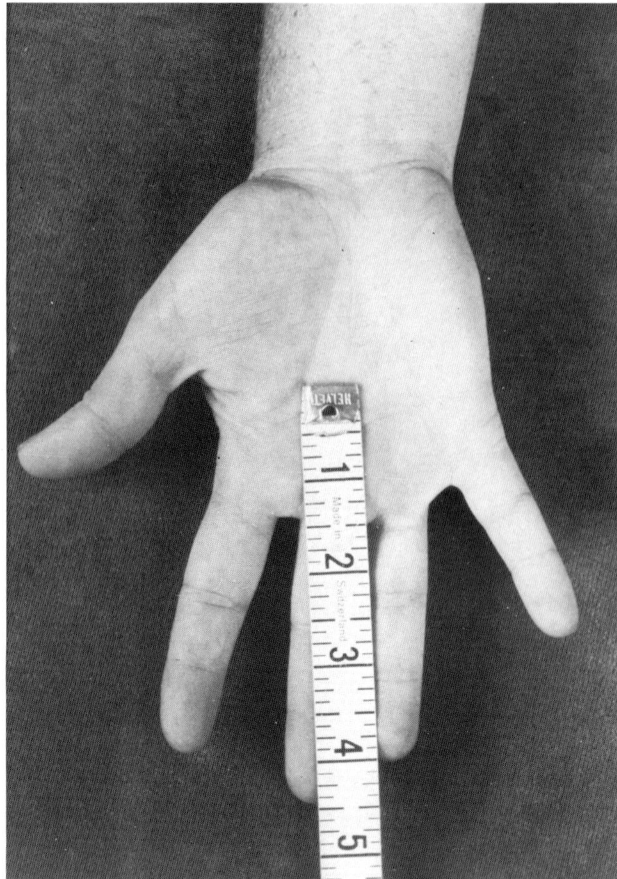

Fig. 22-4. Measurement on size of racket handle.

including the use of clay courts rather than concrete and playing with opponents who do not place a lot of pace on the ball.

Overall in managing these patients, about 95% will respond to this program. It is important that the patient work his way through this condition and have a realistic time scale. If progress in a patient with grade I and II symptoms is limited after 3 or 4 months, injections are utilized. Restricting this to two injections has been our routine. In grade III involvement we may use steroids sooner but often are confronted by patients who have already had several injections without relief. In this setting the exercise program combined with orally administered anti-inflammatory agents is utilized. Surgery is reserved for patients who have complied with this approach for approximately 6 months.

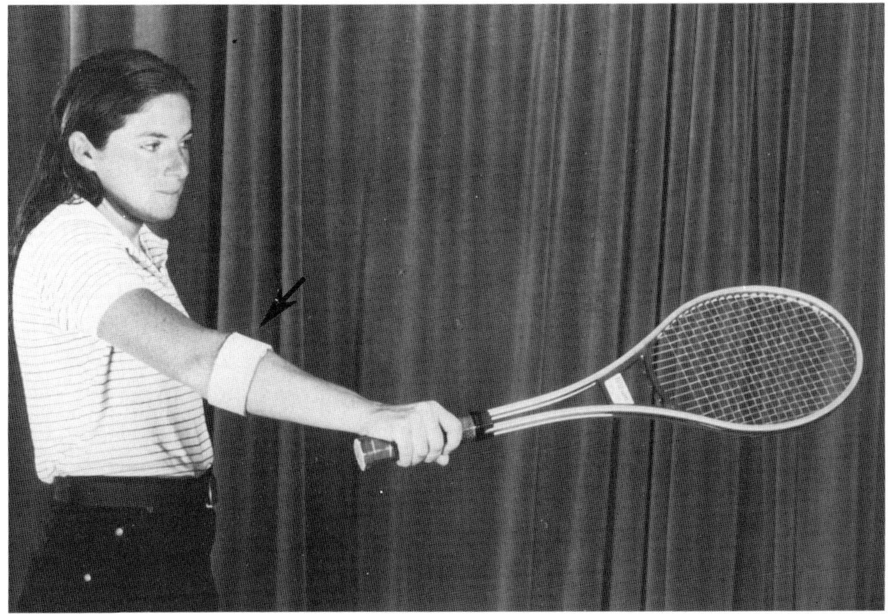

Fig. 22-5. Counterforce brace.

REFERENCES

1. Bernhang, A.M.: The many causes of tennis elbow, N.Y. State J. Med. **79**(9):1363-1366, Aug. 1979.
2. Bernhang, A.M., Dehner, W., and Fogarty, C.: Tennis elbow: a biomechanical approach, J. Sports Med. **2**:235, 1974.
3. Boyd, H.B., and McLeod, A.C., Jr.: Tennis elbow, J. Bone Joint Surg. **55**(A):1183-1187, 1973.
4. Clarke, A.K., and Woodland, J.: Comparison of two steroid preparations used to treat tennis elbow, using the Hypospray, Rheumatol. Rehabil. **14**:47-49, July 1975.
5. Coonrad, R.W., and Hooper, W.R.: Tennis elbow: its course, natural history, conservative and surgical management, J. Bone Joint Surg. **55**(A):1177-1182, 1973.
6. Cyriax, J.H.: The pathology and treatment of tennis elbow, J. Bone Joint Surg. **18**:921-940, Oct. 1936.
7. Goldie, I.: Epicondylitis lateralis humeri (epicondylalgia or tennis elbow): a pathogenetical study, Acta Chir. Scand. Suppl. **339**:1+, 1964.
8. Gruchow, H.W., and Pelletier, D.: An epidemiologic study of tennis elbow: incidence, recurrence and effectiveness of prevention strategies, Am. J. Sports Med. **7**:234-238, 1979.
9. Heyse-Moore, G.H.: Resistant tennis elbow, J. Hand Surg. **9**(B):64-66, Feb. 1984.
10. Lister, G.D., Belsole, R.B., and Kleinert, H.E.: The radial tunnel syndrome, J. Hand Surg. **4**:52-59, Jan. 1979.
11. Nirschl, R.P.: Tennis elbow, Primary Care **4**:367-382, June 1977.
12. Nirschl, R.P., and Pettrone, F.A.: Tennis elbow: the surgical treatment of lateral epicondylitis, J. Bone Joint Surg. **61**(A):832-839, Sept. 1979.
13. Roles, N.C., and Maudsley, R.H.: Radial tunnel syndrome: resistant tennis elbow as a nerve entrapment, J. Bone Joint Surg. **54**(B):499-508, Aug. 1972.
14. Runge, F.: Zur Genese und Behandlung des Schreibkrampfes, Berl. Klin. Wochenschr. **10**:245, 1873.

Surgery and rehabilitation of the professional athlete

Robert P. Nirschl

The historical account of tennis elbow is first noted in the late 1800s.[18,31] The true pathologic aspects of the malady were first alluded to by Goldie[10] and Coonrad[5] and further defined by Nirschl in 1979.[26] Our present observations clearly define tennis elbow as a tendinitis.

The causes of tennis elbow do not vary appreciably from those of other areas of tendinitis, with the common ingredients of repetitive work loads to specific tendon areas in persons primarily over 35 years of age who are often of insufficient conditioning for repetitive activity. Certain subgroups (such as mesenchymal syndrome[24] and gout) seem predestined to tendinitis and often have multiple areas of symptoms including shoulder and elbow in association with carpal tunnel and finger tendinitis.

PATHOLOGY

Tendinitis about the elbow characteristically occurs in the following three areas:
1. Lateral tennis elbow (origin of extensor carpi radialis brevis with encroachment onto extensor communis)
2. Medial tennis elbow (origin of pronator teres, palmaris longus, and flexor carpi radialis with occasional encroachment onto flexor carpi ulnaris)
3. Posterior tennis elbow (olecranon insertion of triceps)

In my experience, lateral tennis elbow is approximately five times more common than medial tennis elbow. Posterior tennis elbow tendinitis is relatively rare (except in competitive baseball throwers; often in association with olecranon bone spurs and loose bodies). Combinations of lateral and medial occur in approximately 10% of cases.

The pathologic types of tendinitis vary widely, as follows:
1. Inflammation only (acute state)
2. Angiofibroblastic tendon change (amount varies)
3. Angiofibroblastic change plus rupture
   NOTE: In some areas (notably the Achilles tendon) alterations of the tendon sheath may also accompany intratendon changes or occur independently.

The term "angiofibroblastic change" was introduced by Nirschl and Stay in 1979[26,28] and is reflective of the characteristic microscopic appearance of chronic tendinitis. This appearance is predominated by young vascular elements with secondary fibroblastic aspects and has a distinctive appearance not related to granulation or more typical scar formation. Interestingly, inflammatory cells are not usually present in microscopic specimens, a finding leading us to some speculation that tendinitis may not be a true inflammatory process.

Two popular theories currently exist concerning the causation of chronic tendinitis:

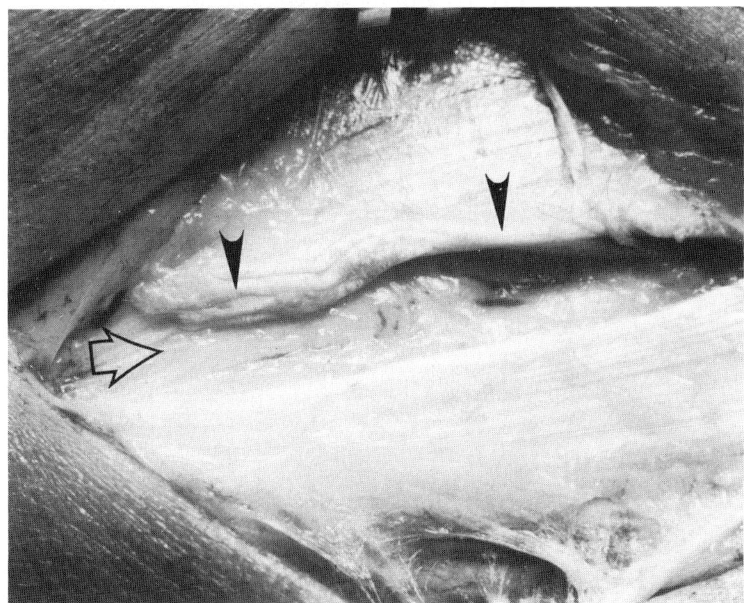

Fig. 22-6. Nirschl tennis elbow, characteristic gross appearance. Pathologic angiofibroblastic hyperplasia appears as a grayish, homogeneous edematous and friable tissue.

1. Vascular deprivation resulting in an actual "infarction of tendon"[19,20]
2. Microrupture causing a physical alteration with the observed pathologic changes merely being a reparative process[3]

Although both concepts may occur and perhaps concurrently, the microscopic findings favor the vascular theory as the predominant factor. Undoubtedly other factors both physical and biochemical play roles in this puzzling phenomenon (Figs. 22-6 and 22-7).

SIGNS AND SYMPTOMS

The average tennis elbow patient is between 35 and 55 years of age and is commonly involved in heavy repetitive forearm activity (such as tennis, throwing, carpentry, lifting, meat cutting),[25,27,29] and 10% of patients will suffer in multiple areas (such as bilateral elbows, medial and lateral elbow, shoulder, de Quervain's disease, finger tendinitis, and neuropraxia of the ulnar and median nerves).[26]

Activities that aggravate the symptoms are essentially musculotendinous stress tests of the involved areas. Thus stress testing of the extensor brevis and finger extensors invariably incite lateral elbow symptoms, and stress testing of the pronator teres and flexor carpi radialis incites the medial elbow. Full elbow extension at the time of stress testing increases the symptoms.

In lateral tennis elbow, localized tenderness is predominantly at the origin of the extensor brevis just anterior and distal to the lateral epicondyle with migration into

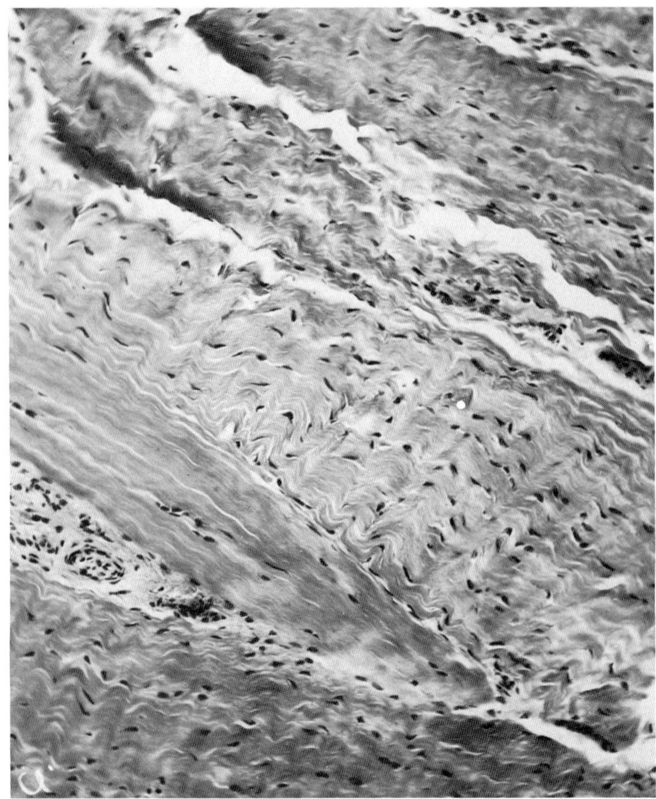

Fig. 22-7. Photomicrograph of pathologic angiofibroblastic hyperplasia. The microscopic appearance is characterized by a predominance of young vascular elements. Inflammatory changes are rarely present. (Courtesy Dr. E. Stay, Department of Pathology, Arlington Hospital, Arlington, Va.)

the lateral epicondylar areas as well as distally along the muscle mass of the extensor brevis.[21]

In medial tennis elbow, localized tenderness is predominantly at the tip of the medial epicondyle and distally approximately 1 inch along the track of the pronator teres and the flexor carpi radialis.[21] Associated ulnar nerve neuropraxia usually manifests with a positive Tinel's sign at zone 3 of the medial epicondylar groove.

In posterior tennis elbow, localized tenderness is present at the triceps insertion into the olecranon just proximal to the olecranon tip. Pain is exaggerated with stress testing of the triceps.

It should be noted that elbow tendinitis may not occur as an isolated phenomenon. On occasion, associated intra-articular alterations may be present. The most common associated alterations include loose bodies of the olecranon and lateral compartments, osteoarthritic traction spurs of the medial compartment, osteochondritis dissecans of the capitellum, medial collateral ligament instability, and ulnar nerve neuropraxia.[23,25,28,33] Signs and symptoms of these possibilities should be sought so as not to overlook adjunctive pathologic changes.

TREATMENT

The treatment concepts are directed to the pathologic stages. Thus a phase I (inflammation only) stage will respond to inflammatory control and preventive maintenance of avoiding future abusive force overload. Phase II or greater pathologic changes will require a promotion of healing or possibly surgery.

The overall treatment algorithm is as follows:[23,25,28]

1. Control of inflammation
2. Promotion of healing
3. Conditioning exercise
4. Control of abusive force loads
5. Surgery

Control of inflammation

The standard concepts of rest, ice, elevation, and anti-inflammatory medications are appropriate.

Keep in mind that there are no scientific data to indicate that anti-inflammatory medications have a biological healing stimulus. Pain relief under the influence of medications no matter how encouraging is not a valid indicator of healing. There are no scientific data to support the concept that rest initiates biologic healing. Rest is best perceived as absence from abuse (so that the independent healing process is allowed to progress without recurrent injury). Appropriate rest therefore in my view is absence from abuse to the injured tissue, not total inactivity.

Promotion of healing

As noted, the relief of inflammation is a separate and distinct issue from the promotion of healing. If pathologic angiofibroblastic change occurs (the rule in chronic tendinitis), biologic healing must occur if the treatment plan is to be successful. My observations in treating approximately 4000 clinical cases of tennis elbow indicate that the following concepts have the potential to stimulate healing.

Rehabilitative exercise. The goal of rehabilitative exercise is to restore injured tissue to normal. The practical expression of this goal includes a healing stimulus to the injured tissue as well as protection of injured tissue by restoring of proper balance and support from surrounding uninjured tissue.

Rehabilitative exercise is designed to stimulate biologic healing to injured tissue by the following three means:

1. Enhancement of "peripheral aerobics" (such as oxygenation, nutrition, collateral circulation)
2. Collagen induction, strengthening, and alignment
3. Enhance biochemical changes associated with endurance training

Present observations of Sobel,[27] Nirschl, and Stanish,[32] indicate that combina-

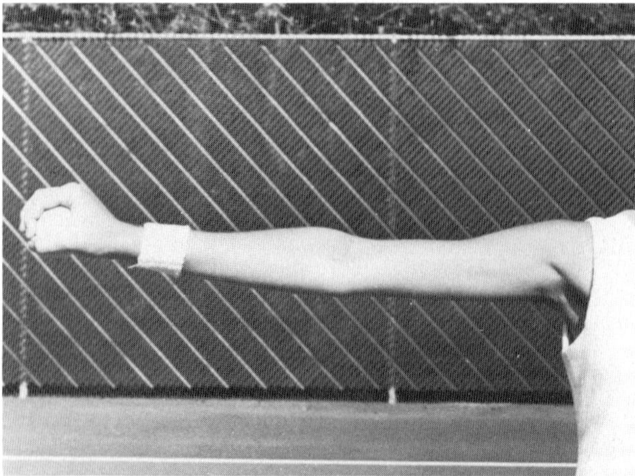

Fig. 22-8. Isometric exercise. Active intrinsic muscle tension without change in muscle length is especially helpful in early rehabilitation.

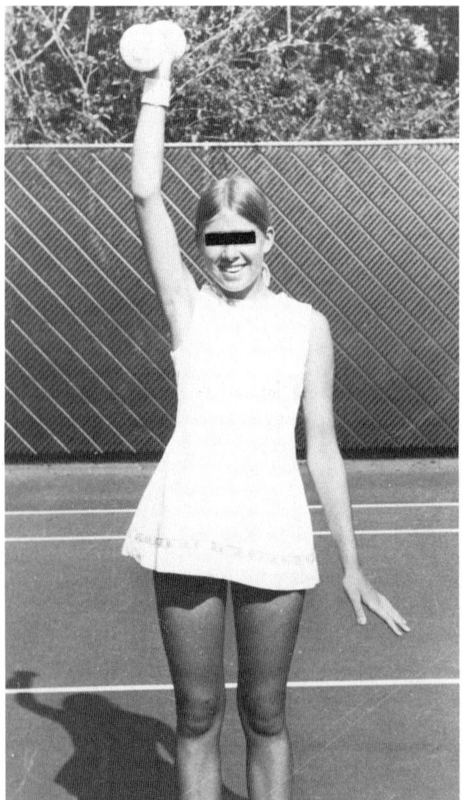

Fig. 22-9. Isotonic exercise. Free-weight isotonic exercise has the advantage of imposing no restrictions on arcs of motion. Because in most local injuries full arm strength is lost, a complete rehabilitation program for the upper extremities and trunk is usually indicated.

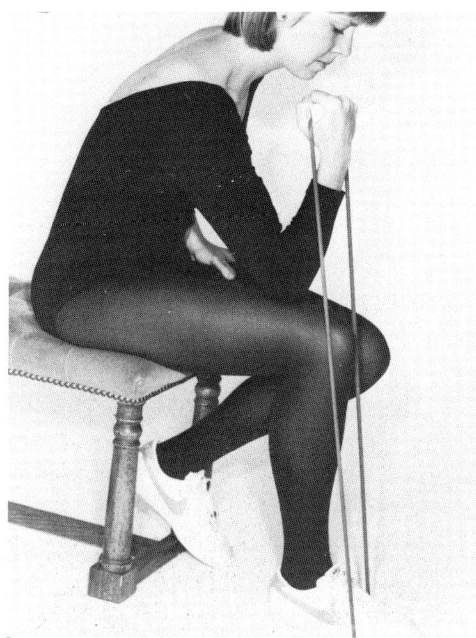

Fig. 22-10. Isoflex exercise. Convenient, effective exercise system utilizing elastic tension cord resistance allows unlimited arcs of motion with both high concentric and eccentric muscle training. Favorable patient compliance has made this exercise concept extremely valuable.

tions of eccentric and concentric resistance exercise offer the best opportunity for this to occur. To accomplish this, our present treatment program includes properly staged combinations of isometric, isotonic, Isoflex, and isokinetic exercise systems.[12,21,22,27] Full-range flexibility exercise is reserved as a last stage, but functional-range flexibility to allow proper progression of the resistance systems is introduced as indicated.

Rehabilitative exercise (Figs. 22-8 to 22-11) to enhance and balance supporting uninvolved tissue includes the following:

1. Strength
2. Endurance
3. Flexibility

In tennis elbow programs, these exercises include shoulder, biceps, triceps, and forearm muscle groups not injured (as in lateral tennis elbow: the flexors, pronators, supinators, and radial and ulnar deviators). Exercise to the uninjured areas is more aggressive, and full-range flexibility is sought early. The resistance systems of isometric, isotonic, Isoflex, and isokinetic are the same but with higher intensity and duration.

High-voltage electrical stimulation. Our present observations are anecdotal, but clinical enhancement appears to occur with this modality of physical therapy. It is my theory that the piezoelectric effect noted with bone healing likely also occurs with

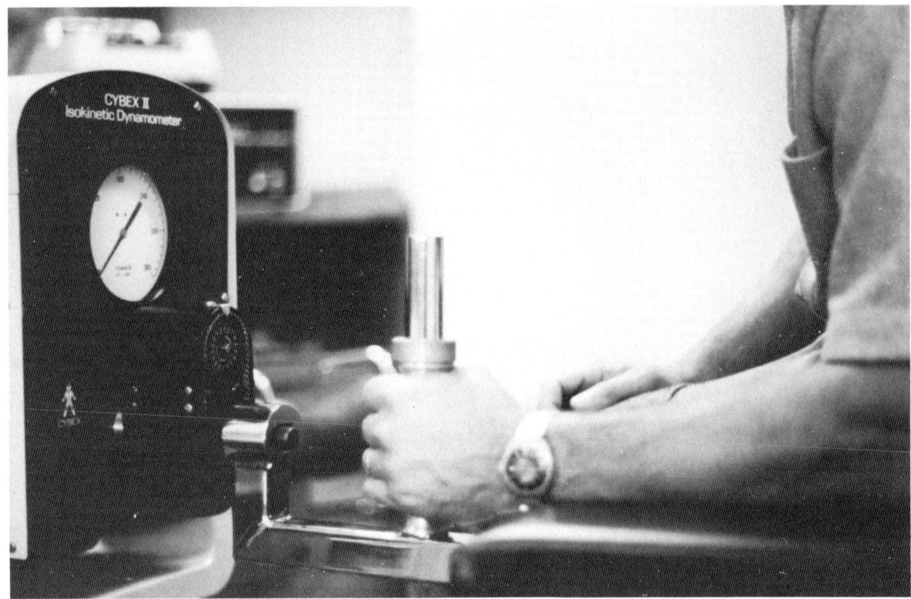

Fig. 22-11. Isokinetic exercise. Fixed-speed variable resistance makes this a valuable rehabilitation exercise tool.

tendon healing.[1,2] I further theorize that the piezoelectric effect is an end stage of rehabilitative exercise that stimulates the biologic cellular healing response.

Exogenous sources of high-voltage electrical stimulation (Fig. 22-12) appear to do the following:

1. Encourage the piezoelectric effect
2. Enhance vascular regeneration
3. Provide an analgesic effect in the majority of patients
4. Stimulate involuntary muscle contraction (that is, provide some activity to injured tissue)
5. Enhance dissemination of edema and hemorrhage

Conditioning exercise

Maintenance of central aerobics with total body conditioning clearly has positive psychologic and physiologic effects on injured patients. It is my observation that by general body support of uninjured areas the rehabilitative process to the injured areas is enhanced.

Full conditioning programs are implemented as appropriate to the individual patient including central aerobics, strength, endurance, flexibility, and fat weight control.

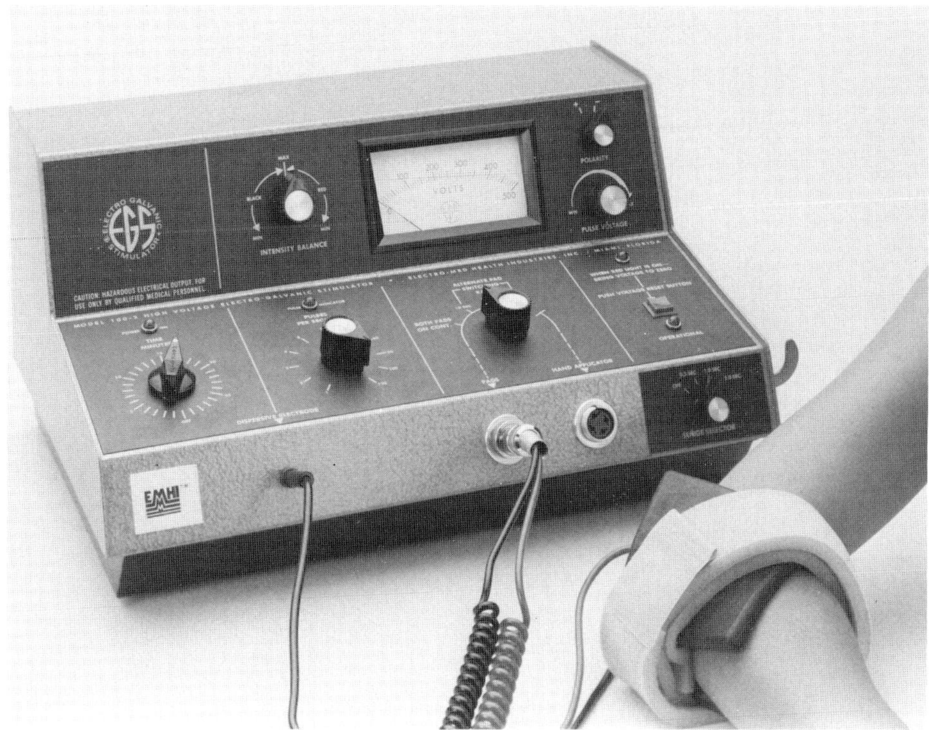

Fig. 22-12. High-voltage electrical stimulation. This most helpful modality appears to enhance healing while providing an analgesic effect. (Courtesy Electromed Industries, Miami, Fla.)

Control of abusive force overloads

It is evident that musculoskeletal tissue must be capable of accepting force loads. To avoid injury, these tissues must have proper capabilities. In sport, injury occurs because these loads exceed tissue capacity. Highly conditioned athletes have better resistance to injury, but the goal of sport is to win, and even the best of tissue often succumbs to injury. In recreational sports, chronic repetitive overload is most common, resulting in tendinitis. Proper conditioning of tissue to accept the physical pressures of sports is critical. Equally important is the effective control of the intensity and technique of the activity to minimize these forces.[21]

Tennis elbow commonly occurs in tennis, squash, racquetball, baseball throwing, and occupations requiring heavy forearm use including carpentry, plumbing, meat cutting, playing instruments by musicians, luggage handling, and even the handshaking of politicians. A review of specific forearm activities and the means of protection are therefore crucial to the diminution of force loads below injury potential.

Counterforce bracing (Figs. 22-13 and 22-14). It has been clinically noted by Ilfeld,[14] Froimson,[8] and Nirschl[25] that constraint of the forearm muscles by nonelastic

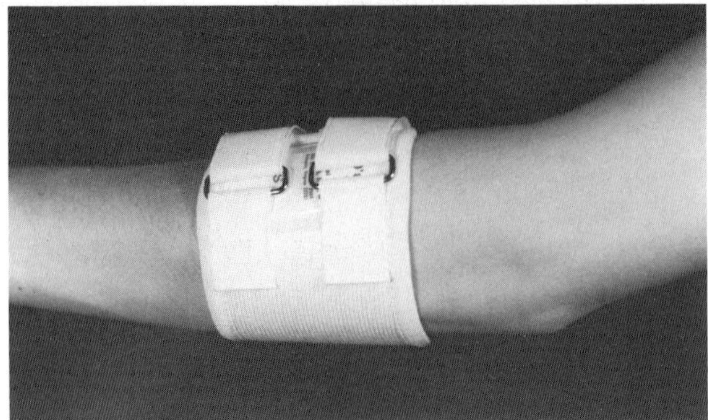

Fig. 22-13. Lateral elbow counterforce brace. Wide nonelastic muscle constraint decreases elbow angular acceleration and decreases forearm EMG activity. The brace demonstrated has advantage of dual tension straps designed for full control over the conical forearm. (Courtesy Medical Sports Inc., Arlington, Va.)

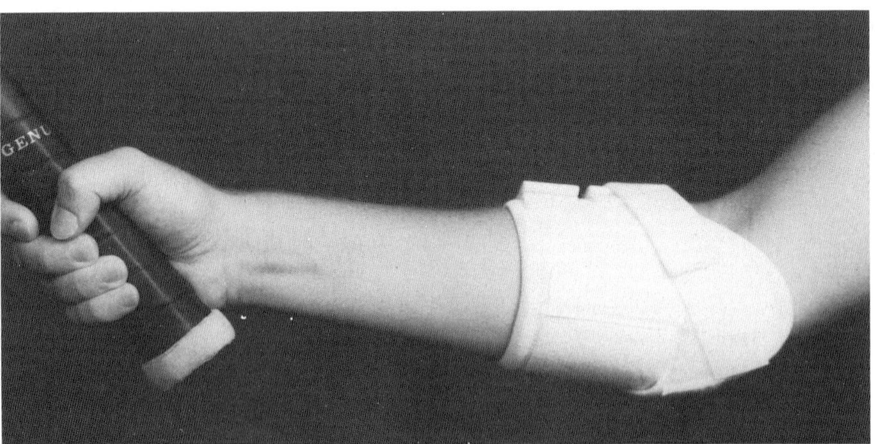

Fig. 22-14. Medial elbow counterforce brace. Extended projection of brace provides additional counterforce support to a key pathologic area. (Courtesy Medical Sports Inc., Arlington, Va.)

compression will diminish the pain of tennis elbow tendinitis. Biomechanical analysis[11] has revealed that counterforce bracing alters angular acceleration and electromyogram muscle responses in sequences that lower mechanical force loads to the braced areas.

Alteration of technique. It is commonly observed that alteration of technique often decreases the pain of the injured area. In lateral tennis elbow, shifting the muscle-tendon activity away from the wrist extensors is effective in controlling symp-

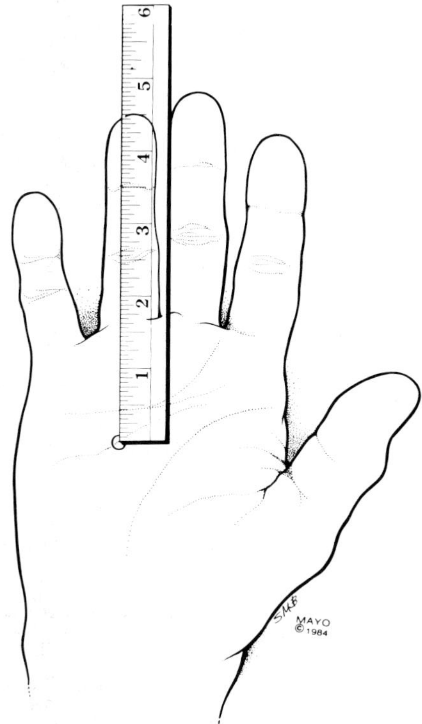

Fig. 22-15. Nirschl technique for proper handle size. Measure from proximal palmar crease to tip of ring finger. Place measuring rule between ring and long fingers for proper ruler placement on palmar crease. The measurement obtained is the proper handle size; that is, if this distance is 4½ inches, the proper grip size is 4½ inches. (From Nirschl, R.P.: Orthop. Clin. North Am. 4(3):787, 1973.)

toms. Likewise, decreasing pronator and wrist flexor activity or elbow extension minimizes the symptoms of medial and posterior tennis elbow respectively.[21]

In sports and occupational activity, many technique changes can be implemented to decrease force loads. The racket sports are perceived as upper body sports. In fact, the majority of power in properly executed racket sports comes from the lower part of the body. A transfer of the power source from the forearm to the lower part of the body is critical in decreasing the potentials of force overloads.

Proper equipment. Hand-held implements can increase force dramatically, especially if improperly sized or shaped. Materials that absorb energy and thereby decrease transfer of abusive forces to the arm are important as well. Proper grip size is especially helpful. Much biomechanical work needs be done to establish the best designs and materials in the racket sports. In tennis, on the basis of clinical observations, I presently recommend the following to minimize the force loads for the average adult:

1. Midsize graphite frame.

2. Twelve to 12½ oz. racket weight. A heavier racket offers the potential of greater momentum but is a disadvantage with the usually weak muscles and poor playing techniques of recreational athletes.
3. Handle size as determined by the Nirschl technique of anthropometric measurement[25] (Fig. 22-15). Too small a handle increases the leverage disadvantage, that is, torque on the arm.
4. String tension of 2 to 3 lb less than the manufacturer recommends for the racket frames in question.
5. Quality synthetic strings are acceptable because the consistency of their mechanical properties are maintained. Gut strings seem to offer an initial resiliency advantage, but this advantage appears to dissipate in a few months.

Activity intensity and duration. Since the common mechanical factor in tendinitis is multiple repetition, the intensity and duration of activity will play a direct role in the causations of overload. Priest and Braden in an analysis of 2500 tennis camp participants observed that those afflicted with tennis elbow on average played tennis twice as much as their asymptomatic counterparts.[28-30]

Modification of activity in combination with the other three factors can be helpful. Practical expression of this concept is defined by number of ball impacts per unit of time, not the amount of time standing on a racket court. In this context, it should be appreciated that racket sport activity varies widely between singles and doubles competition, soft or hard playing surface, quality of competition, practice sessions, and so on. *Caution:* For symptomatic elbows it is not recommended to practice against a practice backboard.

SURGERY INDICATIONS

Much confusion has occurred concerning the indications and technical aspects of surgical intervention. At present, my indications for approaching tennis elbow tendinitis surgically are as follows:

Evidence of major pathologic change in the tendon

1. Persistent inactivity or night pain.
2. Persistent weakness after blockage of pain by local injection.
3. Ease of injection flow (indicative of major distortion of tendon tissue)
4. Adequate trial of a first-class conservative treatment plan. (Most patients who consult me have had inadequate and fragmented prior treatment plans.)
5. Roentgenographic evidence of extra-articular calcification or other evidence of associated joint distortion. Calcification has been present either in the form of epicondylar exostosis or tendon deposition in approximately 20% of our surgical cases. Calcification is not a prerequisite of major tendon alteration but often is suggestive of this, and its presence usually portrays a more difficult prognostic sign for the success of conservative nonsurgical treatment.

Associated intra-articular problems must be dealt with as presented and do not seem to be a specific aggravating factor of the tendinitis.

Mesenchymal syndrome

Approximately 10% of tennis elbow patients present with clinical evidence of multiple areas of tendinitis (as in elbows, shoulders, hands, carpal tunnel, and hip and even with associated plantar neuroma).[24,26] This type of patient is often refractory to conservative treatment plans.

In women, low estrogen levels may contribute to tendinitis, and there appears to be some association with high uric acid levels in both sexes. The majority of multiple-tendinitis patients, described as the mesenchymal syndrome by Nirschl in 1969, have no demonstrable rheumatologic laboratory changes.

SURGICAL TREATMENT
Historical review

The recent literature concerning the surgical treatment of tennis elbow might be considered to have begun with Hohmann in 1927, who described release of the extensor aponeurosis at the level of the lateral epicondyle,[13] a technique now commonly referred to as a muscle slide procedure. Modifications of Hohmann's procedure have included percutaneous approaches as well as destruction of the extensor aponeurosis by electrical cautery. Actual pathologic changes were not recognized or described by Hohmann.

Cyriax published an extensive review article in 1936,[7] correctly concluding that the orgin of the extensor brevis was the major site of the disorder. Interestingly, he theorized that the extensor brevis origin was often partially torn, and he reported success in treating it by closed manipulation of passive forceful elbow extension and forearm supination, there by presumably converting a partial to a complete tear.

Bosworth in 1955 reported a series of 27 elbows utilizing four different techniques.[4] He suggested that his third technique, which included a release of the extensor aponeurosis as well as the orbicular ligament in and about the radial head, was seemingly curative though only four patients had been so treated. Bosworth also correctly observed the intimate relationship between the orbicular ligament and the subtendinous layers of the finger and wrist extensors. With release of the extensor aponeurosis and generous removal of the orbicular ligament, he undoubtedly released or removed the origin of the extensor brevis. Curiously, Bosworth performed the Hohmann operation in 17 instances, but "all" still had some complaints.

After surgery, "the duration of disability postoperatively extended from 8 days to 6 weeks except in two cases." Although Bosworth's definition of disability is vague, such a statement is difficult to accept by present standards or observations.

In a fascinating application of the conviction that the origin of the extensor brevis was the source of the lesion, Garden reported 50 instances in which the extensor brevis tendon was lengthened in the distal part of the forearm.[9] He concluded, as had others,[7] that active muscular contraction of the extensor carpi radialis brevis causes pain, but he theorized that the initimate relationship of the origin of the brevis to the orbicular ligament may also be part of the problem. He appreciated the potential of a much higher morbidity with the Bosworth technique of resecting a portion of the annular ligament than was reported by Bosworth.[4] In 44 cases treated by open Z-plasty lengthening at the musculotendinous junction, no operative-site problems occurred. In six cases the extensor carpi radialis brevis was lengthened at wrist level with significant postoperative wrist pain. Full relief was apparently obtained in all cases, a result not duplicated by others.[6] Obtaining grip and wrist extensor dynamometer data, Garden concluded that "this operation causes diminution neither of the power of wrist dorsiflexion nor in the efficiency of the grip." However, a critical review of his data reveals 20 cases (49%) in which strength had not returned to normal.

Goldie in 1964 presented a comprehensive thesis that for the first time detailed pathologic changes in the subtendinous tissue in and about the lateral epicondyle in 49 patients.[10] He described tendinous tissue that was invaded in "many places" by cellular infiltration of round and fibroblastic cells as well as vascular infiltrates. He described this tissue as granular in nature.

Kaplan reported three cases of resection of the radial nerve to the lateral epicondyle and lateral articular areas with no attempt to identify or remove pathologic tissues.[16] He noted excellent pain relief, but interestingly denervation of a motor branch to the extensor brevis probably occurred with this technique. The length of the surgical incision was approximately 6 inches, and the hospital stay was 5, 6, and 7 days in the three cases. Roles and Maudsley[31] described 33 patients who responded to surgical decompression of the radial nerve. The surgery was performed by 11 different surgeons over a 10-year period. Careful review of the article reveals that the origin of the extensor brevis was released in these cases as a necessary component of decompression of the distal canal of the radial nerve as it enters the forearm.

Surgical pathology

A basic principle of any orthopedic surgery is that a clear definition of the pathologic condition is essential for a well-conceived surgical procedure that will provide consistently reliable results. In many of the prior surgical procedures described, except for those reported by Goldie and Coonrad, this principle has not been strictly followed. Because the extensor brevis origin is largely covered by the muscle belly of the extensor carpi radialis longus, a thorough release of the common extensor origin may correct the pathologic condition even if it is not directly visualized.

Coonrad described gross pathologic changes (including tears) in and about the tendinous structures in both medial and lateral tennis elbow but did not comment on histologic changes.[5] Blazina et al, have suggested that the major pathologic tendon changes in chronic tendinitis occur by moderate but repetitive overload that results in microrupture of the normal tendinous tissue and secondary replacement by the resulting pathologic healing process. Although this theory is attractive, I believe that a more likely sequence of events is similar to that described by McNab in the rotator cuff region of the shoulder[19,20]; that is, a vascular compromise, an altered nutritional state, and force overload cause angiofibroblastic changes with ultimate rupture of these vulnerable tissues.[27,28] In any event, actual disruption of tissue, usually incomplete, occurs in approximately 35% of cases.

Surgery—Nirschl's general concepts

The basic concept of all surgery including tendon surgery is to identify the pathologic problem and deal with it in a constructive manner while avoiding injury to normal structures. In chronic recalcitrant tennis elbow tendinitis requiring surgery for correction, removal of the nonhealing ("nonunion of tendon") angiofibroblastic pathologic nidus is highly successful in eliminating pain while allowing restoration of normal strength. It is critical, of course, to identify the pathologic areas. As noted previously, the most common areas are the origin of the extensor brevis with encroachment on to the extensor communis in lateral tennis elbow, the origin of the pronator teres and flexor carpi radialis in medial tennis elbow, and the insertion of the triceps in posterior tennis elbow.[21]

All excisions are done in longitudinal fashion to avoid injury to normal attachments and thereby reduce weakness and instability (this is especially critical in medial tennis elbow). Since I believe the areas of tennis elbow are relatively avascular, encouragement of vascular supply by drilling three or four holes through cortical into cancellous bone is done before closure.

If additional pathologic findings are present (such as intra-articular calcific cartilaginous loose bodies, osteochondritis dissecans, neuropraxia of the ulnar nerve), these abnormalities can usually be tended to as well at the same surgical sittings.

Surgery—lateral tennis elbow (Nirschl's technique) (Fig. 22-16)

The incision extends from an inch proximal and just anterior to the lateral epicondyle to the level of the radial head. The interface between the extensor longus and extensor aponeurosis is identified, and a splitting incision is made between. The extensor longus is retracted anteriorly bringing the extensor brevis located below into view. The brevis origin normally attaches to the underside anterior edge of the aponeurosis distal to the epicondyle and at the anterior ridge of the epicondyle and distal part of the humerus. In the properly selected case, pathologic change of a dull grayish edematous tissue will be noticed replacing the normal glistening tendon.[26]

This pathologic tissue often encompasses the entire origin of the extensor brevis to the level of the radial head. In approximately 35% of cases pathologic change will be noticed in the anterior underside of the extensor aponeurosis, and this is also removed. Calcific exostosis of the lateral epicondyle is present in 20% of the cases. If these changes are observed, the anterior aspect of the extensor aponeurosis is partially peeled off the lateral epicondyle and the pathologic exostosis is removed. If either situation occurs, it is unusual to have an area greater than 50% of the extensor aponeurosis involved.

A small longitudinal opening is routinely made in the synovium anterior to the radial collateral ligament for inspection of the lateral compartment. In the classical

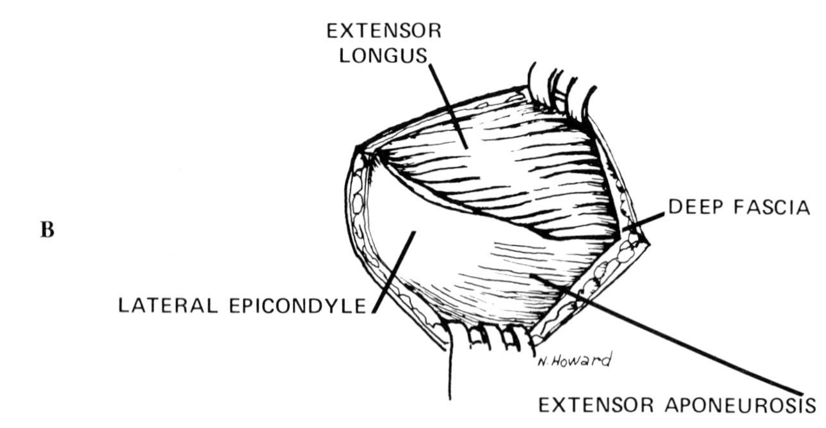

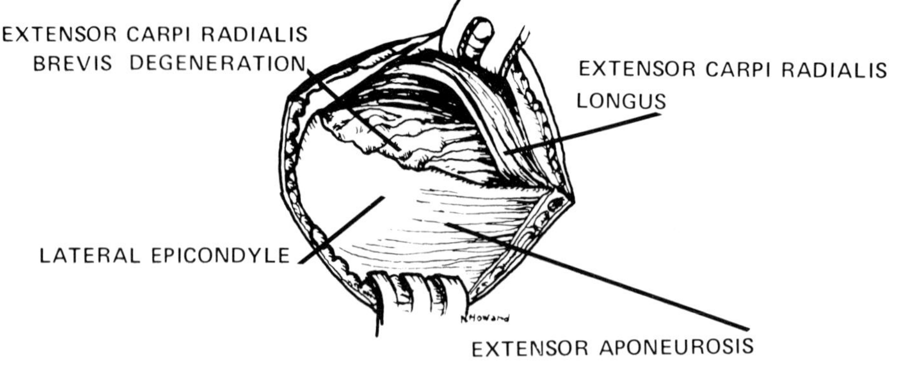

Fig. 22-16. For legend see opposite page.

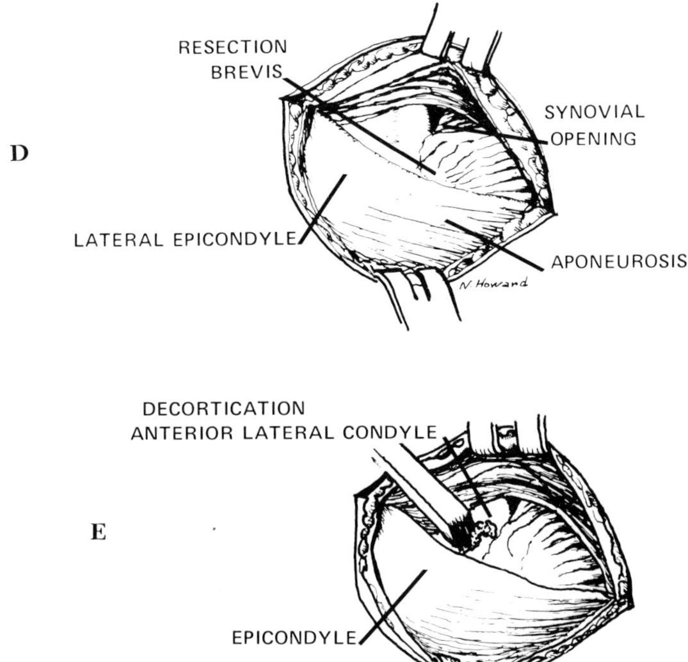

Fig. 22-16. Technique for surgical correction of lateral tennis elbow. **A,** Skin incision. **B,** Incision at interface of extensor longus and aponeurosis. **C,** Anterior retraction of extensor longus exposing synovium for visual inspection of the lateral compartment. **D,** Excision of angiofibroblastic pathologic changes most commonly found in the extensor brevis origin. Encroachment occurs into the anterior edges of the extensor aponeurosis in 35% of cases. The majority of attachment of the extensor aponeurosis is always left intact to maintain strength and stability. **E,** Vascular enhancement is accomplished by osteotome decortication as shown, or three or four holes (5/64-inch diameter) are drilled through cortical bone to cancellous areas for enhancement of vascular supply. Drilling causes less postoperative pain. (From Nirschl, R.P., and Pettrone, F.: J. Bone Joint Surg. **61A:**832, 1979.)

case, it is rare to have any lateral compartment, synovial fringe, or obicular ligament changes.

The wounds are irrigated and three or four drill holes are placed through the exposed cortical bones to cancellous depth to enhance vascular supply. The interface of the extensor longus and extensor aponeurosis are now closed firmly with a 0 gauge absorbable suture. It should be noted that since the extensor brevis is still intimately attached to the underside of the extensor longus at the level of the radial head and distally, no brevis retraction takes place. It is therefore unnecessary to suture the remaining brevis to retain proper mechanical length. This concept is of course pertinent to retaining normal strength after healing has occurred.

Surgery—medial tennis elbow (Nirschl's technique) (Fig. 22-17)

The surgical concepts of medial tennis elbow are the same as those for the lateral (such as excision of angiofibroblastic pathologic tissue without harm to normal structures). In addition, ulnar nerve dysfunction may be associated and surgical treatment may be required to resolve this difficulty as well.[23]

The majority of pathologic changes are present in the origin of the pronator teres and flexor carpi radialis close to their attachment at the medial epicondyle. Encroachment into the flexor carpi ulnaris may occur occasionally. On rare occasion, rupture into the medial joint with secondary pseudobursal formation has been observed.

The incision is longitudinal, approximately 3 inches in length and parallels the medial epicondylar groove starting approximately 1 inch proximal and just posterior to the medial epicondyle. Care is taken to avoid a sensory nerve branch just distal to the epicondyle when the entire medial epicondyle is exposed. A thin muscle layer may mask the pathologic changes underneath, and so it is important to have a clear understanding of the patient's location of primary tenderness before the anesthetic is used.

A longitudinal incision is made in the tendon origins at the prime area of patient tenderness, extending from the medial epicondyle distally for about 2 inches. The tendons are spread and the lesion will come clearly into view if the surgical indications are correct. All excisions of pathologic tissue is done longitudinally and elliptically including resection to the joint in the occasional case as indicated. All normal tissue attachments to the medial epicondyle are left intact. (Caution: The common flexor origin is a key medial stabilizer and indiscriminate release will lead to medial instability.) The resulting elliptical dead space is then closed with absorbable suture (usually 0 or 1 in size).

Surgery—ulnar nerve

For the ulnar nerve, so that a logical treatment sequence is established, the medial epicondylar groove has been divided into three zones: zone 1, Proximal to medial epicondyle; zone 2, at medial epicondyle; zone 3, distal to medial epicondyle.[23,28] (Fig. 22-18). Overall, nerve dysfunction usually occurs by either compression or tension forces. The majority of ulnar nerve symptoms occur by compression in zone 3. Compression from osteophytic spurs, loose bodies, or rheumatoid synovitis can occur in zone 2, and zone 1 compression may be caused by a tight medial intermuscular septum.

Tension forces usually require nerve transfer and can occur with a subluxating or dislocating ulnar nerve (either congenital, traumatic, or iatrogenic), skeletal valgus (usually from fracture malunion), medial ligament rupture with secondary valgus instability (common in throwers), or a scar-hostile environment from prior disease, trauma, or surgery.

My present indications for anterior ulnar nerve transfer are primarily for tension problems and therefore include the following:

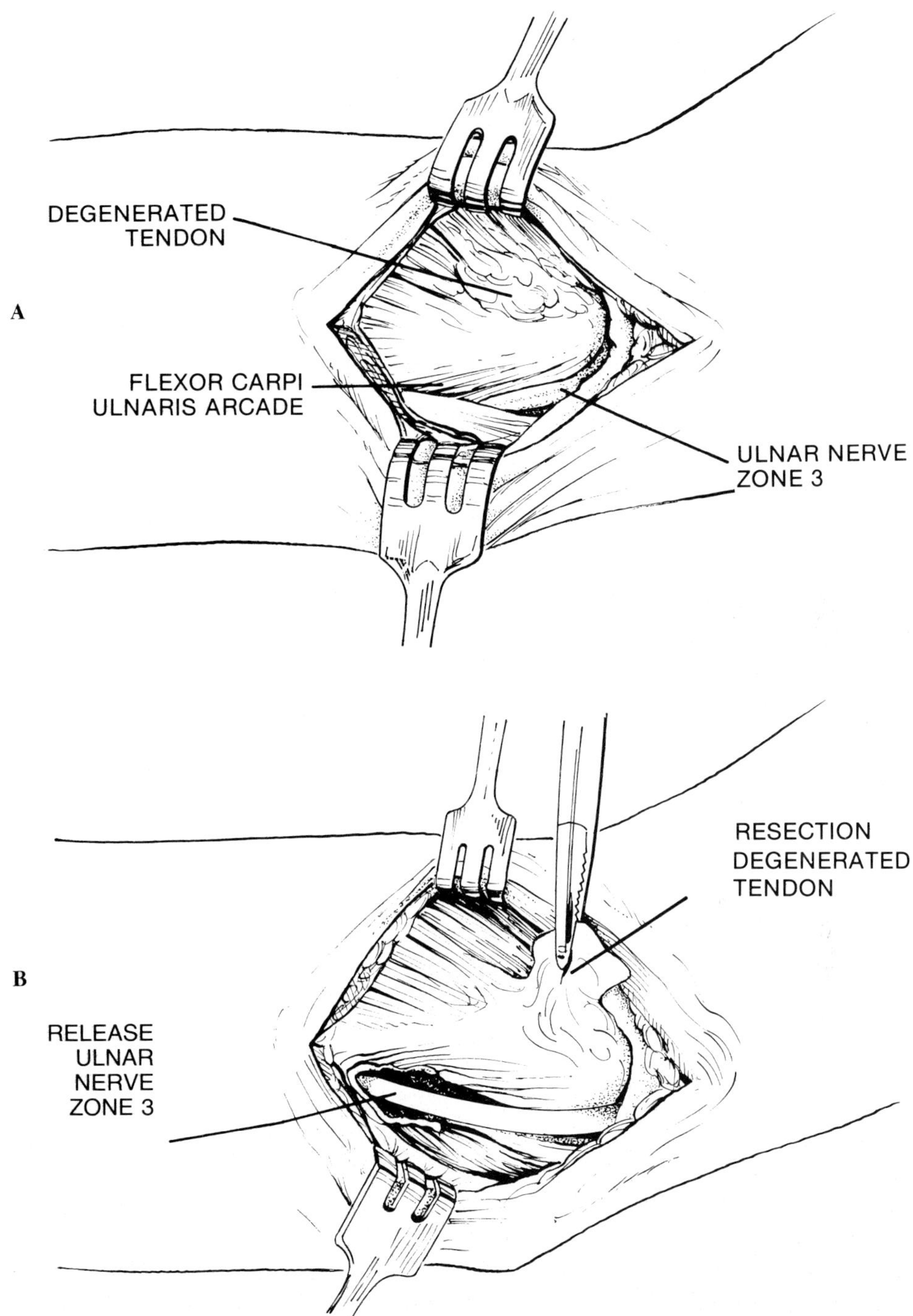

Fig. 22-17. Technique for surgical correction of medial tennis elbow. **A,** Medial tennis elbow surgery. Angiofibroblastic hyperplasia is usually located in the pronator teres and flexor radialis close to the medial epicondylar attachment. **B,** Longitudinal and elliptical excision of pathologic tissue. All normal tissue is left attached because the common flexor origin is an important medial stabilizer. Transverse muscle slides are therefore contraindicated. If ulnar nerve compression neuropraxia is present, decompression of the nerve is done usually at zone 3.

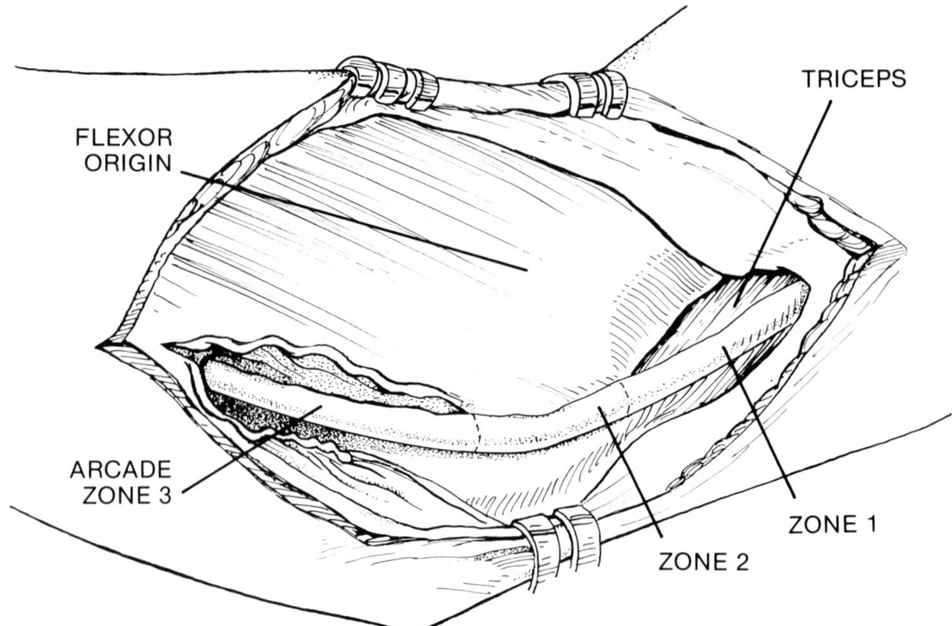

Fig. 22-18. Nirschl classification of ulnar nerve zones at medial epicondylar groove. Ulnar nerve zones at medial epicondylar groove. *Zone 1:* Proximal to medial areas of epicondyle; *zone 2:* at medial epicondyle; *zone 3:* distal to medial areas of epicondyle. Zone 3 includes penetration of the nerve through the flexor ulnaris arcade and is the most common site for compression neuropraxia of the ulnar nerve. (From Morrey, B.F., editor: The elbow and its disorders, Philadelphia, 1985, W.B. Saunders Co.)

1. Nerve subluxation or dislocation from epicondylar groove
2. Skeletal valgus
3. Valgus ligamentous instability
4. Unresolvable hostile environment
5. Necessity of transfer for surgical exposure to medial compartment

In my experience 60% of those patients operated upon for medial tennis elbow will have symptoms reflective of ulnar nerve dysfunction. In most instances, the offending problem is compression neuropraxia at Nirschl zone 3 of the medial epicondylar groove. Decompression of this zone by release of the flexor ulnaris arcade will generally resolve the symptoms.

Posterior tennis elbow

Triceps tendinitis as an isolated entity is relatively uncommon. It is more often associated with posterior compartment osteocartilaginous loose bodies, or lateral tennis elbow. Surgical intervention is quite straightforward with a longitudinal incision in the triceps tendon usually at or close to its olecranon attachment. Elliptical excision

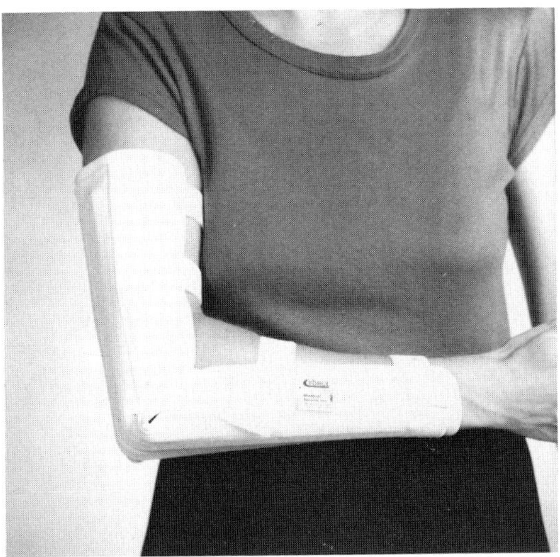

Fig. 22-19. Counterforce elbow immobilizer. Postoperative protection in light supportive comfortable immobilizer with wrist and hand free enhances postoperative rehabilitation. (Courtesy Medical Sports Inc., Arlington, Va.)

of the angiofibroblastic changes similar to the medial tennis elbow approach is undertaken.

Postoperative care

For lateral, medial, and posterior tennis elbow, the postoperative course is similar. The elbow is protected at 90 degrees for 1 week in a counterforce elbow immobilizer (Fig. 22-19). The immobilizer is light and allows active use of the wrist, hand, and shoulder as the patient's tolerance permits. Limbering exercise for 2 weeks is implemented and then followed by strength and endurance resistance exercises starting at approximately 3 weeks from surgery.

Strength resistance exercises include isometrics, isotonics, Isoflex, and isokinetics in proper sequence and intensity. Resistance exercise is continued until full power returns. Full power in the dominant arm is 10% greater in the average person and 20% greater in a competitive racket and throwing sport athlete. Usual full-power return on average requires 4½ months for lateral and posterior tennis elbow and 5½ months for medial tennis elbow. Although full racket and throwing sport competitive activity is not recommended until full-power returns, modified sport technique patterns are often initiated starting at 6 weeks from surgery.

Results

Our present experience with the above surgical techniques is approximately 500 cases, of which 85% experience complete pain relief with full strength return, 12%

are noted to have partial pain relief with or without mild strength deficits but improved over the preoperative condition, 3% of cases experience no pain relief or strength improvements. None of the failure group were noted to have increased pain or strength deficits secondary to the surgery.

Complications have been unusual with the exception of 0.6% temporary superficial infection and 1% of patients have noticed a loss of extension of 3 to 5 degrees.

Other elbow maladies

The classic case of medial tennis elbow may occasionally have associated medial instability. The usual cause is major ligamentous injury from aggressive valgus overload as occurs in baseball or javelin, compression of the lateral compartment, and olecranon shift with secondary formation of osteocartilaginous loose bodies in the lateral and posterior compartments. Stretch neuropraxia of the ulnar nerve may also occur under these circumstances.

With sudden ligamentous rupture, primary repair is indicated. Chronic medial instability may benefit from medial collateral ligament reconstruction utilizing a palmaris longus free tendon graft. Osteocartilaginous loose bodies are best removed when present, especially if joint locking occurs.

If ulnar nerve tension neuropraxia occurs in association with valgus instability, anterior transfer may be indicated.

REFERENCES

1. Bassett, C.A.L.: Pulsing electromagnetic fields: a new method to modify cell behavior in calcified and non-calcified tissues, Calcif. Tissue Int. 34(1):1-8, Jan. 1982.
2. Bassett, C.A.L., Choksh, H.R., Hernandez, E., Pawlik, R.J., and Strap, M.: The effect of pulsing electromagnetic fields on cellular calcium and calcification of non-unions. In Brighton, C.T., Black, J., and Pollack, S.R., editors: Electrical properties of bone and cartilage: experimental effects and clinical applications, New York, 1979, Grune & Stratton.
3. Blazina, H.E., Kerlan, R.K., Jobe, F.W., Carter, J.S., and Carlson, G.J.: Jumper's knee, Orthop. Clin. North Am. 412:665, 1973.
4. Bosworth, D.H.: The role of the orbicular ligament in tennis elbow, J. Bone Surg. 37A:527, 1955.
5. Coonrad, R.W., and Hooper, W.R.: Tennis elbow: its course, natural history, conservative and surgical management, J. Bone Joint Surg. 55A:1177, 1973.
6. Carroll, R.E.: Personal communication, New York, 1968.
7. Cyriax, J.H.: The pathology and treatment of tennis elbow, J. Bone Joint Surg. 18(4):921, 1936.
8. Froimson, A.I.: Treatment of tennis elbow with forearm support band, J. Bone Joint Surg. 43B:100, 1961.
9. Garden, R.S.: Tennis elbow, J. Bone Joint Surg. 43B:100, 1961.
10. Goldie, I.: Epicondylitis lateralis humeri (epicondylalgia or tennis elbow): a pathogenetical study, Acta Chir. Scand., Suppl. 339, 1964.
11. Groppel, J.L., Nirschl, R.P., Pfantsch, E., and Greer, N.: A mechanical and electromyographical analysis of the effects of various joint counterforce braces on the tennis player. Unpublished data, 1984.
12. Groppel, J.L., Nirschl, R.P., Sholes, J., and Sobel, J.: A mechanical comparison of an Isoflex exercise device to the use of free weights. Unpublished data, 1984.
13. Hohmann, G.: Das Wesen und die Behandlung des sogenannten Tennissellenbogens, Munch. Med. Wochenschr. 80:250, 1933.
14. Ilfeld, F.W., and Field, S.M.: Treatment of tennis elbow: use of special brace, J.A.M.A. 195(2):67, 1966.

15. Indelicato, P.A., Jobe, F.W., Kerlan, R.K., Carter, V.S., Shields, C.L., and Lombardo, S.J.: Correctable elbow lesions in professional baseball players: a review of 25 cases, Am. J. Sports Med. **7**(1):72, 1979.
16. Kaplan, E.B.: Treatment of tennis elbow (epicondylitis) by denervation, J. Bone Joint Surg. **41A**:147, 1959.
17. Michele, A.A., and Krueger, F.J.: Lateral epicondylitis of the elbow treated by fasciotomy, Surgery **39**:277, 1956.
18. Major, H.P.: Lawn-tennis elbow, Br. Med. J. **2**:557, 1883.
19. McNag, I.: Rotator cuff tendinitis, Ann. R. Coll. Surg. Engl. **53**(5):271, 1973.
20. Moseley, H.F., and Goldie, I.: The arterial pattern of the rotator cuff of the shoulder, J. Bone Joint Surg. **45B**:780, 1963.
21. Nirschl, R.P.: Arm care, Arlington, Va., 1983, Medical Sports Publishing.
22. Nirschl, R.P.: Isoflex exercise system, Arlington, Va., 1983, Medical Sports Publishing.
23. Nirschl, R.P.: Medical tennis elbow: the surgical treatment. Read at the annual meeting of the American Academy of Orthopaedic Surgeons, Atlanta, Ga., March 1, 1980.
24. Nirschl, R.P.: Mesenchymal syndrome, Va. Med. Monthly **96**:659, 1969.
25. Nirschl, R.P.: Tennis elbow, Orthop. Clin. North Am. **4**(3):787, 1973.
26. Nirschl, R.P., and Pettrone, F.: Tennis elbow: the surgical treatment of lateral epicondylitis, J. Bone Joint Surg. **61A**:832, 1979.
27. Nirschl, R.P., and Sobel, J.: Conservative treatment of tennis elbow, Phys. Sports Med. **9**:42, 1981.
28. Nirschl, R.P., and Stay, E.: Chapter 28 in Morrey, B.F.: The elbow and its disorders, Philadelphia, 1985, W.B. Saunders Co.
29. Priest, J.D., Braden, V., and Gerberich, J.G.: The elbow and tennis (Part I), Phys. Sports Med. **8**(4):80, 1980.
30. Priest, J.D., Braden, V., and Gerberich, J.G.: The elbow and tennis (Part II), Phys. Sports Med. **8**(5):77, 1980.
31. Roles, N.C., and Maudsley, R.H.: Radial tunnel syndrome: resistant tennis elbow as a nerve entrapment, J. Bone Joint Surg. **54B**:499, 1972.
32. Runge, R.: Zur Genese and Behandlung des Schreibkrampfes, Berl. Klin. Wochenschr. **10**:245, 1873.
33. Stanish, W.D., and Curwin, S.: Tendinitis: its etiology and treatment, Lexington, Mass., 1984, The Collamore Press.

23. Fractures of the proximal humerus, clavicle, and scapula

Robert J. Neviaser

Of the fractures in this anatomic area, those involving the scapula are fortunately very uncommon. Although more common than scapular fractures, those involving the proximal humerus are far less frequent than dislocations of the glenohumeral joint. Clavicular fractures are seen frequently but require the least amount of treatment on the part of the physician. In the overall picture of fractures in this region, the indications for open reduction with internal fixation are few. As a basis for comparison, my series of reconstructive procedures on the rotator cuff numbers over 700 whereas operations for fractures in and about the shoulder do not exceed 100. Each area will be dealt with individually.

FRACTURES OF THE PROXIMAL HUMERUS

Originally the concept of classifying fractures of the proximal humerus based on the number of displaced parts was professed by Codman[1] in his classic book on the shoulder published in 1934. He detailed an extensive classification of proximal humeral fractures on this basis. This concept was refined and modified in 1970 into the version that is now commonly used.[3] Since the classification is in such wide usage, it is employed in this discussion. There are several important features to remember. First, this classification is based on displaced, not undisplaced, fractures. Second, there are some fractures and fracture-dislocations about the shoulder that do not lend themselves easily to this classification. A morphologic description may be easier to understand.

Two-part fractures

Injuries that fall into this category include displaced surgical neck fractures, displaced greater tuberosity fractures, and displaced anatomic neck fractures. Fortunately, the last is an extremely rare injury.

Surgical neck fractures are probably the most common of those in the proximal end of the humerus. When displaced, they are usually only moderately malaligned. There are many ways to treat these fractures. One of the most effective ways has been

266

to use a collar and cuff keeping the arm in a dependent position. The weight of the arm and gravity reduce the fracture. Sometimes small, gentle pendulum motions can help to restore length and reduce the fracture satisfactorily. Immobilization is rarely required longer than 14 days. At that time, increasing the pendulum activity and progressing to full rehabilitation over the next several weeks should result in a satisfactory outcome. In the rare instance when a surgical neck fracture cannot be treated in this manner, open reduction may be indicated.[4] This is usually in the severely displaced, irreducible fracture in a younger patient. Of the many fixation devices available, the simplest but most secure is the best. The use of clover-leaf plates requires excessive dissection, and they often must be placed directly over the biceps tendon. This is not a good device to use for most fractures around the shoulder. In a similar vein, Rush pins do not control the fracture fragments even when more than one is used. They have to be inserted through a hole in a rotator cuff and often protrude into the subacromial space. Again, this technique should not be used for fractures of the proximal humerus. Our preference is to use oblique cancellous screws or the tension-band technique.

The next most common displaced two-part fracture is the greater tuberosity. The degree of displacement is often the guideline used to determine whether open reduction is indicated.[2] It is important to obtain an axillary view, since large greater tuberosity fragments are usually rotated externally and posteriorly by the infraspinatus and teres minor (Fig. 23-1, *A* and *B*). As a result, what may appear to be a satisfactory position on an anteroposterior roentgenogram may prove to be inadequate on the axillary view. Of course, greater tuberosity fragments that are retracted superiorly under the acromion by the pull of the supraspinatus also require surgical replacement. The critical point is that displaced greater tuberosity fractures represent a tear of the rotator cuff.[6,7] As such, simple replacement of the fragment without attention to the cuff is inadequate. The cuff must be repaired as well and a decompression performed as part of the surgical approach (Fig. 23-1, *C* and *D*).

Anatomic neck fractures, as previously indicated, are rare as isolated entities. When present, they may remain intracapsular, they often retain satisfactory soft-tissue attachment, and as a result they often will not undergo osteonecrosis. It is reasonable therefore to perform a careful open reduction through a split in the interval between the supraspinatus and subscapularis and fix the head to the shaft with a cancellous screw. If the displaced head has extruded through a rent in the capsule and cuff and is devoid of soft tissue, a prosthetic humeral head replacement should be considered. Whether internal fixation or prosthetic replacement has been performed, the security of fixation should be such that passive motion can be performed within the first week. After 3 to 4 weeks of passive mobility, active motion can be started.

Three-part fractures

The category of three-part fractures encompasses fractures of the humeral neck with associated fracture of either the greater or the lesser tuberosity. The more com-

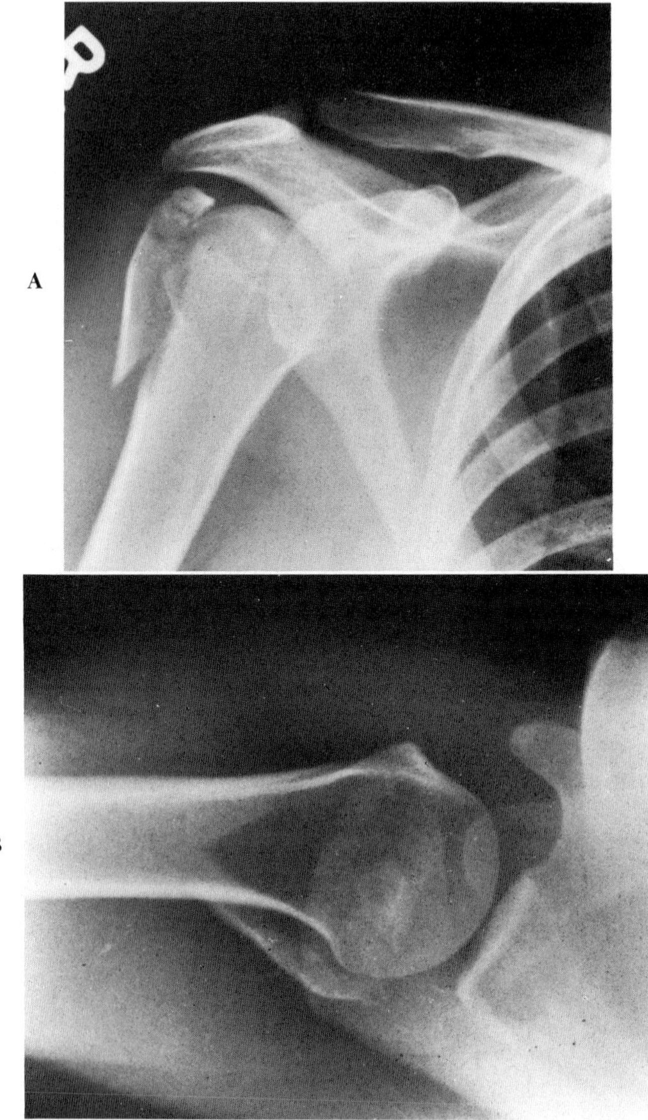

Fig. 23-1. A, Anteroposterior roentgenogram of a fracture of the greater tuberosity. The necessity for open reduction is unclear in this view. **B,** Axillary roentgenogram reveals the greater tuberosity to be rotated and displaced posteriorly, a condition significantly necessitating an open reduction.

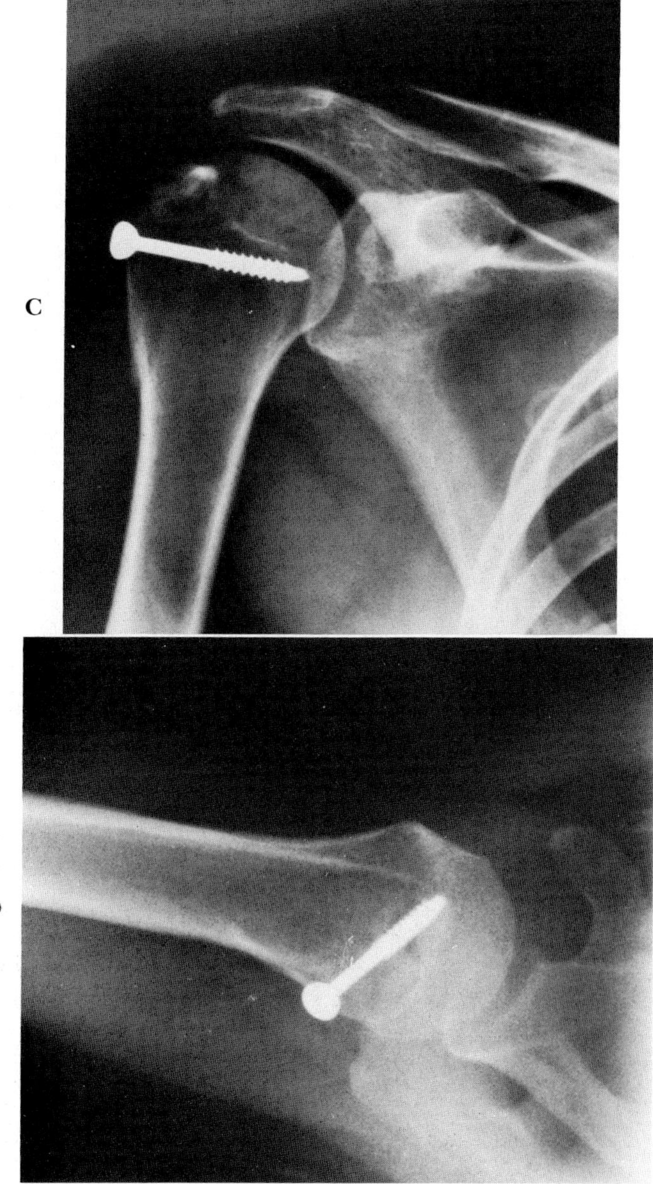

Fig. 23-1, cont'd. C, Anteroposterior roentgenogram of the tuberosity postoperatively, which has been secured with a cancellous screw. The rotator cuff was repaired as well. **D,** Axillary roentgenogram shows the tuberosity to be seated in its normal anatomic position and secured with a cancellous screw. This was done in association with a subacromial decompression and rotator cuff repair.

mon combination is a fracture through the surgical neck with a fracture of the greater tuberosity (Fig. 23-2, *A* and *B*). The lesser tuberosity is usually attached to the head. The head will often be found rotated superiorly so that the articular surface is pointing toward the undersurface of the acromion. The roentgenographic picture of the humerus then appears as a scoop of ice cream on top of a cone with the greater tuberosity displaced.

In an otherwise healthy patient, regardless of age, an open reduction is usually required. The head fragment almost inevitably has soft-tissue attachment and, as a result, is not likely to undergo osteonecrosis. This fragment must be rotated so that the articular surface of the head points toward the glenoid fossa. Then seemingly there is a large defect laterally, and it appears that the head cannot be supported. This, however, is the normal site for the greater tuberosity. When the tuberosity is replaced and transfixed to the head with a cancellous screw, it provides good support for the head (Fig. 23-2, *C* and *D*). The two-screw technique provides secure fixation and allows the patient to undergo an early rehabilitation program. There are occasions when the tension-band technique is useful. The Kirschner wires should be placed from the shaft into the head in as nearly a vertical fashion as possible. The wire loop passes around the greater tuberosity, crosses over its lateral aspect, and loops around the protruding end of the wires inferiorly.

Four-part fractures

Despite the plethora of discussion about four-part fractures, they are uncommon. Many fractures believed to be four part are in fact three part. This is fortunate since three-part fractures have a far lesser frequency of osteonecrosis than four-part fractures have. Again, it is important to remember that roentgenographic interpretation in two planes, preferably anteroposterior and axillary, is necessary in order to establish whether a fracture is three or four part (Fig. 23-3). The four-part fracture usually is associated with a fracture-dislocation, though not always. The fracture fragments include the head from the anatomic neck fracture, the shaft, and each tuberosity as an individual fragment.

This injury generally requires an open reduction. Only if undisplaced can closed treatment be expected to yield a good result. If there is a fracture-dislocation, of course the dislocation should be reduced. If the head remains intracapsular, it usually has adequate soft-tissue attachment and therefore runs only a small risk of undergoing osteonecrosis. If the head is extracapsular, the incidence of osteonecrosis is significantly higher. The complication of posttraumatic osteonecrosis of the humeral head is not so disastrous as that of posttraumatic osteonecrosis of the femoral head. The reason is that the shoulder is not a weight-bearing joint. It has inherently a great deal more motion than the hip does, and as such may not be sufficiently disabling or symptomatic to justify further reconstructive procedures. Therefore, if possible, open reduction with internal fixation is preferred over prosthetic replacement. If the head is completely devascularized and extracapsular, prosthetic replacement is a reasonable option (Fig. 23-4). The technique for open reduction and internal fixation is

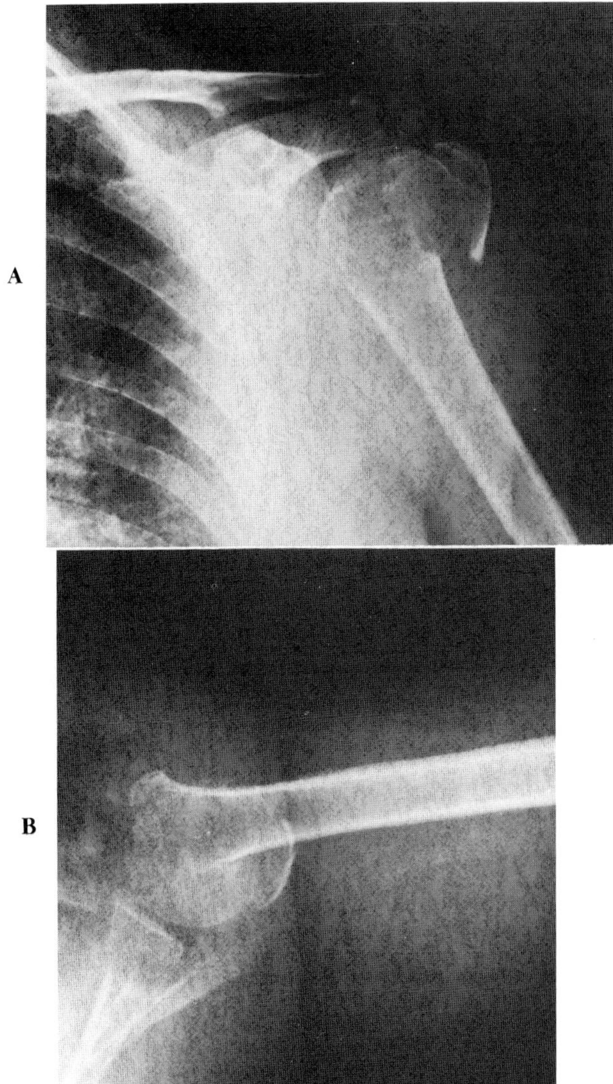

Fig. 23-2. A, Anteroposterior roentgenogram of a three-part fracture with the surgical neck and the tuberosities. **B,** Axillary roentgenogram showing the rotation of the head and tuberosity fragments.   *Continued.*

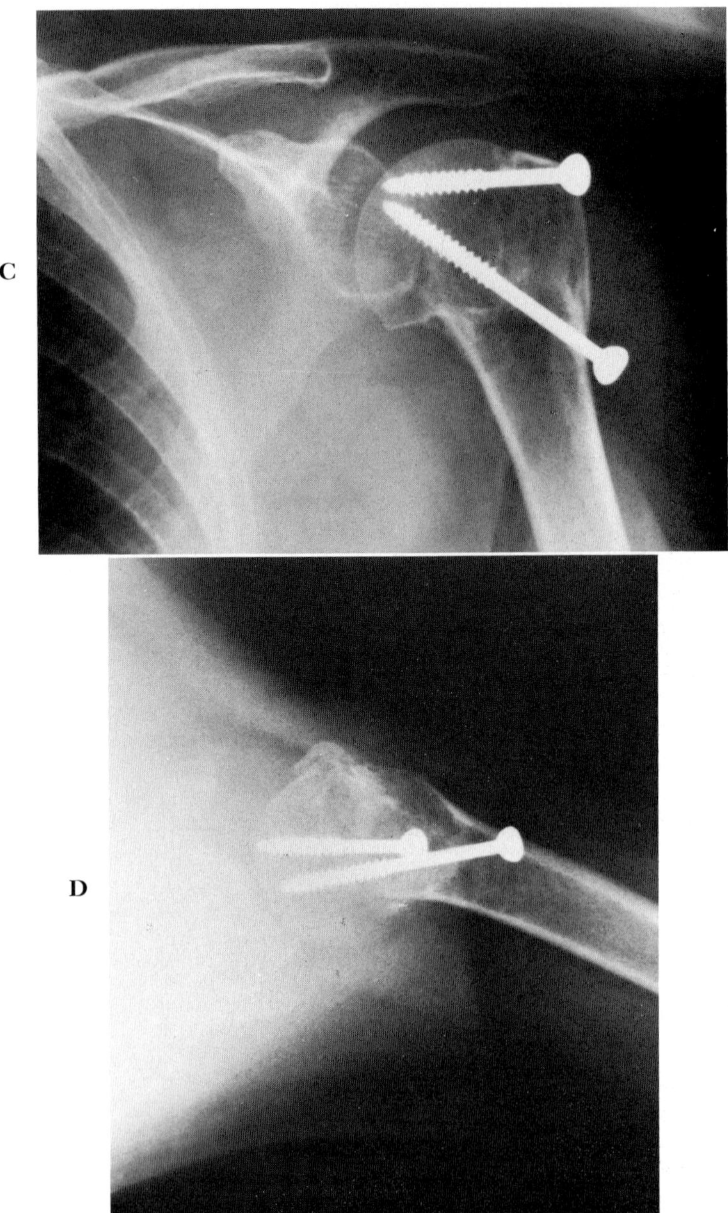

Fig. 23-2, cont'd. C, Postoperative anteroposterior roentgenogram demonstrating fixation of the shaft to the head with an oblique cancellous screw and of the tuberosities to the head with a transverse cancellous screw. **D,** Axillary roentgenogram of the same postoperative case.

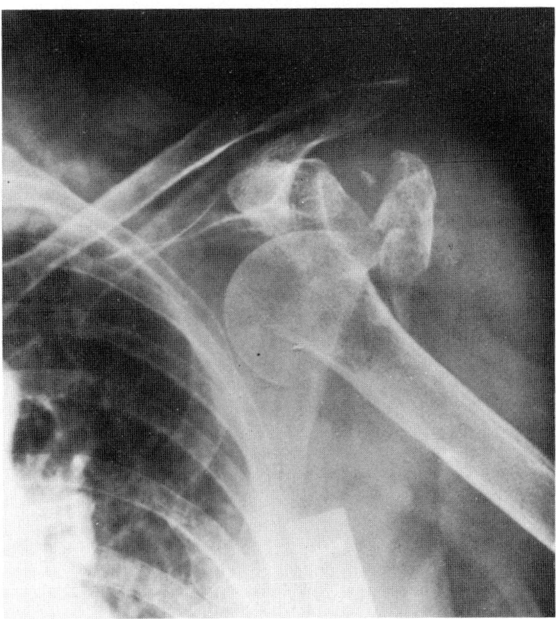

Fig. 23-3. Four-part fracture-dislocation of the humeral head and tuberosities.

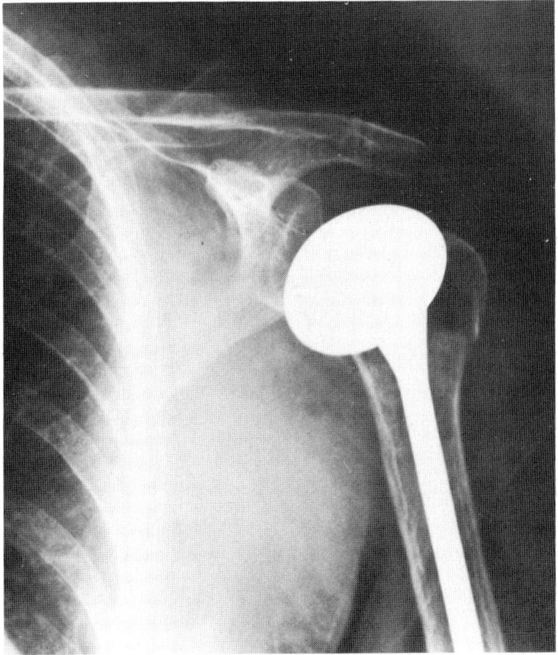

Fig. 23-4. Hemiarthroplasty with the tuberosity secured to the flange by heavy sutures.

identical to that of the three-part fractures. An extra screw may be required to fix the lesser tuberosity to the head fragment. Again, in both instances, early postoperative mobilization is important.

Head-splitting fractures

This group of patients, of course, does not fit perfectly into the two-, three-, or four-part classification. The head-splitting can be from direct trauma longitudinally along the axis of the humerus or can be an anteroposterior fracture-dislocation. The anterior dislocation with humeral head fracture is often the Hill-Sachs type, and the problems associated with this injury are far different from that of other injuries. It is rare to find a large humeral head defect associated with an anterior dislocation. More often than not, the anterior dislocation in the older patient is either associated with a rotator cuff tear or a displaced fracture of the greater tuberosity with a rotator cuff tear. The treatment of these fractures or rotator cuff injuries is as described under two-part fractures (displaced tuberosity fractures). The remaining two entities, head-splitting fractures and posterior fracture-dislocations, are therapeutic problems.

Head-splitting fracture without dislocation usually occurs in the younger patient. Motorcycle accidents, surfing injuries, and other athletic endeavors in the young adult are often the cause for this problem (Fig. 23-5, *A* and *B*). As a result, one is loathe to place a humeral head prosthesis into someone so young. These fracture fragments usually have good soft-tissue attachment, and, if they can be restored to a congruous articular surface of the humeral head, they will survive. It is therefore often possible to piece these fragments together and fix them with Kirschner wires and cancellous screws and produce quite satisfactory results (Fig. 23-5, *C* and *D*).

The posterior fracture-dislocation is important because it is commonly misdiagnosed (Fig. 23-6, *A*). An axillary view is mandatory to establish the posterior dislocation (Fig. 23-6, *B*). Experienced observers, of course, can often make the diagnosis on an anteroposterior roentgenogram, but the confirmation of the axillary view is necessary to avoid missing the diagnosis. Physical findings include a locked internal rotation deformity, a prominent coracoid and anterior acromion, and a history of seizure (epileptic, alcoholic, or head trauma). Because this diagnosis is frequently missed in emergency rooms or by treating physicians, many of these patients will have a long history of a stiff, painful shoulder after a seizure and failure to respond to physical therapy.

If seen early, closed reduction may be successful. The arm can then be immobilized posterior to the coronal plane of the body, and the reduction is usually stable. If it is not stable, open reduction may be necessary. Occasionally transfer of the subscapularis with or without a block of bone will be needed to provide stability. In some cases transfixion of the humeral head to the glenoid with a Steinman pin or a wood screw is also of use. In the early phases, if closed reduction is unsuccessful, open

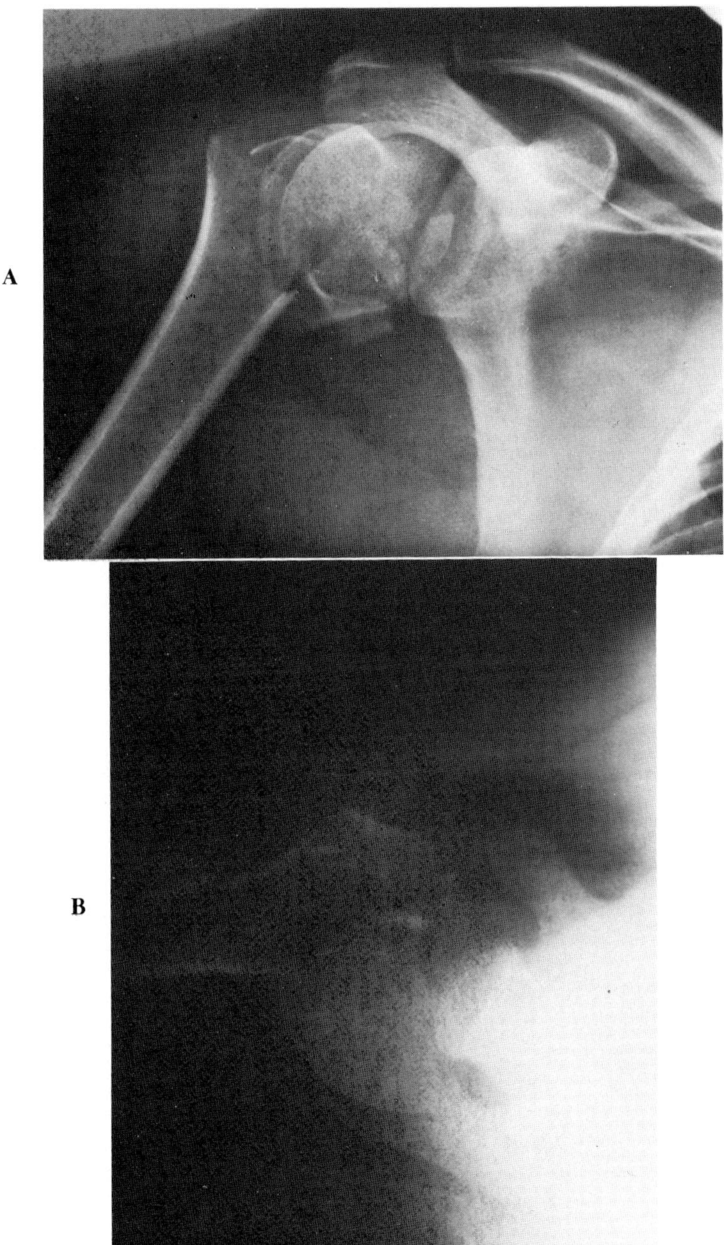

Fig. 23-5. A, Anteroposterior roentgenogram of a head-splitting fracture without glenohumeral dislocation. **B,** Axillary roentgenogram showing the extent of a comminution of the head.

Continued.

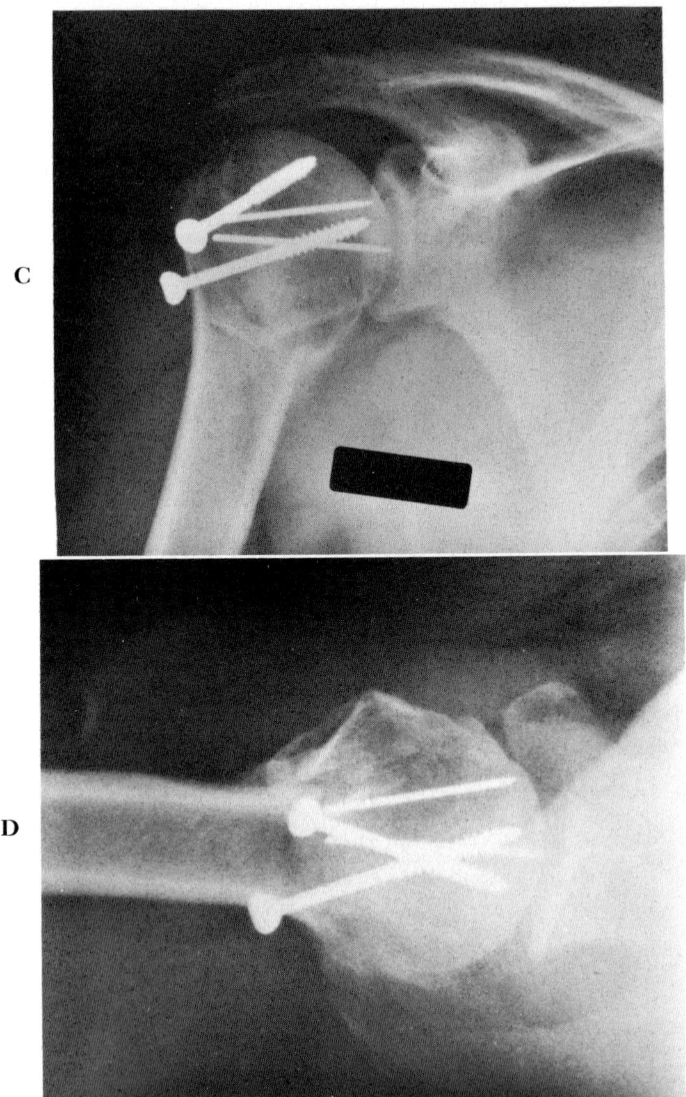

Fig. 23-5, cont'd. C, Anteroposterior roentgenogram postoperatively with the humeral head configuration restored and fixed internally. **D,** Axillary roentgenogram of the same postoperative shoulder.

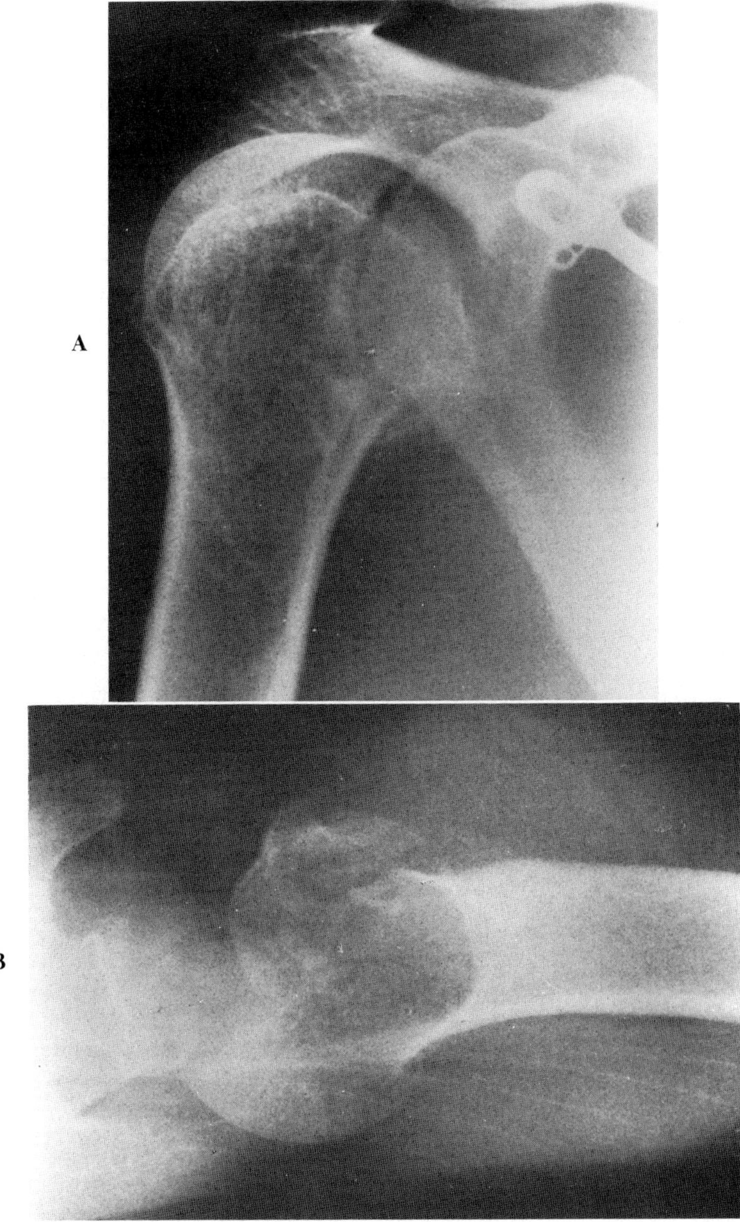

Fig. 23-6. A, Anteroposterior roentgenogram of a posterior fracture-dislocation. The diagnosis is more difficult to make on the anteroposterior projection. **B,** Axillary roentgenogram shows the posterior dislocation of the head with an impaction fracture of the anterior surface at the humeral head.   *Continued.*

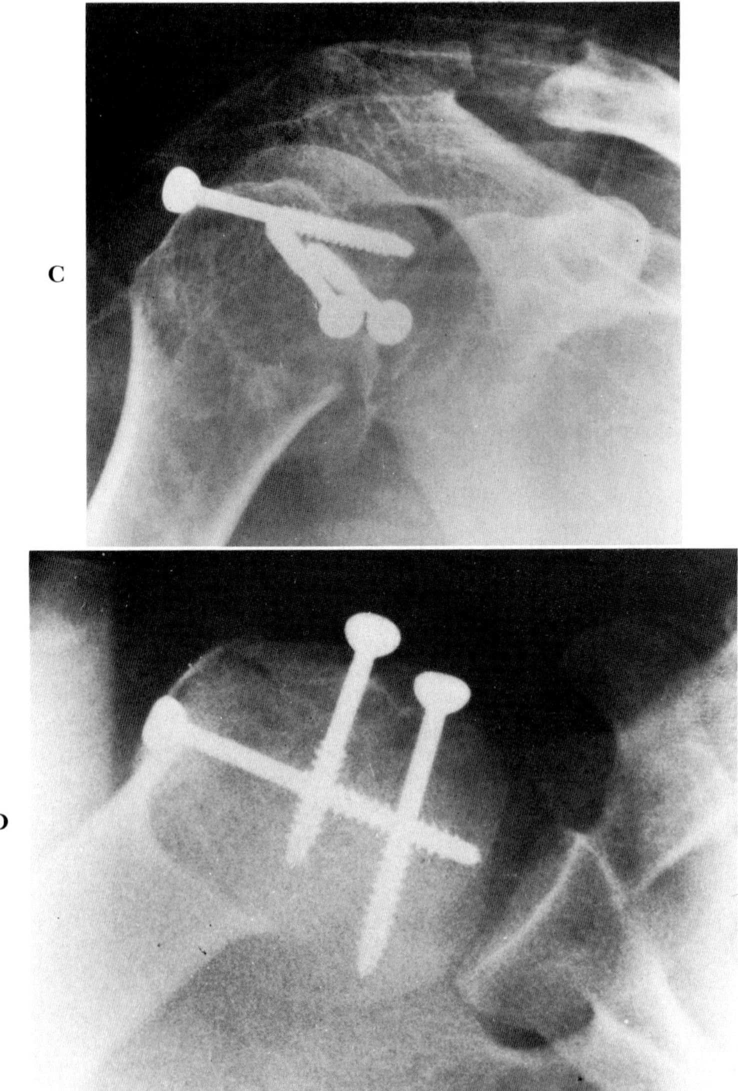

Fig. 23-6, cont'd. C, Anteroposterior roentgenogram showing the posterior fracture-dislocation reduced, the head reconstituted in an anatomic fashion, and the fragments fixed with cancellous screws. **D,** Axillary roentgenogram of the same case postoperatively.

reduction can be carried out with elevation of the compressed articular fragments, which can then be fixed in anatomic position by appropriate fixation devices (Fig. 23-6, *C* and *D*).

FRACTURES OF THE CLAVICLE

Fractures of the clavicle occur with significant frequency. They usually involve the diaphyseal or midshaft portion of the clavicle but occasionally will involve the lateral third. Those involving the outer third constitute a special problem, which will be discussed.

Diaphyseal clavicular fractures

Diaphyseal clavicular fractures occur from a fall on the posterosuperior aspect of the shoulder. This causes a buckling phenomenon that produces the midshaft fracture. These can all be treated by a simple figure-of-eight harness. Anatomic reduction is not necessary and rarely indicated. Open reduction is virtually never necessary except under extremely rare circumstances. Perhaps the only indication for open reduction would be a compromise of the brachial plexus or subclavian artery, which cannot be improved by closed treatment. The figure-of-eight strap has been most useful in treating patients with these injuries. It generally requires 6 to 8 weeks before healing is sufficient to allow free motion of the shoulder. In that interval, forward flexion and abduction of the arm in a 30-degree range is permissible and usually helps prevent any posttraumatic stiffness of the shoulder joint itself. Although better control can be obtained with a plaster jacket, this is rarely necessary. Most patients do not complain about the mild shortening with which most clavicular fractures heal, nor do they complain about the occasional prominence of a small spike of bone at the fracture site. If the latter proves to be a problem, a small incision can be made under local anesthesia and the spike removed with a rongeur.

Probably the most common reason for failure of union with the midshaft fractures is early open reduction and internal fixation. The devices advocated for this include a threaded Steinman pin introduced retrogradely and a compression plating, but both are fraught with danger. The Steinman pin will tend to distract the fragment, since it is threaded throughout its entire length. If not threaded, it has the potential to migrate and in any case must be removed. The plate has the possibility of fracturing if used improperly and, of course, must be removed because it is prominent underneath the skin. A technique described in 1975 has been used with success in treating nonunions of clavicular fractures as well as the rare, occasional primary open reduction.[5] A Knowles pin is placed through the medullary cavity of the straight portion of the clavicle. It is introduced immediately behind the lateral third. It has been used with and without a bone graft. It provides secure, compressive fixation and satisfactory healing for both acute fractures and nonunions (Fig. 23-7) and does not need to be removed.

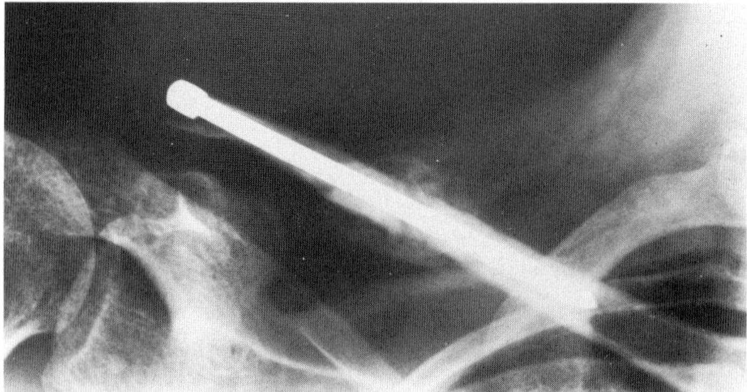

Fig. 23-7. Clavicular fracture that has been bone grafted and fixed internally with a Knowles pin.

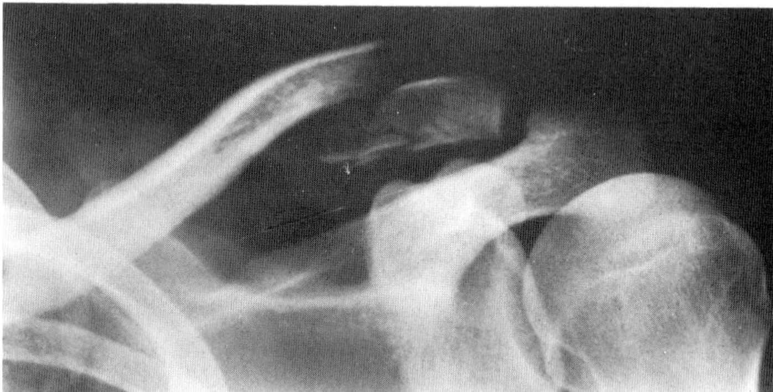

Fig. 23-8. Fracture of the outer third of the clavicle with disruption of the coracoclavicular ligaments.

Fractures of the lateral third

Fractures of the lateral third are either short, oblique fractures with rupture of the coracoclavicular ligaments (Fig. 23-8) or intra-articular fractures in which the cora-coacromial ligaments are intact and attached to the remaining inferior articular fragment (Fig. 23-9). In both instances, primary open reduction should be undertaken unless otherwise contraindicated. These fractures will not unite satisfactorily otherwise and not only will leave a deformity, but can also cause pain. The technique for stabilizing the nonarticular lateral third clavicular fractures has usually been through the introduction of the transarticular medullary smooth pin, which is crimped on the lateral end to prevent migration (Fig. 23-10). Although this technique has been performed successfully, it can leave a slight, bony prominence and a scar at the site of pin introduction. In those who are concerned about esthetics, when the obliquity of the fracture permits, cerclage wiring is also useful and avoids the cosmetic problems of the intermedullary pin. This can be done through a short, vertical skin incision, which

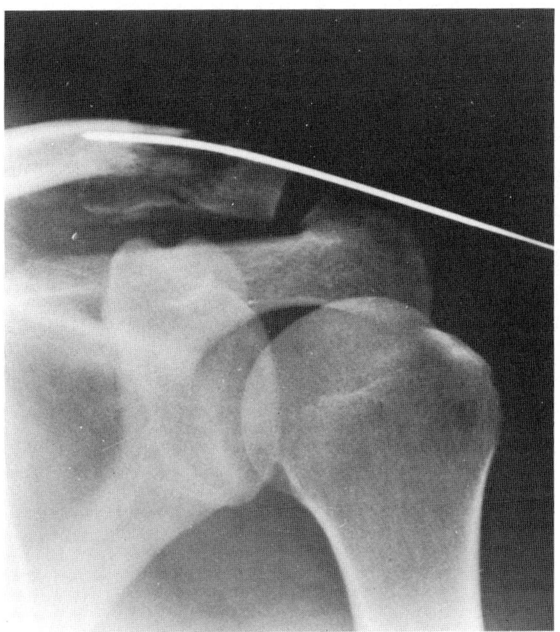

Fig. 23-9. Avulsion fracture of the clavicle involving the acromioclavicular joint with the coracoclavicular ligaments attached to the inferior fragment.

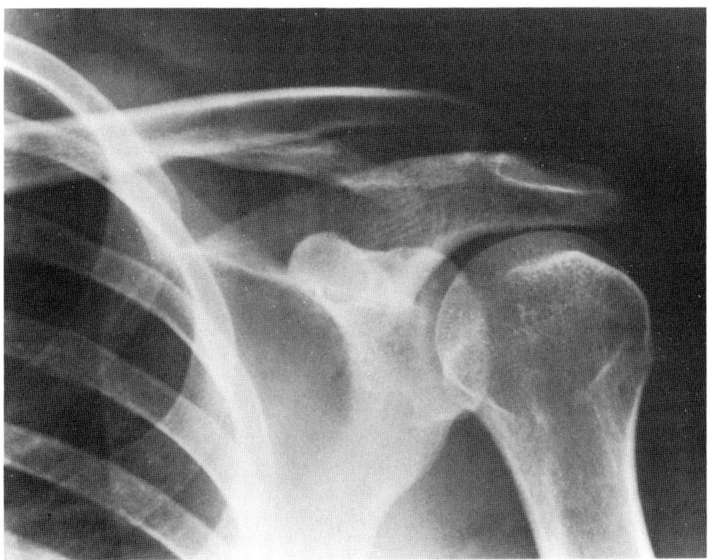

Fig. 23-10. Internal fixation of the lateral third fracture seen in Fig. 23-8.

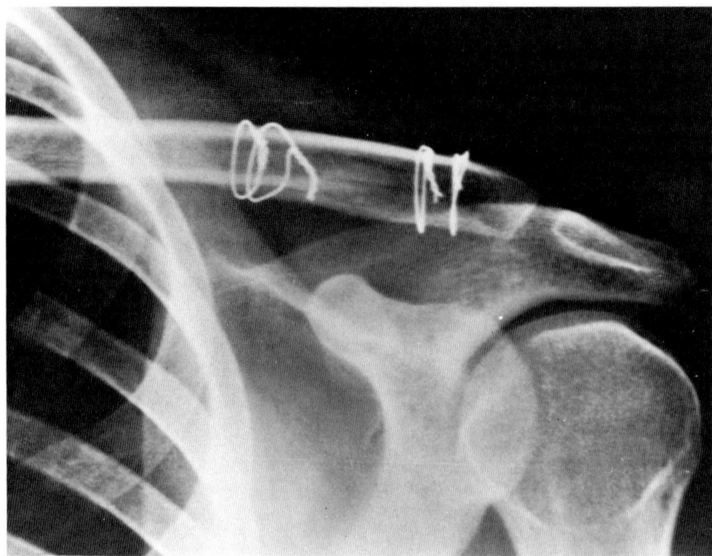

Fig. 23-11. Alternative fixation techniques for oblique fractures in this area, same as that in Fig. 23-9.

is far preferable to the transverse incison, which leaves a very unsightly scar.

The articular fractures with the intact ligaments also should be treated by open reduction and internal fixation. This can readily be accomplished through a vertical esthetic skin incision with cerclage wires for fixation (Fig. 23-11).

FRACTURES OF THE SCAPULA

Fractures of the scapula can either be of the glenoid, scapular neck, or the body. Fortunately these are very uncommon and rarely require anything more than immobilization for comfort. The scapula is encased in a muscular envelope, which provides support for the fractures allowing them to heal quite readily.

Fractures of the glenoid

Fractures of the glenoid usually occur from longitudinal, direct impact in line with the humerus. Multiple fracture lines are often seen in the glenoid, but rarely are they significantly displaced. This is a result of the attachment of the glenohumeral capsule as well as the surrounding rotator cuff, which tends to keep the fracture fragments from separating widely. As a result, open reduction with internal fixation should be done only with a single major fragment that is depressed and has the potential to lead to either posttraumatic arthrosis or instability.

Fractures of the body and neck of the scapula

As already indicated, although these are seen with more frequency than those in the glenoid, they rarely require anything more than immobilizaton for comfort. Since they are surrounded by a muscular envelope, this provides adequate support and a generous blood supply to provide healing. A sling and swathe for comfort is often used until the acute effects of the injury have passed. At that time progressive motion is encouraged so that posttraumatic stiffness will not occur.

REFERENCES

1. Codman, E.A.: The shoulder, Boston, 1934, Thomas Todd & Co.
2. McLaughlin, H.L.: Trauma, Philadelphia, 1959, W.B. Saunders Co.
3. Neer, C.S.: Anterior displaced proximal humeral fractures: 1. Classification and evaluation, J. Bone Joint Surg. **54A:**1077, 1970.
4. Neviaser, J.S.: Injuries in and about the shoulder joint, American Academy of Orthopaedic Surgeons: Instructional Course Lectures **13:**187, Ann Arbor, Mich., 1956, J. W. Edwards.
5. Neviaser, R.J., et al.: A simple technique for internal fixation of the clavicle—a long term evaluation, Clin. Orthop. (109):103, 1975.
6. Neviaser, R.J.: Tears of the rotator cuff, Orthop. Clin. North Am. **11:**295, 1980.
7. Neviaser, R.J., and Neviaser, T.J.: Lesions of the musculotendinous cuff and capsule of the shoulder—diagnosis and management, Part A: Tears of the rotator cuff, American Academy of Orthopaedic Surgeons: Instructional Course Lectures **30:**239, St. Louis, 1981, The C.V. Mosby Co.

24. Acromioclavicular joint injuries in athletes

Jay S. Cox

Acute injuries of the acromioclavicular joint are quite common in sports. They occur usually from a direct fall on the point of the shoulder driving the acromion down away from the clavicle. The amount of force involved will determine what ligaments are injured. The acromioclavicular ligament and joint capsule are the first to fail followed by the coracoclavicular ligaments. There is another type of injury that occurs from a fall on the elbow or the outstretched hand that drives the humeral head upward against the acromion causing damage to the acromioclavicular joint capsule and ligament. This does not tear the coracoclavicular ligament and is a rare injury.

The amount of displacement of the distal clavicle depends on the injuries to the various supporting structures. The extent of rupture of the acromioclavicular ligament and capsule, the extent of rupture of the coracoclavicular ligaments, and the extent of rupture of the trapezius and deltoid musclature determines the position and displacement of the distal end of the clavicle. In the acromioclavicular joint, horizontal stability of the distal end of the clavicle depends on the acromioclavicular ligament and the vertical stability depends on the coracoclavicular ligament. Anteroposterior roentgenograms of acromioclavicular joints with and without weights hung on the wrists are obtained to determine the position of the distal end of the clavicle. Injured and uninjured sides are compared. The roentgen beam should be angled slightly upward in taking the films to offset the clavicular shadow from the acromial shadow. The intensity of the beam should be less than in a regular shoulder roentgenogram.

CLASSIFICATION OF INJURIES (Fig. 24-1)

Rockwood[6] has a new classification for acromioclavicular injuries. Type I has not been changed and is a partial tear of the acromioclavicular ligament with no upward displacement of the distal end of the clavicle. The roentgenograms are normal. The type II injury is a complete rupture of the acromioclavicular ligament and capsule and a partial tear of the coracoclavicular ligament. This allows slight upward displacement of the distal end of the clavicle, and by definition of type II the clavicle is not elevated

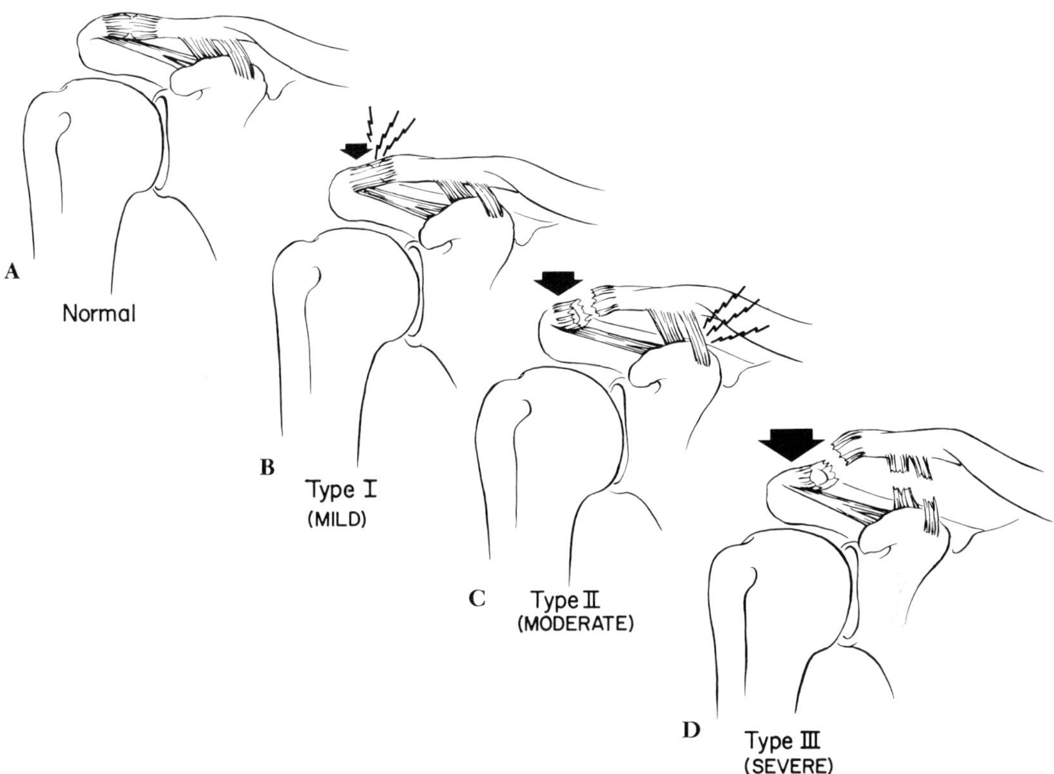

Fig. 24-1. These schematic drawings illustrate the ligamentous injuries that occur to the acromioclavicular joint. **A,** Normal anatomic relationships. **B,** In type I injury, a mild force is applied to the point of the shoulder, which stretches only the acromioclavicular joints but does not disrupt the fibers of the joint. **C,** In type II injury, a moderate force applied to the point of the shoulder displaces the acromion process distally, disrupts the acromioclavicular ligaments, and may partially stretch the coracoclavicular ligaments. **D,** In type III injury, the severe force applied to the point of the shoulder drives the acromion and accompanying coracoid process downward, disrupting both the acromioclavicular and coracoclavicular ligaments. (Modified from Allman, F.L.: J. Bone Joint Surg. **49A:**774, 1967. In Rockwood, C.A., and Green, O.P., editors: Fractures in adults, ed. 2, Philadelphia, 1984, J.B. Lippincott Co.)

above the acromion. This type II injury classification is also not changed.

The type III injury is a rupture of the acromioclavicular and the coracoclavicular ligaments with upward displacement of the distal end of the clavicle above the acromion. Measurement of the distance between the coracoid and the clavicle in both the injured and the uninjured shoulders on the roentgenogram will show any upward displacement of the clavicle. Normally this distance is 11 to 13 mm.[6] A difference of 5 mm between the injured and uninjured shoulder is very significant, and probably a difference of 3 mm of upward displacement is significant. The coracoclavicular ligament is really the prime suspensory ligament of the upper extremity. When it is ruptured, the distal end of the clavicle is not elevated—the shoulder is depressed.

Rockwood[6] has added new classifications of the more severe acromioclavicular injuries. In the type IV injury the distal clavicle ruptures through the deltoid or trapezius muscles. This may occur superiorly or posteriorly. The distal end of the clavicle can usually not be reduced because of the muscle entrapment. This is essentially an irreducible type III injury. In this injury the physical examination may be a better indicator than the roentgenogram. The distal end of the clavicle can be palpated posteriorly. On the roentgenogram, the distal end of the clavicle may not be elevated, and the diagnosis will be missed. Type IV injuries may be misclassified as type II because of the appearance on the standard anteroposterior roentgenogram. A special view as described by Alexander[1] will help to clarify this injury and will show the posterior position of the clavicle.

The type V injury is a complete acromioclavicular dislocation with rupture of the deltoid-trapezius musculature. The distal end of the clavicle is covered only by skin and subcutaneous tissue and is easily palpated under the skin.

The type VI injury is very unusual and very rare. It involves an injury to the sternoclavicular joint and the acromioclavicular joint with the distal end of the clavicle displaced under the coracoid over the tendons of the biceps and the coracobrachialis.

TREATMENT OF ACROMIOCLAVICULAR INJURIES

Treatment of type I injuries involves symptomatic treatment only. This includes temporary immobilization with a sling, ice application, analgesics and anti-inflammatory medications for symptomatic relief, and early rehabilitation of the musculature.

In the type II injury, two methods of treatment are available. The first is symptomatic treatment similar to the treatment of the type I injury. The second is treatment with an acromioclavicular immobilizer for 4 weeks. At the U.S. Naval Academy, 32 of these type II injuries were treated symptomatically and 20 were treated with the immobilizer for 4 weeks.[2] The results were that 62.5% of those treated by symptomatic treatment had residual symptoms. Only 25% of those treated in the immobilizer had residual symptoms. It is my opinion that the reason for this is that with an unreduced distal end of the clavicle the forces across the acromioclavicular joint will be abnormal and produce symptoms of pain and crepitus. In the type III injury the distal end of the clavicle is elevated above the acromion and so there is no articulation at the joint. These unreduced type III injuries may have less residual symptoms than the type II injuries. When the anatomy is restored by reduction and immobilization in the type II injuries the patients had less late symptoms.[2]

Treatment of the type III injury has long been controversial. Three different types of treatment utilized are symptomatic treatment similar to type I injuries, reduction and immobilization with an acromioclavicular immobilizer, and surgical open reduction and fixation of the acromioclavicular joint. If the distal end of the clavicle cannot be reduced manually, the acromioclavicular immobilizer should not be used. Problems with the immobilizer are patient compliance, loss of position, skin irritation and maceration, and stiffness of the shoulder, particularly in older patients. The treatment of these type III injuries is discussed in more detail later in this chapter.

Treatment of the type IV and type V injuries is surgical. The surgical procedures available are (1) acromioclavicular joint repair, fixation, or reconstruction with or without the coracoclavicular repair, and (2) coracoclavicular ligament repair, fixation , or reconstruction. Dynamic muscle transfers with fixation of the tip of the coracoid and the muscle origins of the short head of the biceps and coracobrachialis to the clavicle are not used very often.

Temporary fixation across the acromioclavicular joint with pins or wires has been a popular method during surgical repair. If wires are used, they should be bent at the exposed end to prevent migration and the wires should be of sufficient width to prevent breakage. Wires may damage the articular cartilage of the acromion or the distal end of the clavicle. Fixation of the clavicle to the coracoid process can be accomplished with a screw, wire, tape, fascia, or suture. Complications of the screw are loosening, breakage, or rarely injury to the brachial plexus or brachial arteries or veins. Complications of fascia, wire, or tape are fractures through the drill hole in the clavicle or erosion through the clavicle.

Although the treatment of the type IV and type V injuries is generally regarded as surgical restoration of the anatomy, the uncomplicated type III injury has been a subject of some controversy. In 1974 Powers and Bach[5] sent a questionnaire to all the orthopaedic training programs in the United States to determine the current method of treatment of the type III injury. They did not differentiate between the simple type III injury or the complicated injuries now classified as types IV and V. The majority of the program chairmen in 1974 were treating the type III injury by surgery. Ninety-five percent recommended surgical repair and fixation, with 60% recommending acromioclavicular fixation with wires or pins and 35% recommending coracoclavicular fixation usually by a screw. Nonoperative treatment was rarely advocated. In 1976 Imatani et al.[4] reported very good results using nonoperative treatment in complete dislocations of the acromioclavicular joint. In 1977 Glick[3] reported successful results with nonoperative treatment in professional football players in type III injuries.

To determine the current method of treatment in an uncomplicated type III injury, questionnaires were sent to several sports medicine–oriented orthopaedic surgeons and also the chairmen of the orthopaedic residency training programs. Of the sports medicine–oriented surgeons, almost 75% recommended nonoperative treatment for the uncomplicated type III acromioclavicular injury. The majority of those who did recommend surgery utilized some type of fixation between the coracoid and the clavicle. Many of these sports physicians qualified their recommended treatment by stating that in athletes playing sports such as football, hockey, lacrosse, and rugby the majority of them would recommend the nonoperative treatment. However, in a throwing athlete with an injury to the dominant shoulder, most recommended restoration of anatomy by surgical repair.

The orthopaedic surgeons in charge of residency training programs also had a majority recommending nonoperative treatment, but this was only 58% as compared to the 75% of the sports physicians recommending the nonoperative treatment. Thirty-three percent of this group were using symptomatic treatment for type III, and 25% were using an acromioclavicular immobilizer for 4 to 6 weeks. Of those 42% recommending surgery, more recommended wires or pins across the acromioclavicular joint than some type of fixation between the coracoid and the clavicle. Therefore the surgical choice of the sports medicine surgeons was tape, wire, or fascia fixation between the coracoid and the clavicle, but in the orthopaedic training programs there is a slight tendency to favor acromioclavicular fixation. In response to a question about excision of the distal end of the clavicle in an acute repair, approximately 25% in each group recommended excision.

The general principles of surgical repair are reduction and fixation of the distal clavicle, débridement of the acromioclavicular joint, repair of the coracoclavicular ligaments, repair of the acromioclavicular ligaments, and repair of the deltoid and trapezius musculature. The distal end of the clavicle is not excised unless damaged or unless there are existing changes in the joint at the time of surgical repair.

Deltoid and trapezius muscle aponeurosis repair is very important. This musculature across the superior surface of the clavicle and acromion is frequently damaged and if not repaired may cause residual pain and weakness. Excision of the distal end of the clavicle is rarely indicated in acute repairs, but it is recommended if the surfaces are damaged.

The surgical treatment of chronic pain in the acromioclavicular joint involves excision of approximately 1.5 cm of the distal end of the clavicle. If too much of the distal end of the clavicle is excised, a floating unstable clavicle will result. If too little is excised, impingement of the clavicle on the acromion may cause persistent pain.

The recommended surgical treatment of the chronic dislocation is excision of the distal end of the clavicle and reconstruction of the coracoclavicular ligament. One excellent method of reconstruction described by Rockwood[6] involves the surgical incision in Langer's lines across the acromioclavicular joint. The coracoacromial ligament is identified and cut at its attachment on the acromion. Sutures are placed through this severed end of the ligament, and drill holes are made in the distal clavicle for fixation. Thus the coracoacromial ligament is used to reconstruct the coracoclavicular ligaments. A screw for temporary fixation is placed between the clavicle and the coracoid, and the distal end of the clavicle is excised.

Late roentgenographic changes in the acromioclavicular joints that have been injured are present in a high percentage of patients regardless of the type of injury.[2] These changes included resorption of the distal end of the clavicle, blunting, osteophyte formation, and irregularities of the acromioclavicular joint. These changes were not correlated with symptoms or physical findings and appear to be posttraumatic changes rather than degenerative arthritis.

In summary, the horizontal stability of the distal clavicle depends on the acromioclavicular ligament, and vertical stability depends on the coracoclavicular ligament. Type I injuries are treated symptomatically. Type II injuries can be treated symptomatically or with an immobilizer. Those treated with the immobilizers did have decreased symptoms and physical findings.[2] Type III injuries are controversial, but there is the choice of symptomatic treatment, joint immobilizer, and surgery to correct the deformity. The majority of orthopaedic surgeons seem to favor nonoperative treatment for these type III injuries at the present time. In the type III injuries of the dominant extremity of a throwing athlete, most surgeons recommend surgical restoration of the anatomy. Treatment of the type IV and V injuries is in most instances surgical correction and repair of the trapezius deltoid musculature.

The Alexander roentgenographic view will help show posterior displacement of the distal end of the clavicle in the type III or type IV injury.

Methods of surgical correction include pin or wire fixation across the joint with repair of ligaments or fixation between the coracoid and the clavicle with either a screw, wire, fascia, or tape with or without the repair of the coracoclavicular ligaments.

Surgical treatment of chronic pain involves excision of the distal 1.5 cm of the clavicle. Excision of too much gives a floating unstable clavicle, but excision of too little may give continued impingement. For chronic painful dislocation of the distal end of the clavicle, surgery involves excision of the distal end of the clavicle, reconstruction of the coracoclavicular ligament, and temporary fixation of the distal end of the clavicle with pins across the acromioclavicular joint or a screw between the clavicle and the coracoid. Roentgenographic changes are very common after acromioclavicular joint injuries but may be entirely asymptomatic.

REFERENCES

1. Alexander, O.M.: Radiography of the acromioclavicular articulation, Med. Radiography Photography **30**:34-39, 1954.
2. Cox, J.S.: The fate of the acromioclavicular joint in athletic injuries, Am. J. Sports Med. **5**:258-263, 1977.
3. Glick, J.M., Milburn, L.J., Haggerty, J.F., and Nishimoto, D.: Dislocated acromioclavicular joint: follow-up study of 35 unreduced acromioclavicular dislocations, Am. J. Sports Med. **5**:264-270, 1977.
4. Imatani, R.J., Hanlon, J.J., and Cady, G.W.: Acute complete acromioclavicular separations, J. Bone Joint Surg. **57A**:328-331, 1975.
5. Powers, J.A., and Bach, P.J.: Acromioclavicular separation: closed or open treatment, Clin. Orthop. (104):213-223, 1974.
6. Rockwood, C.A., and Green, O.P.: Fractures in adults, ed. 2, Philadelphia, 1984, J.B. Lippincott Co., Vol. 1.

25. Anterior subluxation and dislocation of the shoulder

Bertram Zarins

This chapter deals with anterior instability of the glenohumeral joint in athletes: incidence of injury, classification of shoulder instability, diagnosis, pathologic findings in anterior instability, treatment of anterior subluxation and dislocation, recurrent instability after surgical repair, and rehabilitation.

INCIDENCE IN SPORTS

The overall incidence of shoulder injury sustained in 21 common sports (excluding football) at a college was reported to be 16%.[10] In studies of high school and professional football, 10% of injuries were to the shoulder.[16,23] The injuries were not broken down into percentage of dislocation or subluxation.

The incidence of anterior subluxation or dislocation as a percentage of all injuries in specific sports was found to be as follows: baseball, 4%[5]; wrestling, 4%[24]; and skiing, 2.5%.[6,25] Shoulder dislocations accounted for 10% of all upper extremity injuries in skiing.[15]

CLASSIFICATIONS OF GLENOHUMERAL INSTABILITY

The term "instability" is used in this chapter as a general term to include both dislocation and subluxation. Glenohumeral instability can be classified as follows:
1. *Direction* of instability: anterior, posterior, inferior, or multidirectional
2. *Severity* or degree of instability: subluxation (the humeral head momentarily slips in and out of the joint) or dislocation (humeral head stays out of the socket)
3. *Time:* primary (first time dislocated), recurrent, or chronic[21] (unreduced)
4. *Cause:* traumatic, atraumatic, voluntary, or neuromuscular

Adjectives from all four categories are used to completely describe shoulder instability. Thus a first-time dislocation can be termed "primary, traumatic anterior glenohumeral dislocation." A shoulder that momentarily slips out of joint without having sustained an injury can be called "recurrent atraumatic anterior glenohumeral subluxation" and so forth.

"

This chapter deals with anterior glenohumeral subluxation and dislocation, acute and recurrent.

MECHANISMS OF INJURY

In order for the humeral head to be subluxated or dislocated anteriorly the elbow and hand must move posteriorly. In other words, the arm must go behind the coronal plane of the body. The most common mechanism of injury is the arm being forced into excessive abduction, extension, and external rotation as in cocking the arm to throw a baseball or serve in tennis.[2] If the arm is already maximally externally rotated in a position of abduction and is forced into further external rotation or extension, the force drives the humeral head anteriorly. This can avulse the anterior capsule and labrum from the glenoid rim (Bankart lesion).[4] As the humeral head comes out of the socket, compression of the posterior humeral head against the anterior glenoid rim can result in injury to the posterior humeral head (Hill-Sachs lesion).

A less common mechanism of injury is hyperextension of the arm behind the body. It is also possible to dislocate the humeral head anteriorly by direct trauma if a blow comes from the posterior aspect of the shoulder.

Electromyographic studies have been done by Jobe et al.[11] showing the activity of various muscles in different phases of pitching. There is a "silent phase" characterized by a relative absence of electrical activity in the shoulder muscles when the arm is in the overhead position (windup or preparation stage and also early acceleration phase). This absence indicates that the rotator cuff may function to stabilize the humeral head rather than to move it during throwing.

DIAGNOSIS OF ANTERIOR SHOULDER INSTABILITY

In obtaining the history of injury, a description of the exact position of the arm at the time of the initial injury will lead to an understanding of the direction of motion of the humeral head. In cases in which the inciting event was atraumatic, determine the motion causing the onset of the symptoms. For example, determine which phase of the pitching act caused symptoms: windup, cocking, acceleration, ball release and deceleration, or follow-through. The same type of information is needed when the history is elicited in cases of recurrent instability.

It is important to know how much trauma caused the initial dislocation or subluxation. Determine the amount of force that causes recurrent symptoms, and whether the patient can voluntarily recreate the instability using muscular action. Other factors that will influence decision making are whether the dominant shoulder is involved, the sport in which the athlete participates, and the position played if it is a team sport.

In performing a physical examination, try to reproduce the position of the arm causing symptoms and apply stress in the direction that will tend to force the humeral head out of the joint. For anterior instability, the position of the arm is typically 90 degrees of abduction, extension, and external rotation. In this position, externally rotate the arm while pushing forward on the posterior aspect of the humeral head. A

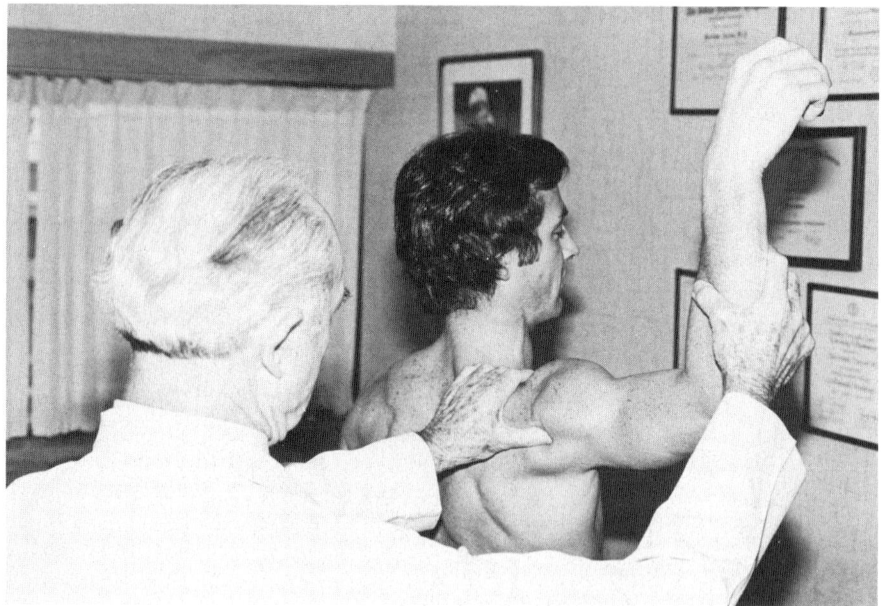

Fig. 25-1. Examination of right shoulder for anterior instability. The arm is in a position of extension, 90 to 120 degrees of abduction, and maximal external rotation. The patient's shoulder is externally rotated further while the examiner pushes forward on the posterior aspect of the humeral head ("apprehension test").

positive "apprehension test" is suggestive of anterior shoulder instability[20] (Fig. 25-1).

Always check the opposite shoulder, and compare the degree of external rotation on both sides. A baseball pitcher will typically have increased external rotation and slight limitation of internal rotation of the throwing shoulder compared to the non-dominant shoulder.[14] This is the physiologic pattern for the pitcher.

With the arm in the neutral position and the patient bending forward slightly at the waist, grasp the humeral head with one hand and try to move it in an anteroposterior direction. The patient's shoulder muscles should remain relaxed (Fig. 25-2). Compare the amount of laxity with the contralateral (normal) shoulder.

In patients in whom anterior shoulder subluxation is suspected because of symptoms and confirmed by a positive apprehension test, check the shoulder for stability in other directions. With the arm in abduction push down on the humeral head to look for inferior instability (Fig. 25-3). To detect posterior instability, apply a posteriorly directed force to the arm in a position of adduction, internal rotation, and 90-degree forward flexion (Fig. 25-4). These tests will help detect multidirectional instability.

Routine roentgenograms are taken in the anteroposterior projection with the arm in neutral rotation, 60-degree internal rotation, and 60-degree external rotation. One of the projections should be on a large film to include a portion of the chest and spine

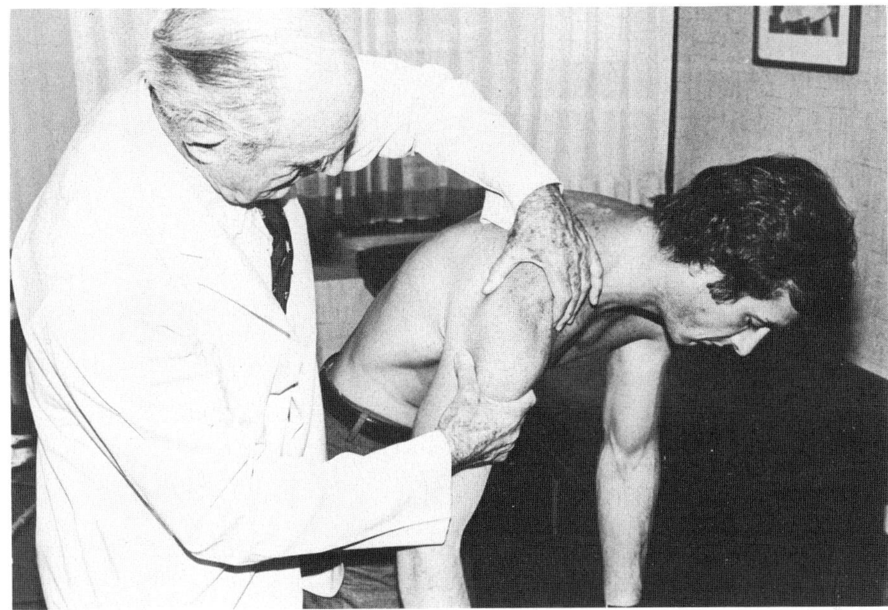

Fig. 25-2. Determining anteroposterior humeral head laxity. The patient bends forward at the waist and relaxes the shoulder muscles. The examiner grasps the patient's scapula with one hand and the humeral head with the other and translocates the humeral head in an anteroposterior direction.

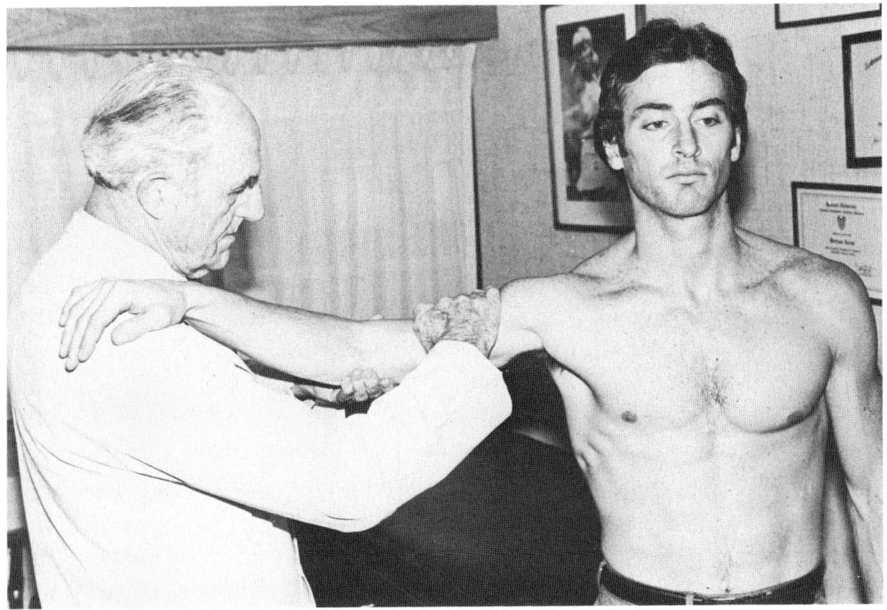

Fig. 25-3. Examination for inferior instability. With the patient's shoulder abducted 90 degrees, push downward on the humeral head and upward on the elbow.

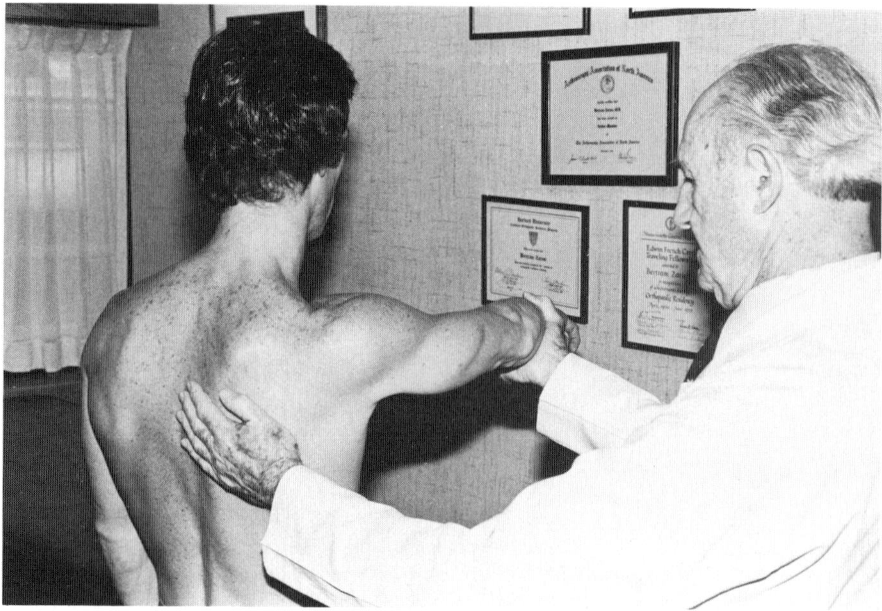

Fig. 25-4. To detect posterior instability, apply a posteriorly directed force to the shoulder in a position of adduction, internal rotation, and 90 degrees of forward flexion.

to look for possible causes of referred pain to the shoulder. A 30-degree oblique view is excellent for showing a tangential view of the glenoid cavity. An axillary view should always be taken. Look for a Hill-Sachs lesion of the posterior humeral head and a defect in the anterior glenoid rim. Arthrography is ordinarily not useful to diagnose instability though axillary views might outline the glenoid cavity and labrum. For better visualization of the glenoid rim axillary arthrotomography is usually most useful.[8] Computerized tomography scans occasionally give additional information.[7]

Arthroscopy can be very useful by allowing visualization of the entire glenoid labrum as well as the posterior half of the humeral head. This will allow localization of tears in the glenoid rim or labrum giving indirect evidence of direction of the humeral head subluxation. For example, avulsion of the anterior labrum from the glenoid rim (Bankart lesion) is consistent with anterior instability. Visualization of a Hill-Sachs lesion is further evidence to support this diagnosis. Arthroscopy is especially useful in cases in which the direction of dislocation has never been documented or in patients with suspected multidirectional instability.

Electromyography is ordinarily not useful in diagnosing anterior instability. It can be revealing in patients who have voluntary instability as a means of determining the muscle pattern causing the dislocation.[13]

In evaluating the patient's shoulder symptoms, keep in mind other pathologic conditions that refer pain to the shoulder. The symptoms of thoracic outlet syndrome can be reproduced when one holds the arm in the abducted, externally rotated over-

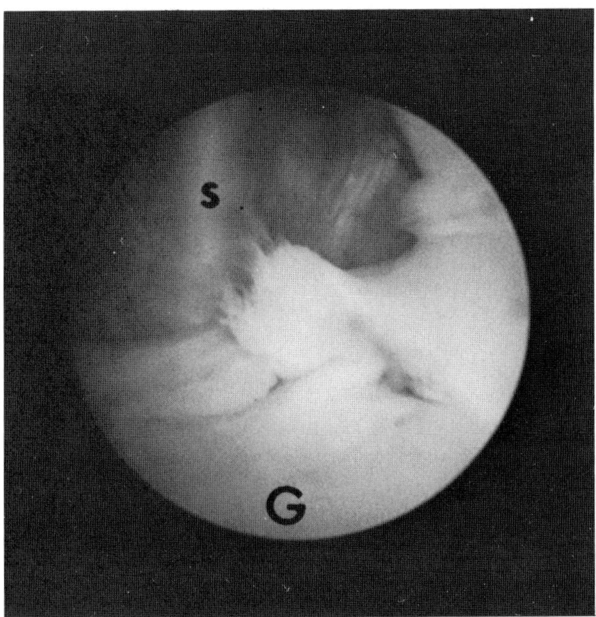

Fig. 25-5. Arthroscopic view of torn anterior superior labrum from the glenoid rim, left shoulder. There is no tearing or detachment of the capsule. *G,* Glenoid cavity; *S,* subscapularis tendon; *upper right,* biceps tendon.

head position. Also consider other shoulder derangements such as impingement syndromes, rotator cuff lesions, acromioclavicular joint injury, and other neurovascular syndromes.

PATHOLOGY OF ANTERIOR SHOULDER INSTABILITY

Excessive laxity of the anterior shoulder capsule is a common cause of anterior instability and is frequently the primary lesion.[20,22] This is especially true in cases of atraumatic subluxation or in shoulders in which minimal trauma was responsible for the shoulder instability. Excessive capsular laxity can be estimated at the time of shoulder surgery after the subscapularis tendon has been dissected from the underlying capsule. Rotate the arm into complete external rotation and pick up the anterior shoulder capsule with tissue forceps. The amount of slack in the capsule can be graded based on the distance the capsule can be lifted from the humeral head.

The anterior capsule and labrum can be avulsed from the glenoid rim without bony injury. Also the capsule and labrum can remain attached to the glenoid rim, but the rim itself can be fractured at various distances from the anterior edge of the glenoid cavity. A large fracture of the glenoid rim is usually the result of significant trauma causing the initial shoulder dislocation.

It is possible to tear the labrum itself without detaching the capsule from the glenoid rim (Fig. 25-5). It is also possible to tear the labrum in a way that it remains attached at its upper and lower ends similar to a "bucket-handle" tear of a meniscus. Such a labral tear can cause additional symptoms of catching or popping in a shoulder that has humeral head instability.

The posterior humeral head can be damaged from contact against the anterior glenoid rim in anterior dislocation. This Hill-Sachs lesion is usually visible on roentgenograms.

TREATMENT OF ANTERIOR SHOULDER SUBLUXATION

Nonoperative. Avoidance of forceful throwing or other overhead activities is an effective way of eliminating the symptoms caused by subluxation. However, this may not be acceptable to the patient, especially the athlete. There are certain exercises commonly used to condition and strengthen the shoulder that can aggravate subluxation; these should be avoided. The most common one is overhead weight lifting with the grip too wide on the bar or with the weight too far posterior. If the weight drops behind the coronal plane, the arm goes into excessive hyperextension or external rotation. The Nautilus machine that allows the shoulder to go into extreme abduction and external rotation has enough inertia to aggravate subluxation and, in fact, can be deleterious to the patient with anterior instability. In overhead weight lifting, the hands should be positioned close to each other on the weight bar and the elbows and hands should be kept forward of the coronal plane.

Rotator cuff–strengthening exercises should be done with the arm below shoulder level. Resistive internal and external rotation exercises should be done with the elbow kept at the side. In performing abduction-strengthening exercises do not abduct the shoulders beyond 60 degrees.

Surgical. If the patient continues to have symptoms from subluxation despite nonoperative measures and will not accept modification of activities as an alternative, surgical treatment can be considered. An adequate trial of nonoperative treatment including adherence to an exercise program should be attempted in all cases of shoulder subluxation.

If surgery is performed, elimination of the primary cause of the shoulder instability should be the goal. If the capsule is lax, anterior shoulder capsulorrhaphy is the treatment of choice. If a Bankart lesion is present, this should be repaired by use of the Bankart technique.[19,20] All tissues should be returned to their normal anatomic position including the coracoid process if detached. Procedures that rely on limitation of external rotation for effectiveness (such as Magnuson-Stack or Putti-Platt) should not be performed in the athlete who needs full range of shoulder motion. This is especially true in the throwing athlete. The Bristow procedure should not be performed in throwing athletes in my opinion, since transferring the coracoid process to the anterior glenoid interferes with the subscapularis muscle function and often limits shoulder motion. Metal should not be used for internal fixation around the shoulder joint, especially in the athlete, because of the extremes of motion required for sports.

Simple excision of a torn glenoid labrum has shown to be effective in certain cases.[17] Arthroscopic resection of a torn labrum has been shown to be effective by Andrews.[3] It is important to know, however, that these shoulders had no apparent subluxation.

Arthroscopic staple capsulorrhaphy is being performed at several centers. Results are still forthcoming. In my opinion, this technique has the potential of causing serious complications because the staple is too large and protrudes beyond the edge of the glenoid rim too far. The staple can damage the humeral head. This arthroscopic technique should be viewed as experimental at this time.

TREATMENT OF ANTERIOR SHOULDER DISLOCATION

Primary dislocation. Closed reduction can be carried out using a number of methods. A simple way to reduce the shoulder is to bring the arm into the overhead position to minimize the stabilizing effect of shoulder muscles. Traction with the arm in this position will usually reduce the shoulder. Another easy method is the Stimson maneuver: hang the arm over the edge of a table with the patient in the prone position. Attach a 5- or 10-pound weight to the wrist to exert traction. Apply gentle manual lateralward pressure on the humeral head through the axilla combined with internal and external rotation. Other methods such as Kocher[12] or Hippocratic[1] require a great deal of force and are usually more difficult to perform.

The optimal length of time the shoulder should be immobilized after initial dislocation has not been proved, but common practice is to hold the shoulder in a sling for about 3 weeks. A study by Henry and Genung[9] showed that the length of time a shoulder was immobilized did not influence the recurrence rate. Older patients, in whom the risk of recurrent dislocation is lower and the risk of stiffness is higher, can be held for shorter periods.

After the immobilization is discontinued, the range of motion should be regained slowly, especially abduction and external rotation. Upon return to sports a harness or brace that limits extremes of motion can be useful. Resistive exercises to strengthen the rotator cuff musculature are important to improve dynamic stabilization of the shoulder.

Recurrent dislocation. The younger the patient, the higher the incidence of recurrent dislocation or subluxation, or both, after the initial dislocation.[19] If major trauma was the cause of the initial dislocation, the incidence of recurrent dislocation is lower than in a shoulder in which minimal or no trauma caused the dislocation.

If the shoulder remains unstable despite conservative measures, surgical repair should usually be performed. The same guidelines used for recurrent dislocation can be applied for subluxation: the Bankart procedure is performed if a Bankart lesion is present; anterior capsulorrhaphy is carried out if the anterior capsule is lax and no Bankart lesion is present. Rowe has shown the Bankart procedure to be effective in correcting instability even if a large Bankart or Hill-Sachs lesion exists.[18] However, the recurrence rate after surgical repair was slightly higher in shoulders that had a large Hill-Sachs lesion compared to shoulders that did not. A large fracture of the anterior glenoid is not necessarily an indication to perform a bone block procedure. Reattachment of the capsule to the glenoid rim through drill holes (Bankart procedure) usually stabilizes the shoulder and still allows full range of motion. I do not recommend the use of the Magnuson-Stack, Putti-Platt, Bristow, Nicola, Eden-Hybennett or duToit procedures in throwing athletes because these procedures commonly limit external rotation. The major drawback of the Bankart procedure is that it is technically more difficult to perform than most of the procedures listed above. Its major advantages, however, are that early range of motion can be instituted after surgery (2 or 3 days), and a full range of stable motion is usually achievable.

Recurrent instability after surgical repair. The shoulder that continues to become dislocated even after a surgical repair has been performed to correct this condition, or the shoulder that sustains a new traumatic dislocation after reparative surgery should be carefully evaluated to determine the cause of the recurrence. Failure to correct the Bankart lesion in shoulders treated with the Putti-Platt, Bristow, Magnuson-Stack, or Nicola procedures was found to be the most common cause of failure.[22] A new Bankart lesion was commonly found in shoulders that dislocated again after a prior Bankart procedure. Most shoulders with recurrent instability after prior surgery can be treated with the Bankart procedure. However, if the prior surgery has excessively scarred the anterior capsule and subscapularis tendon (as with a prior Bristow procedure) a Putti-Platt procedure is usually the best alternative.

REHABILITATION

Gentle active range of motion exercises can be begun as early as 1 or 2 days after surgery if the primary lesion has been corrected and the tissues have returned to their normal anatomic positions (as with the Bankart procedure). If the success of surgery depends on limiting external rotation or the subscapularis tendon is insufficient, the shoulder should be immobilized for 3 to 4 weeks after surgery. In either event, return to contact sports should be delayed until 6 months after surgery. Use of a harness or brace to restrict motion should be considered if the player returns to sports earlier than this time.

The goal of rehabilitation after the Bankart procedure or anterior capsulorrhaphy is full range of motion and normal muscular strength. The strengthening exercises should not be done with the arms in the overhead position, and the position of arms behind the sagittal plane of the body should be avoided for 3 months after surgery.

REFERENCES

1. Adams, F.L.: The genuine works of Hippocrates, vols. 1 and 2, New York, 1886, William Wood & Co.
2. Andrews, J.R.: Shoulder injuries in the athlete, Orthop. Trans. **7:**174, 1983.
3. Andrews, J., and Carson, W.: The arthroscopic treatment of glenoid labrum tears in the throwing athlete, Orthop. Trans. **8:**44, 1984.
4. Bankart, A.S.B.: The pathology and treatment of recurrent dislocation of the shoulder joint, Br. J. Surg. **26:**23-29, 1938.
5. Barnes, D.A., and Tullos, H.S.: An analysis of 100 symptomatic baseball players, Am. J. Sports Med. **6:**62-74, 1978.
6. Carr, D., Johnson, R., and Pepe, M.: Upper extremity injuries in skiing, Am. J. Sports Med. **9:**378-383, 1981.
7. Danzig, L., Resnick, D., and Greenway, G.: Evaluation of unstable shoulders by computed tomography: a preliminary study, Am. J. Sports Med. **10:**138-142, 1982.
8. El-Khoury, G.Y., Albright, J.P., Monzer, A.M., et al.: Arthrotomography of the glenoid labrum, Radiology **131:**333-337, 1979.
9. Henry, J.H., and Genung, J.A.: Natural history of glenohumeral dislocation—revisited, Am. J. Sports Med. **10:**135-141, 1982.
10. Jackson, D., Gurman, W., and Berson, B.: Patterns of injuries in college athletes: a retrospective study of injuries sustained in intercollegiate athletes in the colleges over a two year period, The Mt. Sinai J. Med. **47:**423-426, July-Aug. 1980.
11. Jobe, F.W., Tibone, J.E., Perry, J., and Moyner, D.: An EMG analysis of the shoulder in throwing and pitching, Am. J. Sports Med. **11:**3-5, 1983.
12. Kocher, T.: Eine neue Reductionsmethode für Schulterverrenkung, Berl. Klin. Wochenschr. **7:**101-105, 1870.
13. Leffert, R.D., Rowe, C.R., Kozlowski, B., and Meister, M.: Treatment of voluntary dislocation of the shoulder by therapeutic exercise based on video-electromyography analysis, Orthop. Trans. **7:**141, 1983.
14. Micheli, L.: Overuse injuries in children's sports: the growth factor, Orthop. Clin. North Am. **14:**337-360, 1983.
15. Mogan, J.V., and Davis, P.H.: Upper extremity injuries to skiing. In Symposium on Skiing Injuries, Clin. Sports Med. **1:**295-308, 1982.
16. Olsen, O.C.: The Spokane Study: high school football injuries, Physician and Sportsmedicine **7:**75-82, Dec. 1979.
17. Pappas, A.M., Goss, T.P., and Kleinmann, P.K.: Symptomatic shoulder instability due to lesions of the glenoid labrum, Am. J. Sports Med. **11:**279-288, 1983.
18. Rowe, C.R., Patel, D., and Southmayd, W.W.: The Bankart procedure: a longterm end-result study, J. Bone Joint Surg. **60A:**1-16, 1978.
19. Rowe, C.R., and Sakellarides, H.T.: Prognosis in dislocations of the shoulder, J. Bone Joint Surg. **38A:**957-977, Oct. 1956.
20. Rowe, C.R., and Zarins, B.: Recurrent transient subluxation of the shoulder, J. Bone Joint Surg. **63A:**863-872, 1981.
21. Rowe, C.R., and Zarins, B.: Chronic unreduced dislocations of the shoulder, J. Bone Joint Surg. **64A:**494-505, 1982.
22. Rowe, C.R., Zarins, B., and Ciullo, J.V.: Recurrent anterior dislocation of the shoulder after surgical repair, J. Bone Joint Surg. **66A:**159-168, 1984.
23. Shields, C., and Zomar, V.: Analysis of professional football injuries, Contemp. Orthop. **4:**90-95, 1982.
24. Snook, G.: A survey of wrestling injuries, Am. J. Sports Med. **8:**450-453, 1980.
25. Tapper, E.: Ski injuries from 1939 to 1976: the Sun Valley experience, Am. J. Sports Med. **6:**114-121, 1978.

26. Shoulder arthroscopy

Frank A. Pettrone

Arthroscopy has proved to be a valuable addition to the orthopaedic surgeon's armamentarium in the evaluation and treatment of knee disorders. With the surgeon's increased experience and newer technologic advances in video equipment, arthroscopes, and instruments (manual and motorized) other joints and a wider range of disorders may now be approached arthroscopically. These factors have provided an impetus to increased utilization of shoulder arthroscopy.

HISTORY

Burman, in an early study of arthroscopy in 1931, stated that the shoulder was the easiest joint on which to perform arthroscopy. Other authors have also presented its usefulness in various specific shoulder problems. Wiley studied frozen shoulders, distended the capsule, and manipulated the joint with good results. Haira and Maitland, as well as Conti, also used arthroscopy with manipulation for frozen shoulders. Watanabe presented its use for identifying osteochondral fractures and loose bodies and evaluating rheumatoid arthritis. Bateman commented on its use in rotator cuff tears, snapping shoulders, humeral subluxations, and recurrent dislocations. In his book on arthroscopy,[5] Johnson described its usefulness in the removal of loose bodies, resection of remnants of the biceps tendon, removal of portions of a torn rotator cuff, synovectomy in rheumatoid disease, and staple fixation for subluxating shoulders. Caspari[2] has added improvements in technique and equipment and commented upon additional surgical indications. Andrews and Carson[1] have more recently described partial labral tears in the throwing athlete and the results of arthroscopic resection of this lesion.

Arthroscopy of the shoulder is more demanding and exacting in technique than arthroscopy of the knee. However, with a knowledge of shoulder anatomy (gross anatomic as well as arthroscopic) this useful technique can be mastered.

TECHNIQUE

Local anesthesia may be used, but I believe that general anesthesia provides easier positioning of the patient (in traction) and a more complete level of muscle relaxation. The procedure may still be done on an outpatient basis.

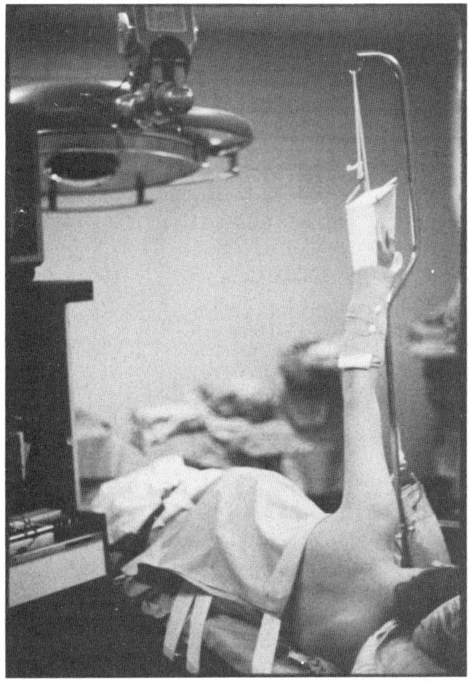

Fig. 26-1. Proper positioning of the patient. Lateral decubitus position with arm abducted.

The patient is placed in the lateral decubitus position with the involved arm abducted (Fig. 26-1). The forearm is held with skin traction and the arm suspended by traction (10 to 15 pounds). The arm position should be between 45 and 70 degrees of abduction and 10 to 20 degrees of forward flexion. Care must be taken not to use excessive traction for distraction because stretch injury to the brachial plexus has been reported. The shoulder should be supported by sandbags and the pelvis secured to the operating table by tape. It is helpful to draw with a marking pen the topographic landmarks (acromion, coracoid, acromioclavicular joint, glenoid, humeral head) after prepping, draping, and creating a sterile field.

The primary viewing portal is posterior. Initially an 18-gauge spinal needle is introduced. The entrance is in the "soft spot," approximately 2 cm inferior to the posterolateral tip of the acromion. The surgeon's other hand should mark the coracoid process and, with this as a spatial guide, introduce the needle (Fig. 26-2). Arm rotation or distraction can help when this space is entered. Thirty milliliters of saline solution are then introduced to distend the shoulder joint. A nick in the skin is made with a scalpel at the soft spot. The sharp trocar, then blunt, and finally the cannula and trocar are introduced into the joint (Fig. 26-3). Backflow of saline solution confirms the correct position. I prefer a larger (4 or 5 mm) arthroscope for clarity of visualization. The joint may be distended and drained through the sidearms of the

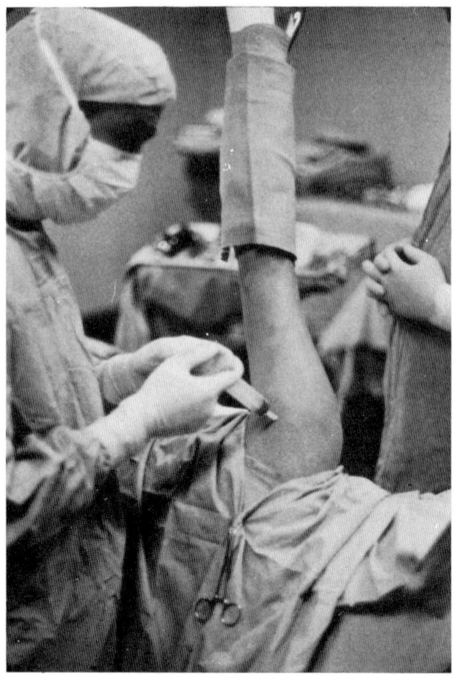

Fig. 26-2. Needle distension of the shoulder joint.

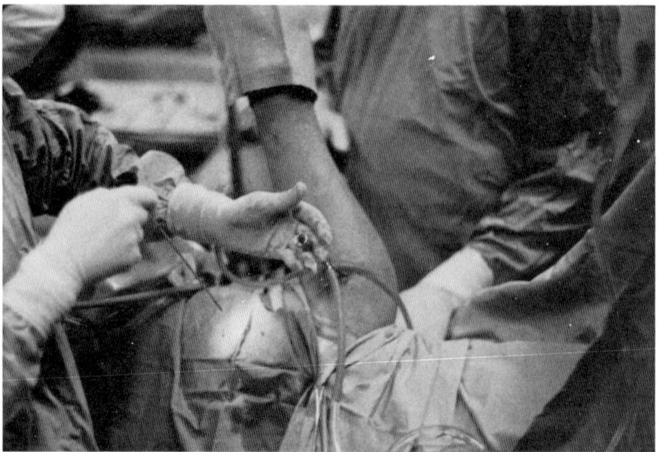

Fig. 26-3. Cannula and trocar introduction into joint.

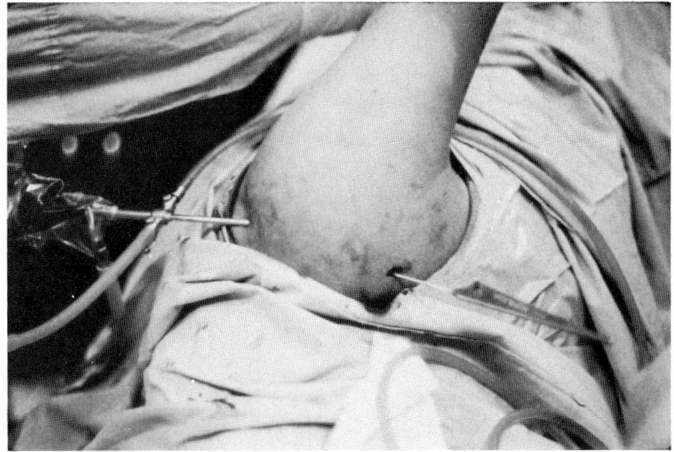

Fig. 26-4. Establishing the anterior portal.

telescope for purely diagnostic viewing. Operative arthroscopy requires other portals for a flow cannula and instrument introduction.

The second portal is anterior, approximately halfway between the acromion (anterolateral edge) and the coracoid. I prefer to achieve this from inside rather than percutaneously. The arthroscope is probed anteriorly into a triangular interval between the humeral head (inferior), glenoid (medial), and biceps tendon (superior). The light from the arthroscope transilluminates the skin. The 18-gauge spinal needle is then introduced from the anterior side (staying lateral to the coracoid process) into the joint at this triangular interval and confined by direct arthroscopic visualization. Sharp and blunt trocars are then used to establish the portal (Fig. 26-4).

For specific arthroscopic surgery, I frequently add a third portal for an inflow cannula. As suggested by Caspari,[2] the superior portal is used. The spinal needle is inserted from above, just posterior to the acromioclavicular joint and proximal to the medial edge of the acromion and confirmed arthroscopically to lie above the humeral head. A Varies needle is then inserted, and an inflow valve is connected to this cannula. One then has excellent flow and distension of the joint from the superior portal, viewing from the posterior portal, and use of the anterior portal for instruments.

ARTHROSCOPIC ANATOMY

The entire shoulder joint must then be methodically evaluated. The first structure to be identified is the biceps tendon. This should serve as orientation for the initiation of arthroscopic examination.

The biceps tendon is nearly vertical with the patient in the lateral decubitus position and arm abducted (Fig. 26-5). It should be inspected from its insertion on the superior aspect of the glenoid down anteriorly into the bicipital groove. Superiorly its attachment continues with the superior aspect of the glenoid labrum.

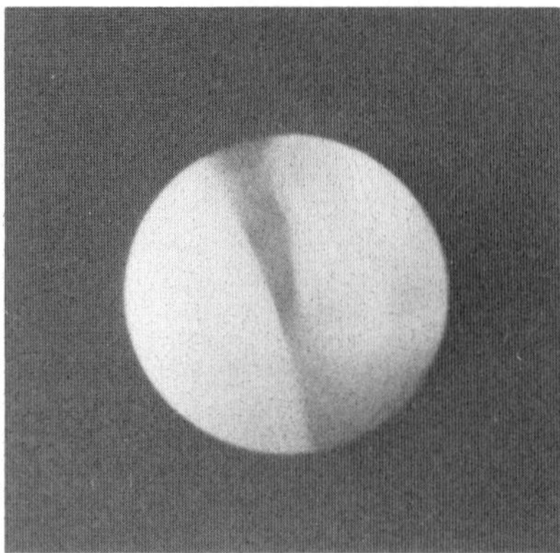

Fig. 26-5. Arthroscopic view. Biceps tendon is superior.

The articular surfaces of the glenoid and humeral head are then inspected. This is facilitated by internal and external rotation of the humeral head as well as rotation of the 30-degree fore-oblique arthroscope.

The glenoid labrum is next evaluated. One should begin superiorly at the biceps tendon insertion and proceed along the inferior rim. If the inferior rim is not seen, further brief distraction of the arm with traction is helpful. The posterior rim is then viewed. Slight position retraction and rotation of the arthroscope is helpful here.

The glenohumeral ligaments are then viewed. These three are thickenings of the anterior capsule and provide stability for the anterior and inferior capsule. The middle ligament is frequently distinct and broad and may be confused with the subscapularis tendon.

The subscapularis tendon is seen in the interval between the superior and middle glenohumeral ligament. Arthroscopically, with the arm abducted, it is not a broad, flat structure but rather cordlike over the anterior aspect of the capsule. This is its posterosuperior edge.

The rotator cuff is visualized next and is located just superior to the biceps tendon. Rotation of the arthroscope is useful to follow the supraspinatus to its insertion on the humeral head.

The synovium itself should be examined in several areas and probed or biopsied as indicated. Inspection of the recesses should be thorough in inspection for loose bodies and to evaluate laxity.

POTENTIAL COMPLICATIONS

The arm is suspended by skin traction of about 10 to 15 pounds. Excessive traction on the forearm can injure neurovascular structures leading to neurapraxia.[3,4] This harmful effect can be achieved when the traction device is fixed to an immovable object and the operating table is lowered.

If fluid leaks out from the shoulder joint capsule, the soft tissues may become distended very quickly. Fluid may also exude from the shoulder along the bicipital groove. This will therefore limit the time available for shoulder arthroscopy.

Not infrequently, bleeding obscures the field of vision in shoulder arthroscopy. This can be remedied by a third inflow cannula to increase the flow rate and also still have continuous drainage. Infiltration of the portals with a local anesthetic and epinephrine may help control this extracapsular bleeding.[4]

SURGICALLY AMENABLE LESIONS

Tears of the glenoid labrum. Glenoid labrum tears are seen in athletically active patients, particularly those engaged in the throwing sports. Fraying lesions of the upper third of the labrum are well suited to resection.[1,6]

Supraspinatus-biceps tendinitis. Partial tears of the supraspinatus and long head of the biceps tendon are amenable to débridement and resection.

Loose bodies. Loose bodies and osteochondral defects of the humeral head and glenoid are viewable and able to be arthroscopically treated.

Other indications. Manipulation under anesthesia with arthroscopic dilatation and observation, synovectomy for rheumatoid arthritis, and resection of full-thickness rotator cuff tears are other indications. This resection has been described, but its indications and results are at present unclear.[4]

Arthroscopic stabilization of the subluxating shoulder has also been described. Although the attractiveness of an arthroscopic procedure is obvious, several complications of this technique have already been presented.

DISCUSSION

Arthroscopy of the shoulder is gaining its place in the treatment of shoulder disorders. From a technical standpoint, it is much more difficult to enter than the knee joint. The two layers of muscle, a tighter and narrower plane of the joint, and nearby neurovascular structures are the major impediments. Attention to detail, familiarity with the anatomy, proper setup of the patient and equipment, and distension of the joint are essential for adequate and safe arthroscopy of a shoulder. Several current surgical indications are presented. The information obtained from a complete diagnostic arthroscopy make this a valuable technique. I believe that with increasing experience, improved scientific equipment, and individual surgical inquisitiveness and ingenuity our surgical capabilities will expand in the future.

REFERENCES

1. Andrews, J.R., Carson, W.G., and Ortega, K.: Arthroscopy of the shoulder: technique and normal anatomy, Am. J. Sports Med. **12:**1-7, 1984.
2. Caspari, R.: Shoulder arthroscopy: a review of the present state of the art, Contemp. Orthop. **4:**523-530, 1982.
3. Cofield, R.: Arthroscopy of the shoulder, Mayo Clin. Proc. **58:**501-508, 1983.
4. Johnson, L.L.: Arthroscopy of the shoulder, Orthop. Clin. North Am. **11:**197-204, 1980.
5. Johnson, L.L.: Diagnostic and surgical arthroscopy: the knee and other joints, ed. 2, St. Louis, 1981, The C.V. Mosby Co.
6. Pappas, A.M., et al.: Symptomatic shoulder instability due to lesions of the glenoid labrum, Am. J. Sports Med. **11:**279-288, 1983.

27. Shoulder examination and diagnosis in the throwing athlete

James R. Andrews
Scott D. Gillogly

The functional anatomy of the throwing athlete's shoulder undergoes changes that make it very different from the nonthrowing shoulder. The extreme stresses placed on the dynamic stability during the throwing act create these adaptive changes in the normal anatomy. It is the extreme acceleration and deceleration of the throwing act that generates the forces that often predispose the shoulder to injury. During the examination of the throwing athlete, the physician must not only have an appreciation of the normal variational anatomy of the shoulder, but must also have an understanding of the mechanics of the throwing act.

The most obvious characteristic of the throwing shoulder is the increased amount of hypertrophy evident in the shoulder girdle. Because of this the physician may have difficulty palpating specific structures or recognizing muscle wasting that may be present with chronic injury or nerve damage.

Another readily apparent characteristic is a pronounced increase in external rotation and relative loss of internal rotation when compared to the nonthrowing shoulder. This physical finding should not be mistakenly diagnosed as an abnormal internal rotation contracture. In fact, a lack of this combination of increased external rotation and decreased internal rotation may indicate abnormalities in the throwing shoulder.

The hyperextensibility of the throwing shoulder may be an adaptive change or may reflect joint hypermobility. This characteristic of the competitive throwing athlete's shoulder contributes to subluxation and dislocation and associated lesions.

The throwing motion is a highly complex and integrated motor function that places maximum stresses on the structures of the shoulder. The competitive throwing athlete performs at a level of stress just under the maximum tolerance of the tissues. When the tolerance of the tissues is exceeded, injury occurs.

This work was supported in part by the Hughston Sports Medicine Foundation, Inc., Columbus, Georgia.

306

Although the repetitive throwing motion has led to gradual adaptive changes and hypertrophy of the tissues about the shoulder, even minor alterations in throwing mechanics can lead to disruption of the balance between maximum stress and maximum tolerance. By having an understanding of basic throwing mechanics the physician can not only diagnose, treat, and guide rehabilitation of the injured throwing shoulder, but also aid in prevention of recurrence.

HISTORY

As with any examination, the patient's history is the first step. The usual questions of duration and location of pain and aggravating factors should be asked. The character of the pain can influence the diagnosis. For example, the dull aching pain that is often felt at night may indicate a rotator cuff tear, whereas a stabbing, burning pain may be suggestive of bursitis or tendinitis.

The patient can sometimes be specific when describing the location of the pain, such as pinpointing the acromioclavicular joint. However, patients often complain of a more generalized area of pain, which usually indicates an injury to a deeper structure, such as a torn rotator cuff. The duration of pain may be vague and chronic indicating lesions such as an attrition cuff tear secondary to impingement. In the case of some acute or specific injuries, further questioning may be helpful in determining the subtleties of apprehension or subluxation. Radiation of pain, paresthesias, or numbness may indicate compressive neuropathy such as a thoracic outlet syndrome or entrapment of specific nerves such as the subscapular nerve on the scapula or axillary nerve in the quadrilateral space.

The history should include assessment of previous subluxations or dislocations that may have produced a Hill-Sachs lesion or Bankart lesion. A quiescent inflammatory condition may recur after an offseason or a break in training. A history of hearing or feeling popping may indicate a glenoid labrum tear or a subluxating biceps tendon. Crepitus, or grinding, can occur with degenerative disease in the acromioclavicular joint or from chronic bursitis.

The patient should be asked or, if possible, should demonstrate where in the throwing act symptoms occur. Other factors such as a change in the throwing style or specific technique or grip changes should be correlated to the onset or type of symptoms.

PHYSICAL EXAMINATION AND DIAGNOSIS

The physician should establish a consistent routine for physical examination of the throwing shoulder. This not only ensures completeness, but also allows the examiner to simplify his diagnostic formulation by logically relating the functional anatomy of throwing to the physical findings on examination. While keeping in mind the normal anatomic characteristics of the throwing shoulder, one should always include the uninjured shoulder in the exam as well.

Initial examination begins with inspection of the various contours of the shoulder. One can usually start this while conversing with the patient, taking the history, and

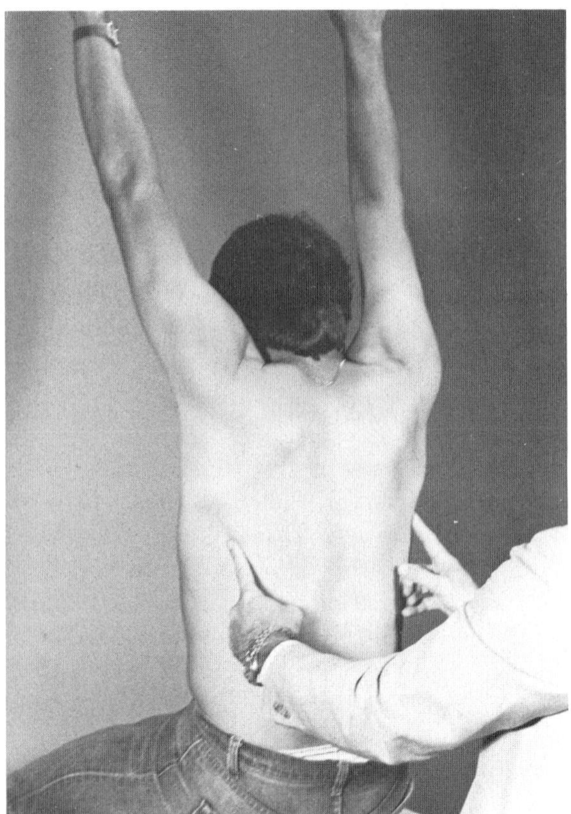

Fig. 27-1. Method of demonstrating overhead abduction. (From Zarins, B., Andrews, J., and Carson, W.: Injuries to the throwing arm, Philadelphia, 1985, W.B. Saunders Co.)

observing the patient undressing and moving to the exam table. Obvious asymmetry, atrophy, hypertrophy, erythema, and swelling can be recognized. The patient's overall functional status can also be observed during this period by the degree of symptoms caused by the simple maneuvers of undressing.

We begin the active portion of the examination from the posterior aspect of the throwing shoulder with the patient sitting. Rotation is first checked with the arm at 90 degrees of abduction, with both external and internal rotation being noted in this position. By comparing this rotation to the contralateral side, we will readily see the excessive external rotation and loss of internal rotation. We then check overhead abduction by having the patient raise his arms directly overhead (Fig. 27-1). It is important to watch the scapula during abduction to ensure that it does not ride out laterally. Next we examine the sternoclavicular joint with the arm in full abduction noting the normal 50 degrees rotation of the clavicle. The sternoclavicular joint is commonly overlooked and can be a source of pain and crepitus in the throwing shoulder. The clavicle is palpated distally for tenderness out to the acromioclavicular joint.

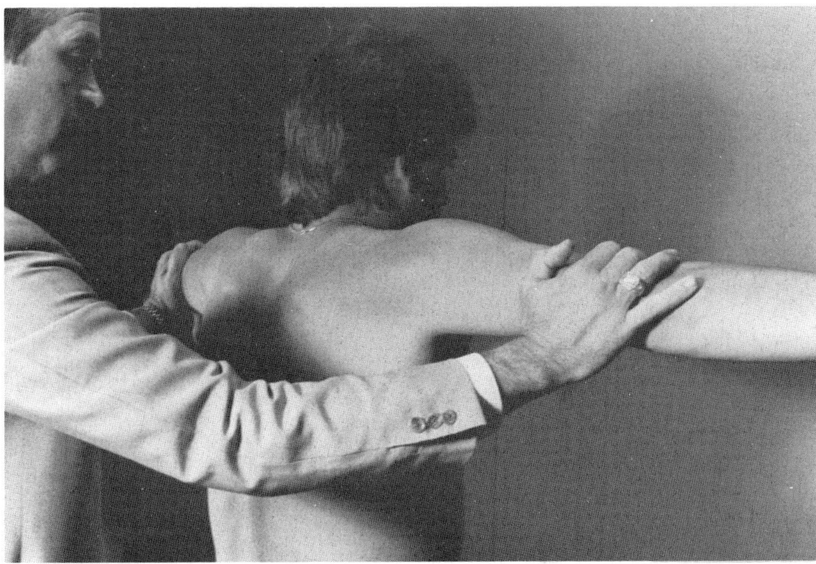

Fig. 27-2. Testing for strength of the supraspinatus. (From Zarins, B., Andrews, J., and Carson, W.: Injuries to the throwing arm, Philadelphia, 1985, W.B. Saunders Co.)

This joint is also palpated for dislocation, pain, and crepitus in various degrees of abduction and flexion. Remember that dislocation in this joint can occur in the anterior or posterior direction, as well as in the superior direction.

Next, we test for strength of the supraspinatus as described by Doctor Frank Jobe by having the shoulder in 90 degrees of abduction and 30 degrees of forward adduction and full internal rotation (Fig. 27-2). The patient maintains this position as the examiner offers downward resistance. Weakness or pain may indicate a superior rotator cuff lesion or neuropathy of the supraspinatus nerve.

An impingement test is carried out with the patient sitting and abducting his arm full overhead. Impingement of the coracoacromial arch can be detected by simultaneous manual depression of the scapula (Fig. 27-3).

Another stability can be examined with the patient in the sitting position. The throwing arm is held by the examiner at 90 degrees of shoulder abduction and 90 degrees of elbow flexion. An increasing, though gentle posterior force is applied to the patient's hand causing external rotation of the shoulder (Fig. 27-4). Patient apprehension alone or with pain indicates subluxation or dislocation. Diffuse pain alone on this apprehension test may indicate rotator cuff tear rather than subluxation. When this test is performed, the anterior glenoid should be palpated, and if reproducible localized pain is produced by palpation, it may indicate anterior subluxation as well. The examiner should always be prepared for actual anterior dislocation to occur with this abduction–external rotation test, particularly with a hyperextensible throwing shoulder and a too vigorous external rotation force.

We then have the patient stand and examine the posterior musculature noting

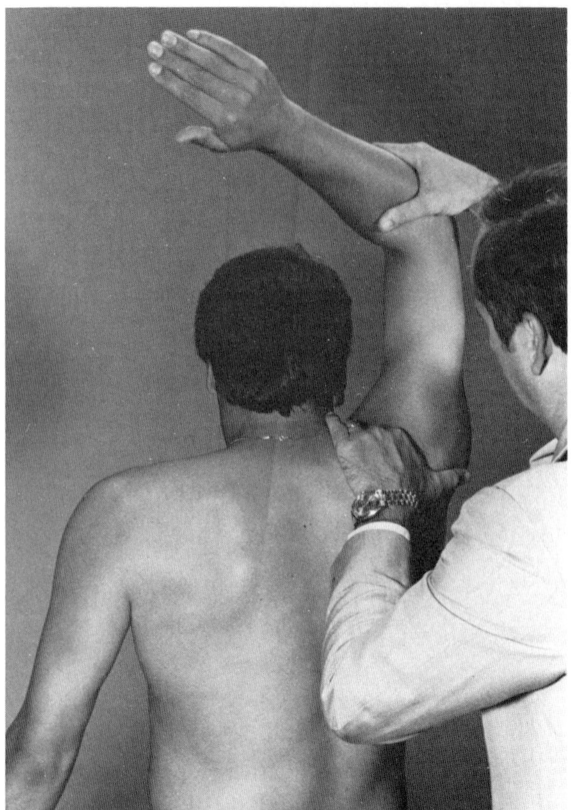

Fig. 27-3. Testing for impingement of the coracoacromial arch. (From Zarins, B., Andrews, J., and Carson, W.: Injuries to the throwing arm, Philadelphia, 1985, W.B. Saunders Co.)

hypertrophy of the teres minor, which is a common finding in the throwing shoulder (Fig. 27-5). The posterior musculature can be accentuated when we have the patient place his hands on his hips and tighten his muscles. The posterior musculature is palpated for any areas of tenderness. We can measure comparatively the internal rotation for both shoulders by recording which thoracolumbar spinous process the patient can touch his thumb to (Fig. 27-6). This measurement will again point out the relative lack of internal rotation on the throwing side. We then have the patient push against the wall checking for winging of the scapula indicating weakness in the serratus anterior muscle or injury to the long thoracic nerve (Fig. 27-7). With the arms overhead the rotation of the scapula on the thoracic wall is checked for asymmetry or tightness. Remember that scapulothroacic motion is an important component of the throwing motion at the shoulder. Inferior stability can also be checked from the standing position when we pull straight down on the arm while palpating and looking for a contour defect on the anterior lateral shoulder. A patient with inferior stability will usually volunteer feeling his glenohumeral joint subluxate.

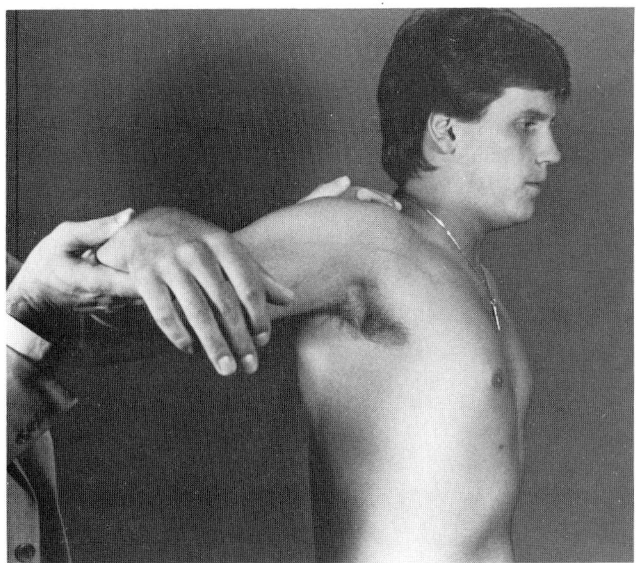

Fig. 27-4. Testing for anterior stability. (From Zarins, B., Andrews, J., and Carson, W.: Injuries to the throwing arm, Philadelphia, 1985, W.B. Saunders Co.)

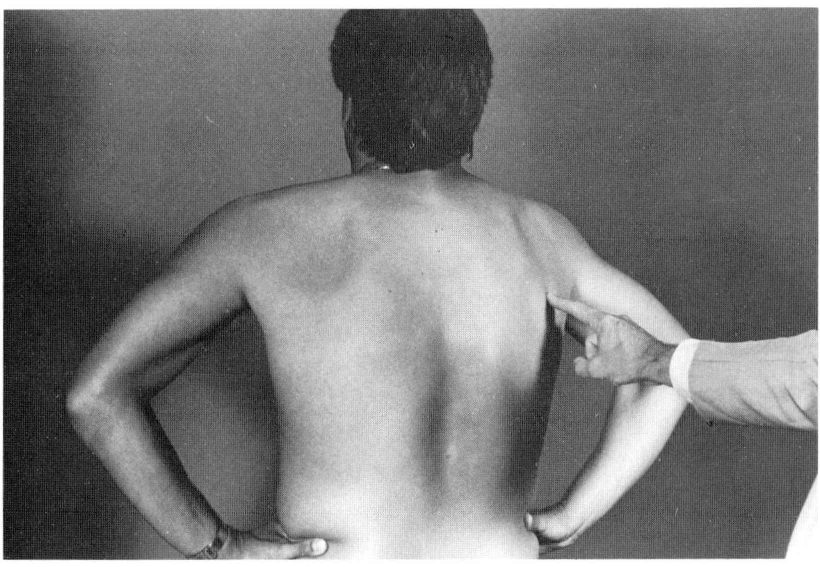

Fig. 27-5. Examine the posterior musculature for hypertrophy of the teres minor. (From Zarins, B., Andrews, J., and Carson, W.: Injuries to the throwing arm, Philadelphia, 1985, W.B. Saunders Co.)

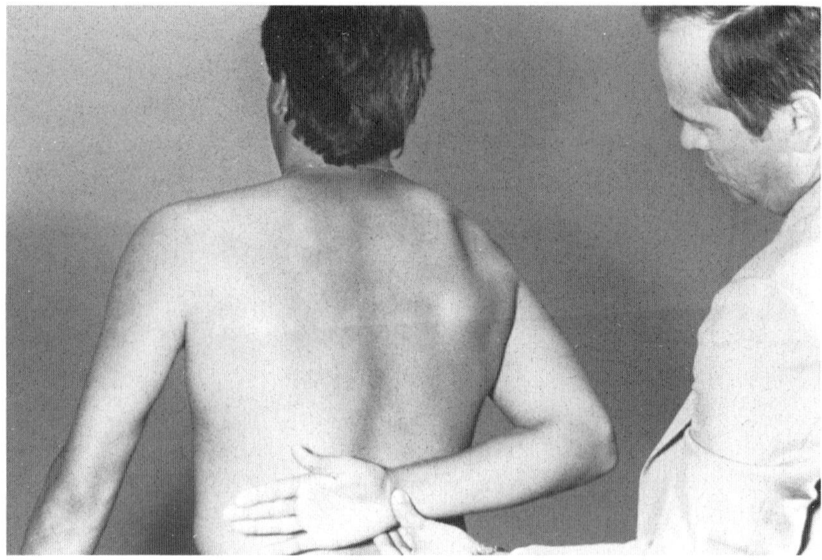

Fig. 27-6. Measuring for internal rotation. (From Zarins, B., Andrews, J., and Carson, W.: Injuries to the throwing arm, Philadelphia, 1985, W.B. Saunders Co.)

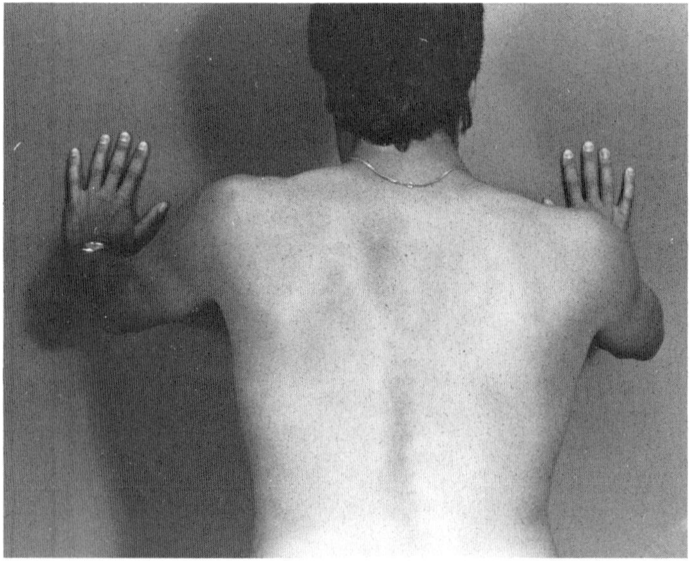

Fig. 27-7. Checking for weakness in the serratus anterior muscle or injury to the long thoracic nerve. (From Zarins, B., Andrews, J., and Carson, W.: Injuries to the throwing arm, Philadelphia, 1985, W.B. Saunders Co.)

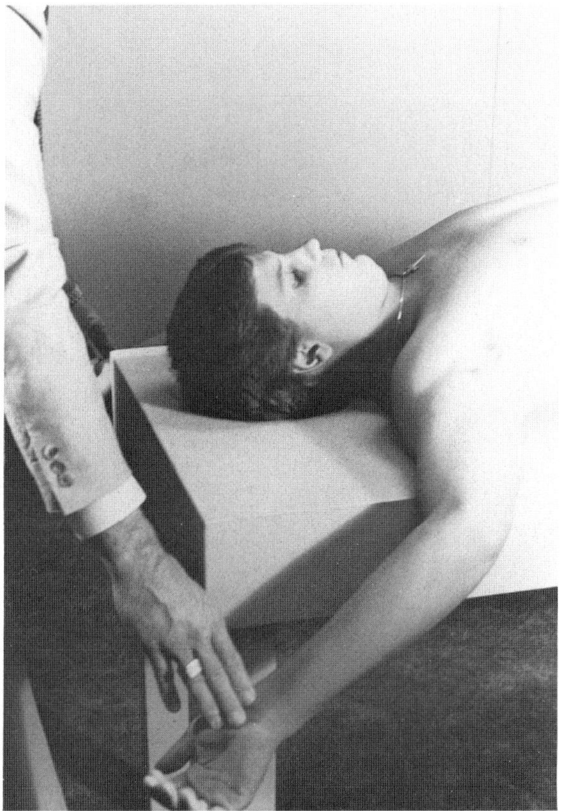

Fig. 27-8. Observing rotation on both sides with the arm abducted 90 degrees. (From Zarins, B., Andrews, J., and Carson, W.: Injuries to the throwing arm, Philadelphia, 1985, W.B. Saunders Co.)

Next, with the patient supine we again observe the rotation on both sides with the arm abducted 90 degrees (Fig. 27-8). Notice the increased external rotation of the throwing shoulder and relative loss of internal rotation. Rotation should also be recorded with the arm in the full overhead position. Horizontal adduction across the body is checked as we look for tightness in the motion necessary for follow-through at the end of the deceleration phase of throwing (Fig. 27-9). Tightness within the glenohumeral joint itself can be checked when the scapula is held posteriorly fixed with one hand while the arm is put through attempted abduction overhead.

While the patient is still in the supine position, subtleness of anterior subluxation can again be examined. Starting with the shoulder at 90 degrees of abduction and the elbow flexed at 90 degrees, the examiner places one hand on the glenohumeral joint with the fingers posterior to the humeral head and the thumb anterior. The examiner supports the arm with the other hand and applies an anteriorly directed stress to the humeral head levering it anteriorly (Fig. 27-10). This maneuver is repeated at various

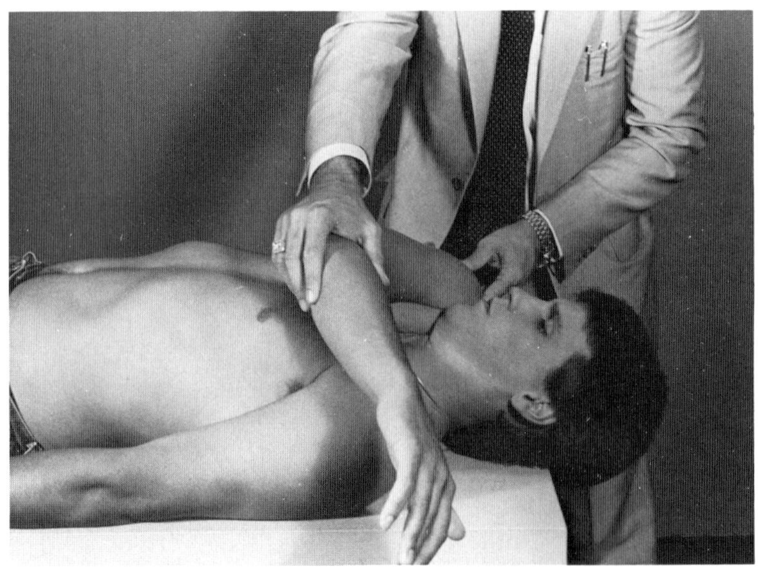

Fig. 27-9. Horizontal adduction across the body is checked. (From Zarins, B., Andrews, J., and Carson, W.: Injuries to the throwing arm, Philadelphia, 1985, W.B. Saunders Co.)

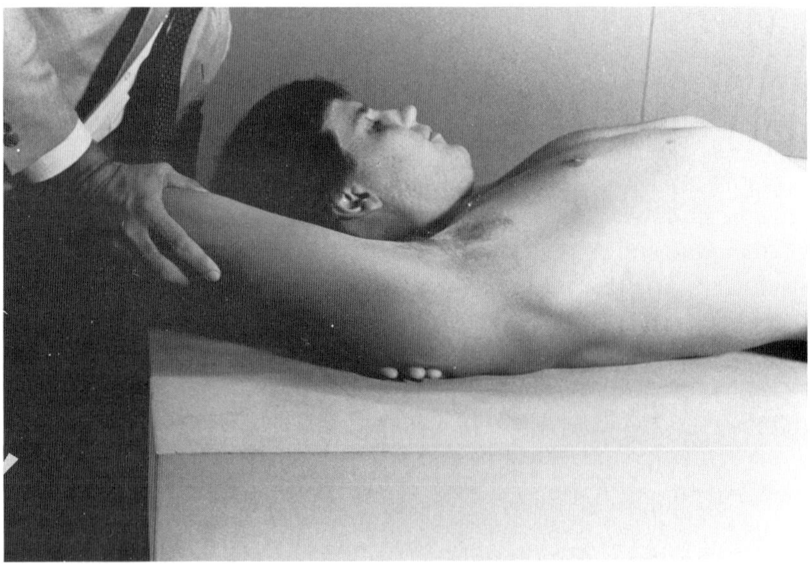

Fig. 27-10. Testing for anterior subluxation. (From Zarins, B., Andrews, J., and Carson, W.: Injuries to the throwing arm, Philadelphia, 1985, W.B. Saunders Co.)

degrees of increasing abduction to the full overhead position while the examiner feels for anterior subluxation. Posterior instability is assessed next. Frequently throwing athletes demonstrate considerable posterior laxity. The throwing arm is forward flexed and adducted while the examiner's hand provides a posteriorly directed stress with the thumb on the humeral head. The examiner will feel the posterior subluxation with his fingers placed posteriorly (Fig. 27-11). Any posterior instability will reduce itself as the arm is brought back to an abducted position. Glenoid labrum tears are prevalent in the throwing shoulder. It is important that this arthroscopically correctable lesion be looked for and diagnosed clinically. We use the "clunk" test to make the clinical diagnosis of an anterior labrum tear, particularly an anterior labrum tear that occurs most commonly in the throwing shoulder (Fig. 27-12). This test is performed with the patient supine. The examiner's hand is placed posteriorly on the humeral head and the opposite hand holds the humeral condyles at the elbow providing a back-and-forth rotating force. The patient's arm is brought into full overhead abduction, and the hand on the humeral head provides an anterior force, while the opposite hand rotates the humerus. You will feel a "clunk" or grinding in the shoulder as the humerus hits or snaps on the labral tear, indicating a positive "clunk" test.

Impingement of the rotator cuff on the acromion complex can occur in throwing shoulders. Impingement of the rotator cuff, particularly of the supraspinatus portion against the undersurface of the anterior third of the acromion and the strong coracoacromial ligament, can lead to primary attrition tears of the rotator cuff and produce inflammation and edema in the subacromial bursa and biceps tendon, or act secondarily to extend, complete, or inhibit healing of true traumatic cuff tears in the throwing shoulder. The physical examination that brings out impingement pain involves bringing the patient's arm into about 120 degrees of forced forward elevation, which is a combination of forward flexion and abduction, while the examiner's other hand fixes the scapula against elevation by firmly holding the scapula at the top of the shoulder. Additionally, impingement can be checked by maximal internal rotation of the forward flexed arm with the scapula fixed. These tests can be done with the patient either sitting or supine, although in a particularly large athlete it may be easier with the patient supine.

It should be emphasized that contrary to what is found in the general patient population, high-performance throwing athletes quite frequently exhibit tears in the rotator cuff that begin on the deep rather than the superficial portion of the rotator cuff. This is apparently produced by the extreme tension placed on the undersurface of the cuff by the throwing motion and the rapid deceleration of the shoulder. It follows then that findings on examination for these types of lesions do not necessarily mimic the typical findings and the examiner must observe closely for subtle clues.

The biceps tendon can also be examined while the patient is in the supine position. With the shoulder in 90 degrees of abduction and neutral rotation, the bicondylar axis of the elbow is grasped in one hand while the other hand palpates the anterior part of the shoulder (Fig. 27-13). The bicondylar axis is then internally rotated 15 degrees so that the biceps tendon and the bicipital groove point directly toward

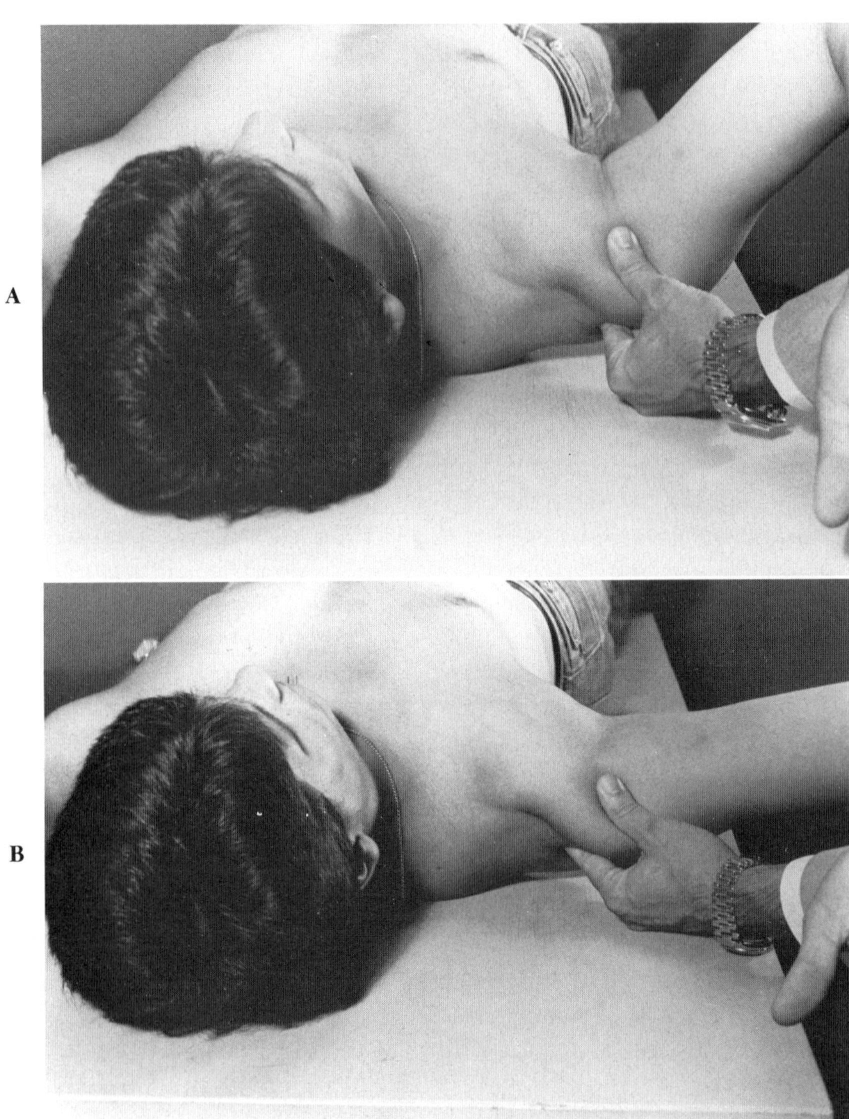

Fig. 27-11. A, Assessing posterior instability. The examiner's hand provides a posteriorly directed stress with the thumb on the humeral head. **B,** Any posterior instability will reduce itself as the arm is brought back to an abducted position. (From Zarins, B., Andrews, J., and Carson, W.: Injuries to the throwing arm, Philadelphia, 1985, W.B. Saunders Co.)

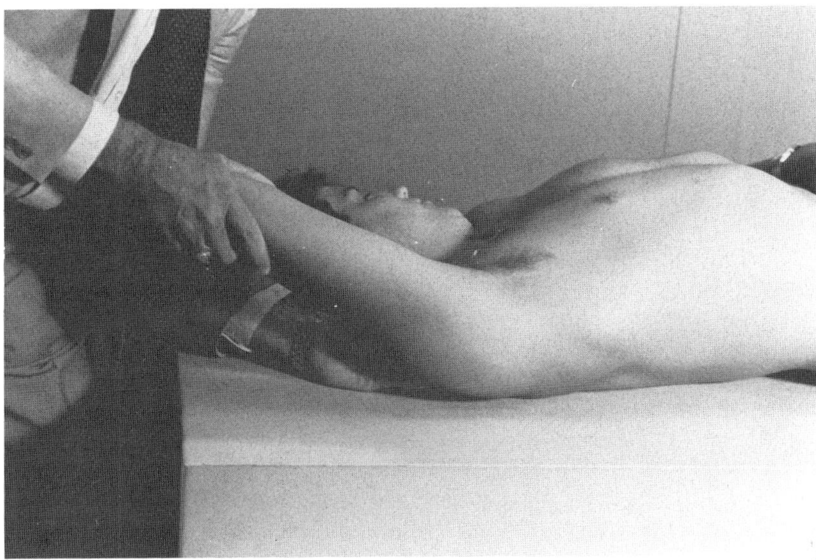

Fig. 27-12. "Clunk test" for diagnosis of the anterior labral tear. (From Zarins, B., Andrews, J., and Carson, W.: Injuries to the throwing arm, Philadelphia, 1985, W.B. Saunders Co.)

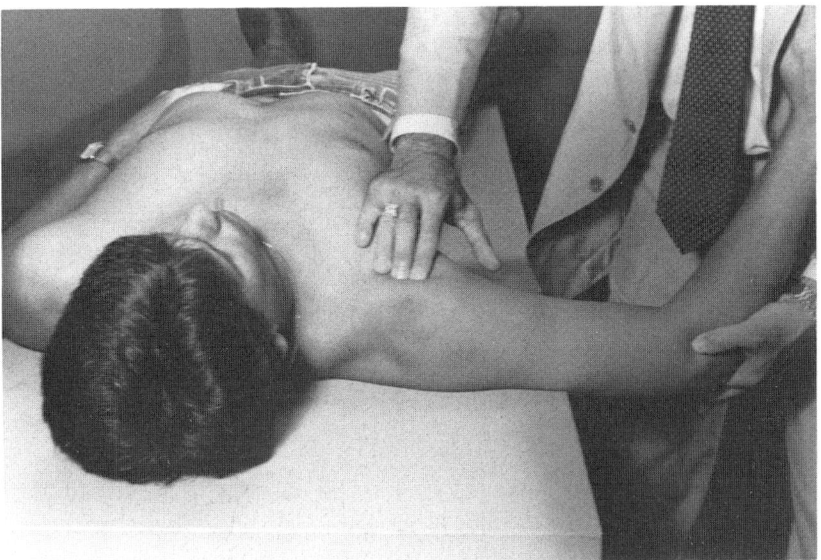

Fig. 27-13. Testing function of the long head of the biceps tendon. (From Zarins, B., Andrews, J., and Carson, W.: Injuries to the throwing arm, Philadelphia, 1985, W.B. Saunders Co.)

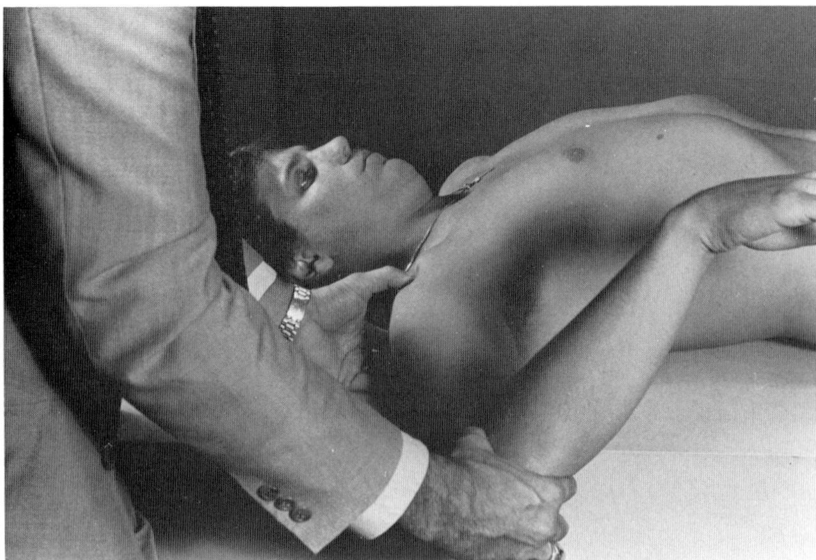

Fig. 27-14. Palpating the anterior muscles for isolated tenderness. (From Zarins, B., Andrews, J., and Carson, W.: Injuries to the throwing arm, Philadelphia, 1985, W.B. Saunders Co.)

the ceiling and are made easily palpable. Palpation of the biceps tendon can be augmented when the arm is dropped off the table toward the floor. This position bowstrings the tendon and makes it more prominent. Next the humerus is internally and externally rotated while the biceps tendon and groove are palpated. This allows the examiner to appreciate any snap or pop if the tendon is subluxating out of the bicipital groove. Pain elicited along the biceps tendon or the groove indicates bicipital tendinitis or injury to the "biceps tendon–labrum complex."

The specific anatomic landmarks are again identified anteriorly. The anterior acromion and coracoid act as reference points to guide further palpation of the anterior muscles for isolated tenderness (Fig. 27-14). The anterior deltoid can be palpated. Next the arm is internally rotated and adducted across the patient's chest to allow palpation of the supraspinatus area just anterior to the acromion. The infraspinatus can also be palpated more posteriorly, as can the teres minor. Rotator cuff tears in throwing athletes more commonly involved the supraspinatus or infraspinatus, or a combination of both, rather than the teres minor.

The final position for examining the throwing shoulder is with the patient in the prone position. The throwing arm is allowed to fully relax and drop over the side of the examining table with the elbow extended and pointing directly toward the floor. This encourages the posterior deltoid to fall anteriorly with the aid of the examining hand and allows further palpation of the posterior cuff musculature, the teres minor, and more superiorly the infraspinatus (Fig. 27-15). The quadrilateral space can also be palpated inferior to the teres minor near its insertion, anterior to the long head of the

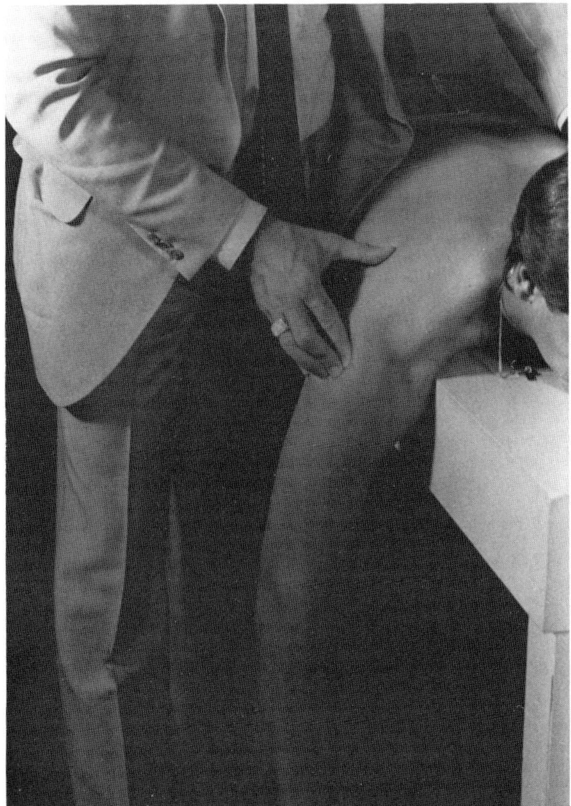

Fig. 27-15. Palpating the posterior cuff musculature, the teres minor, and the infraspinatus. (From Zarins, B., Andrews, J., and Carson, W.: Injuries to the throwing arm, Philadelphia, 1985, W.B. Saunders Co.)

triceps and posterior to the humerus. This area may very rarely be a source of compression on the axillary nerve and posterior humeral circumflex artery as they exit the quadrilateral space.

The posterior capsule can be directly palpated with the patient in the prone position by palpation just superior to the teres minor at the glenohumeral joint. The posterior capsule can be a source of chronic inflammation as it is stretched or even avulsed from its scapula attachment through the repeated trauma of the throwing motion. This finding correlates with roentgenographic evidence of calcification in the posterior capsule in this localized area.

True internal and external rotation of the glenohumeral joint can be confirmed, once again, while the patient is in the prone position. The examiner holds the scapula fixed and maximally internally and externally rotates the humerus while the shoulder is in 90 degrees of abduction (Fig. 27-16). This further identifies contractures acting on the glenohumeral joint.

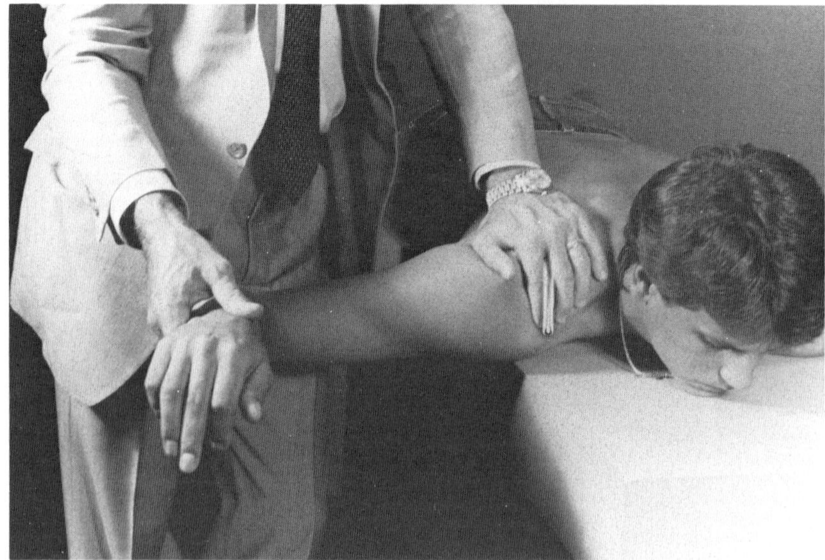

Fig. 27-16. Confirming true internal and external rotation of the glenohumeral joint. (From Zarins, B., Andrews, J., and Carson, W.: Injuries to the throwing arm, Philadelphia, 1985, W.B. Saunders Co.)

ADDITIONAL DIAGNOSTIC PROCEDURES

Physical examination of the throwing shoulder routinely requires further diagnostic aids to confirm and support the physical findings leading to a conclusive diagnosis and to rule out any underlying lesion not evident on examination. Roentgenographic examination should include an anteroposterior view in internal and external rotation and a transaxillary lateral with further views such as the West Point view, as indicated. Other available diagnostic aids include shoulder arthrography with double contrast or with arthrotomography. Diagnostic arthroscopy offers a method of evaluating shoulder disorders in throwing athletes, since it affords an opportunity for examination under anesthesia, as well as simultaneous definitive treatment in many cases.

The physical examination outlined above is aimed directly at shoulder problems in throwing athletes and should act as a guide to the specific tests that should be incorporated into the framework of the physician's routine complete examination. Evaluation should, of course, include a full neurologic assessment and examination of related areas such as the cervical spine and the elbow.

SUMMARY

The repetitive maximal stresses placed on the throwing shoulder make it extremely susceptible to injury. To better tolerate these stresses, the shoulder develops adaptive alterations in its functional anatomy. By having an understanding of basic throwing mechanics, obtaining a specific patient history, and performing a thorough physical examination directed at the functional anatomy of the shoulder, the physician can effectively diagnose and treat shoulder injuries in the throwing athlete.

28. Shoulder tendinitis

Robert P. Nirschl

HISTORICAL INTRODUCTION

The modern concepts of diagnosis and treatment of shoulder tendinitis have gradually evolved, starting with the report of Codman in 1911.[3] As with clinical maladies at the elbow, accurate correlation and identification of the tissues actually involved in pathologic change has occurred only recently and in some circumstances is still evolving. Key milestones from Codman's[4] contributions progress with Moseley,[13] McLaughlin,[11] De Palma,[5] McNab,[29] Neer,[16] and Jobe.[9] Since the classic article of Neer in 1972,[15] it has been common to equate rotator cuff tendinitis with anterior acromial impingement.[17,27]

The more recent experience of Andrews,[1] Fowler,[6] and Nirschl[21-23] working with swimming, racket, and throwing sport athletes has led however to considerations other than impingement as a primary factor in rotator cuff tendinitis.

PATHOETIOLOGY (SECONDARY ROLE OF IMPINGEMENT)

The pathologic phases as noted by Nirschl[19,20] in tennis elbow (such as phase I inflammation only, phase II angiofibroblastic change, and phase III angiofibroblastic change plus rupture) are present in all areas of tendinitis including the compartmentalized rotator cuff. These pathologic changes (angiofibroblastic hyperplasia) appear to be related primarily to repetitive intrinsic tension overload in both the compartmentalized rotator cuff and the commonly injured noncompartmentalized tendons at the elbow, knee, ankle, and foot.

Lindblom and Palmer,[10] Moseley and Goldie,[14] Rothman and Park,[28] and Rathbun and McNab[29] have all identified a critical zone of vascular supply in the rotator cuff. A consensus of these authors was that impingement may further squeeze vascular supply from an already compromised area with resultant devitalization. Nirschl has categorized the devitalization phenomenon as "infarct of tendon."[21]

The mechanical issues however are clearly more sophisticated than this simplistic view. Inman[8] et al. have demonstrated a complex interrelationship of shoulder movement. Saha[31] has stated that "locking of the greater tuberosity against the acromion never takes place in any position of abduction" if healthy relationships exist. He

322

further has noted that a rolling-down movement of the humeral head in the glenoid cavity inevitably takes place with active humeral flexion or abduction. Saha's great contribution to shoulder mechanics was in recognizing the zero position of approximately 165 degrees of elevation and 45 degrees of forward position where the shear and compressive forces are equally balanced.

Sarrafin[32] has noted that compression at the level of the glenohumeral joint is essential for stability. At 90 degrees of abduction and beyond, the pull of the deltoid passes through the glenohumeral joint providing this stability. At less than 90 degrees the deltoid forces pass outside the joint thereby causing upward humeral displacement, unless counteracted by the counterforcing compression forces of the transversely positioned rotator cuff muscles. Sarrafin confirms Saha's report that compression and shear forces are maximum at 90 degrees of elevation and essentially nil at 150 degrees.

Hollingshead[7] states that the supraspinatus is a shoulder abductor. Perry[25] has also identified the role of the supraspinatus as a primary humeral head depressor, as well as possible external rotator. Andrews[1] has also suggested that the long head of the biceps may act as a humeral head depressor. This action maintains the humeral head firmly in the glenoid and controls potential upward humeral head migration when abduction occurs in association with deltoid contractile power.

Eccentric contraction of the supraspinatus to smoothly decelerate the internal rotation and adduction in the swimming, racket, and throwing sports may also be an extremely important function. This action could conceivably be the key causative intrinsic tensile overload factor in rotator cuff tendinitis[30] because these functions often occur in the vulnerable 90-degree high-shear and glenohumeral compression load position.[23]

When fatigue, injury, and intrinsic pathologic changes occur, weakness and muscle imbalance also occur. With this weakness and imbalance, firm humeral head control is lost, resulting in upward humeral migration.

It is clear that control of the humeral head is essential for normal shoulder function. Rotator cuff muscle strength and tendon health are the dynamic keys to this control.[26] This important function likely has passive backup constraints. The size, placement, and position of the coracoacromial ligament makes it ideal for this function, and I openly speculate that this in fact is the true function of this ligament. This being the case, aggressive resection of the coracoacromial ligament may be derogatory to the long-term normal balance and function of the glenohumeral joint and possibly invite rotator cuff injury. If rotator cuff dysfunction results in upward humeral migration, impingement may indeed occur. Unlike Neer,[16,17] however, it is my belief that impingement is secondary to rotator cuff muscle weakness and that the key pathologic change in the supraspinatus tendon occurs primarily by intrinsic tension overload. This concept is extremely important because it shifts the emphasis of treatment to the supraspinatus and rotator cuff tendons and muscles rather than the acromion or the coracoacromial arch space per se. This of course better explains the success of conservative treatment in the Neer[17] clinical stages I and II, since exercise

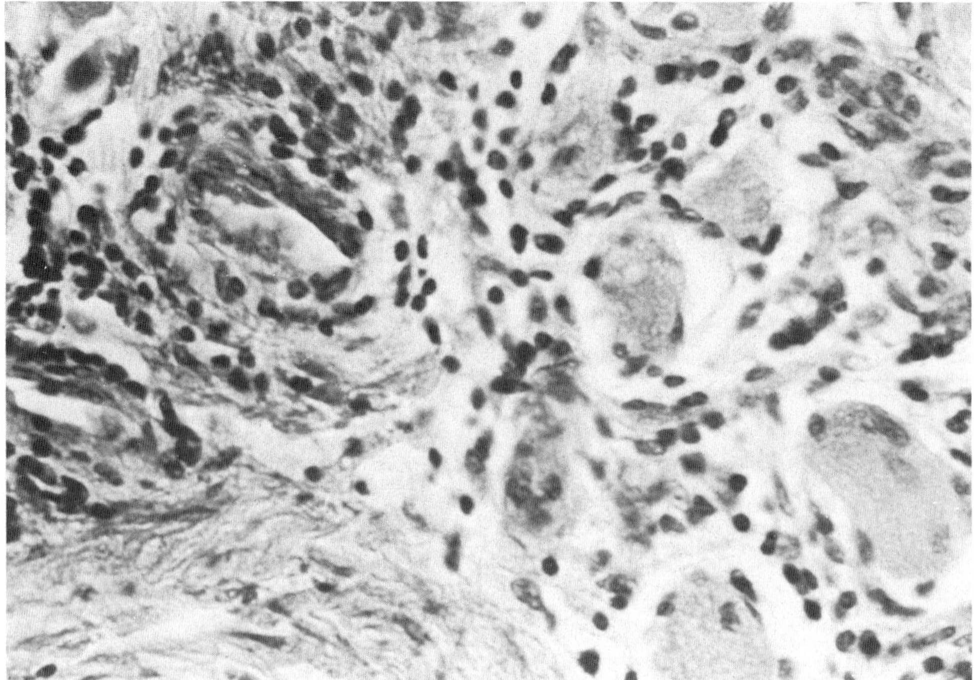

Fig. 28-1. Angiofibroblastic hyperplasia. Characteristic microscopic appearance commonly seen in advanced tendinitis. Young vascular elements are the hallmark of these changes. (Courtesy E. Stay, M.D., Department of Pathology, Arlington Hospital, Arlington, Virginia, 1985.)

and anti-inflammatory modalities will have no effect on the hereditary position, exostosis, or design of the acromion (Fig. 28-1).

SIGNS AND SYMPTOMS

The characteristic symptoms of rotator cuff tendinitis are localized to the supraspinatus (the tendon close to greater tuberosity attachment and muscle in the supraspinatus fossa) region with extension of pain and tenderness to the long head of the biceps. Pain is also perceived in the middeltoid area to its insertion on the proximal end of the humerus. Additional symptoms may also be identified at the posterior shoulder insertion of the infraspinatus and teres minor and at the acromioclavicular joint. The pain is invariably initiated by active abduction to 90 degrees usually in combination with internal-external rotation movement. Constant nonactivity pain can occur, usually indicative of major pathologic change or tear. Crepitus in the acromial arch areas is a common accompanying sign.

Classical signs include the Neer impingement sign (forceful forward elevation to 180 degrees while the scapula is depressed),[17] forceful internal rotation with the shoulder abducted 90 degrees and forward flexed approximately 45 degrees, and

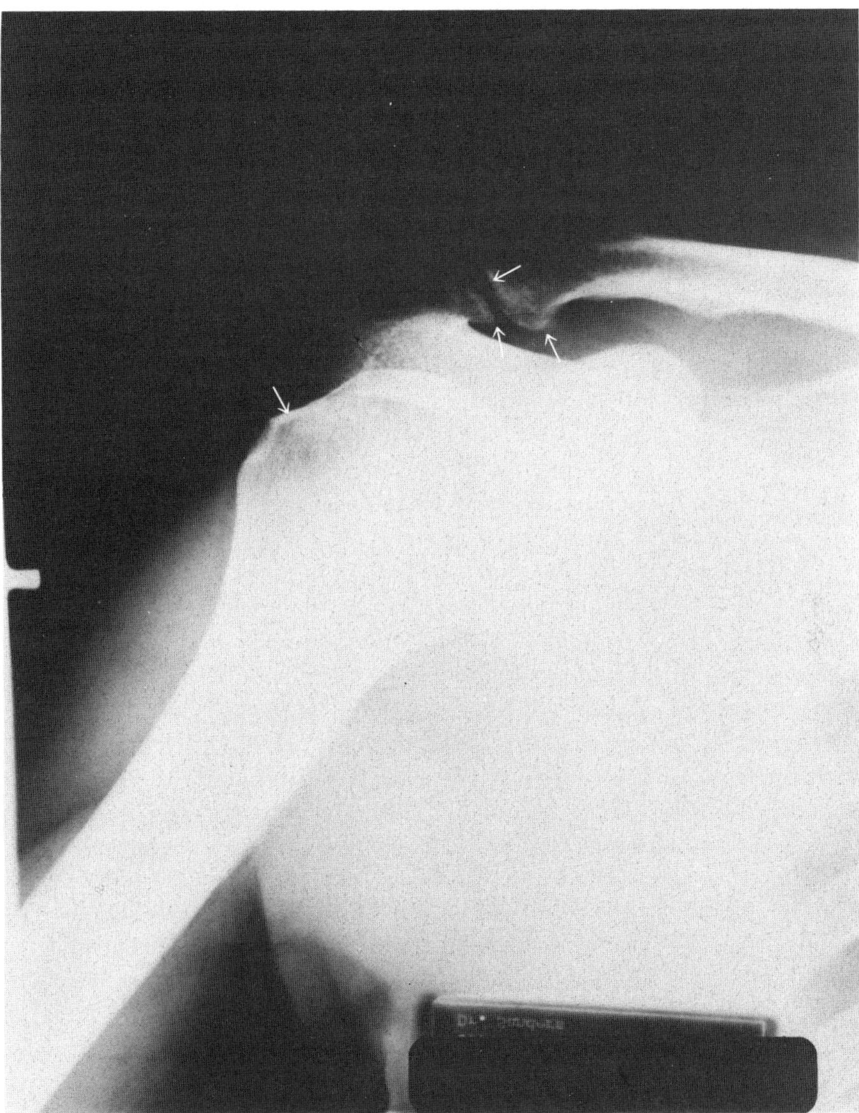

Fig. 28-2. Common roentgenographic changes in rotator cuff tendinitis include acromioclavicular osteoarthritis and bony exostosis or erosion at the humeral greater tuberosity.

supraspinatus stress test in the same position and 90 degrees of lateral abduction. Palpable tenderness is characteristically at the supraspinatus insertion to the greater tuberosity with encroachment onto the bicipital groove.

Tenderness at the acromioclavicular joint indicates acromioclavicular osteoarthritis and at the posterior rotator cuff indicates infraspinatus and teres minor tendinitis. Both acromioclavicular osteoarthritis and posterior cuff tendinitis are common accompanying abnormalities associated with supraspinatus cuff tendinitis.

Roentgenographic changes may present a spectrum from no abnormality to greater tuberosity bony exostosis and erosion, subdeltoid and rotator cuff calcification, acromioclavicular osteoarthritis, subacromial and subacromioclavicular joint exostosis, and upward migration of the humeral head.[33] A normal arthrogram does not rule out major pathologic change, which often occurs before rupture. An abnormal arthrogram is of course indicative of a full rotator cuff rupture (Fig. 28-2).

CONSERVATIVE TREATMENT

The basic treatment concepts of shoulder tendinitis are similar to other tendinitis areas.[23] As in tennis elbow tendinitis, it is critical to establish the pathologic phase if possible (such as inflammation only versus angiofibroblastic change progressing to either partial or complete rupture). Since the rotator cuff encompasses four tendons (supraspinatus, infraspinatus, teres minor, and subscapularis) and the potential exists for adjacent extension of a lesion onto the biceps, subdeltoid bursae, acromioclavicular joint, and the subacromion, accurate diagnosis concerning all symptomatic pathologic areas is critical.

The most common areas of pathologic changes are the supraspinatus tendon segment of the rotator cuff and acromioclavicular osteoarthritis. Supraspinatus weakness or rupture allows upward migration of the humeral head, and secondary impingement may occur. In 25% of older patients (average age 59) Neer has reported an anterior subacromial exostosis.[16] Neer has stated however that this lesion has not been observed by him in patients under 40 years of age.[15] Teres minor and infraspinatus tendinitis are fairly common companions to supraspinatus tendinitis, and on occasion may be identified as an isolated injury (usually in competitive throwers).

With the aforementioned tendinitis changes, loss of motion (abduction plus rotations) is a common problem, and on occasion a true associated adhesive capsulitis may be present (rather than, for example, motion restriction secondary to tendinitis pain).

The basic treatment formula outlined for tennis elbow tendinitis (see p. 247) is utilized:

1. Relief of pain
2. Promotion of biologic healing
3. Rehabilitative exercise to injured tissue
4. Conditioning exercise
5. Force overload reduction
6. Surgery if conservative effort fails

In other areas of tendinitis, I do not advocate early full-range flexibility to injured tissue. In the classical rotator cuff tendinitis, however, the restricted motion is usually attributable to structures other than the supraspinatus (such as adhesive capsulitis). Since full range of motion is essential to a quality rotator cuff rehabilitative resistance exercise program, early flexibility exercises are prescribed. If adhesive capsulitis proves recalcitrant to usual physical therapy methods, manipulation under anesthesia is undertaken.

Relief of pain follows fairly standard approaches, including the use of anti-inflammatory medications (occasional cortisone injection properly placed may be appropriate). Modalities of physical therapy (pp. 247 and 341) and analgesic medications are prescribed as needed.

The rehabilitative strength-endurance resistance program utilizes a closely supervised progression of isometrics, isotonics, Isoflex, and isokinetics.[23] Emphasis is on full-range exercise in multiple diagonal arcs with isolation of all segments of the rotator cuff and alternation of concentric and eccentric exercise modes (pp. 341 to 346).

"Peripheral aerobics" (endurance) is achieved by high repetitions and lower resistance as well as arm pedaling and rowing systems.

The basic goals of the rehabilitative exercises are to enhance oxygenation and nutrition to injured tissue without injury overload and to restore balanced strength, endurance, and flexibility to the injured and adjacent noninjured tissue. It is especially critical to restore supraspinatus strength to control the humeral head and eliminate the potential of compression injury from secondary impingement.

Alterations in sport technique are primarily in the realm of avoidance of those

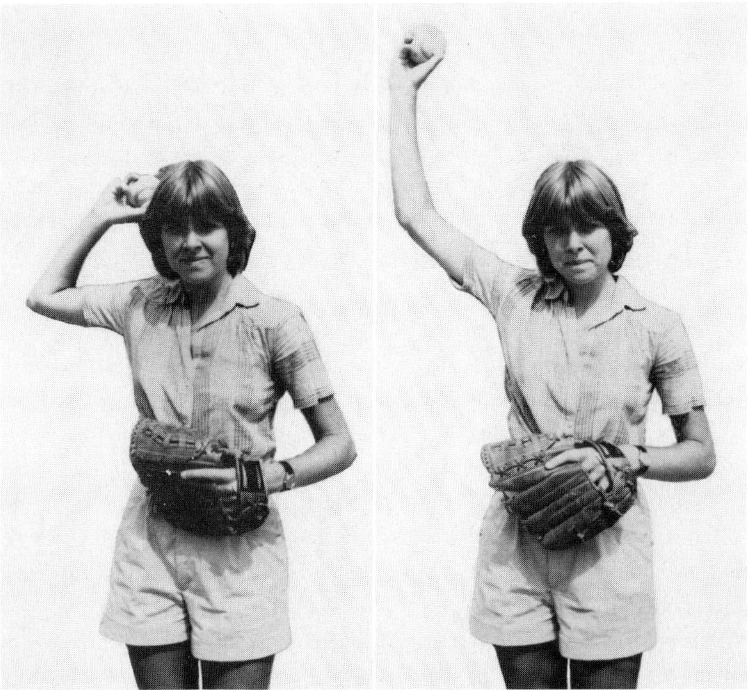

Fig. 28-3. Protective technique. High arm elevation throughout the acceleration phase appears protective to the rotator cuff as elevation above 90 degrees decreases shear and compression forces, which are controlled by the rotator cuff. This is more easily attained in the tennis serve and in football throwing, since the basic motion is up. In baseball pitching, the elevated mound forces a downward acceleration phase increasing tension on the cuff and medial areas of the elbow. (From Nirschl, R.P.: Arm care, Arlington, Va., 1983, Medical Sports Publishing.)

positions of motion that cause Nirschl phase 3 activity pain or greater.[23] This invariably occurs with forceful internal rotation with humeral abduction at approximately 90 degrees, identified as the high-shear and compression load force position. Fatigue also appears to play a role in injury. Therefore intensity and duration of activity may play a critical role, resulting in derogatory technique alteration with the loss of protective supraspinatus and biceps control of the humeral head as fatigue occurs (Fig. 28-3).

SURGICAL TREATMENT: GENERAL CONCEPTS

If conservative treatment fails, surgical care is appropriate and often beneficial. Since the primary tissue involved statistically is the supraspinatus segment of the rotator cuff,[2,4,12] the primary surgical considerations are invariably focused in this region. It must be appreciated, however, that encroachment and independent but associated adjacent pathologic change is often present. These changes may include varying combinations of subdeltoid bursitis, acromioclavicular osteoarthritis, biceps tendinitis, infraspinatus and teres minor tendinitis, anterior subacromial exostosis, greater tuberosity erosion with or without exostosis, adhesive capsulitis, and subscapularis contracture. On lesser occasions anterior labrum tears and anterior shoulder subluxation may also be present. Since all these tissues can be involved in varying degree, the surgical approach must be capable of dealing with these contingencies.

The pathologic changes in the supraspinatus that necessitate surgery vary (such as painful angiofibroblastic invasion of modest degree to partial tears or cuff erosions with progression to full-thickness tears). Full-thickness tears also vary widely from simple vertical tears to large retracted transverse tears. Hydroxyapatite calcifications may occur in the tendon or adjacent subdeltoid bursas and bony exostosis is fairly commonplace at the greater tuberosity.

ACROMIOPLASTY CAUTION

At present, decompression of the coracoacromial arch by resection of the coracoacromial ligament and anterior acromioplasty as reported by Neer are popular approaches to supraspinatus tendinitis. These approaches are predicated on the concept that impingement is the primary pathologic factor in rotator cuff tendinitis. Unless a specific primary hereditary inadequacy of the coracoacromial arch space can be demonstrated however, it is best to ascribe impingement as a secondary and not a primary phenomenon. The success therefore of isolated coracoacromial arch decompression understandably would be expected to be quite inconsistent, and observations have proved this to be true, especially in competitive athletes.

Anterior acromioplasty as described by Neer with the technique often unfortunately exaggerated by others also invites either extended rehabilitation or permanent harm because the deltoid is reflected in varying degree with this procedure.[18]

As noted, it is my opinion that impingement can and does occur but as a secondary not primary phenomenon. If supraspinatus weakness occurs, the humeral head may migrate upward with abduction. In early cases, a quality rehabilitative program generally corrects the problem, reinforcing the concept that impingement occurs secondary to strength deficiency. In those cases in which surgery is indicated, angiofibroblastic pathologic changes have been initiated primarily by intrinsic tension over-load and secondarily by compression overload. Major upward humeral migration with impingement may cause late compensatory anterior subacromial bony exostosis. Neer has noted this to occur in only 25% of his 1972 reported cases and not at all in patients under 40 years of age.[15,17] The distinction between primary tension overload and secondary compression impingement is critical to the surgical concept, since it shifts the surgical emphasis to the rotator cuff itself rather than the coracoacromial space.

Since the anterior acromial lesion as described by Neer is present in the minority of cases, it is unlikely that the anterior acromioplasty is intrinsic to surgical success in the majority of cases and is harmful when deltoid normalcy is disturbed.[16,18] If anterior acromioplasty is indicated, it may be performed by a technique that avoids alteration of the acromial deltoid origin.[23] In addition, since the coracoacromial ligament may in fact be an important passive constraint to upward humeral migration, resection should be limited to the needs of exposure of the rotator cuff.

PREFERRED SURGICAL TECHNIQUE (NIRSCHL)

The hallmark of surgery is to correct pathologic alteration while protecting normal tissue. This is especially true of rotator cuff surgery. To protect the deltoid origin, the traditional anterior acromioplasty is avoided. Adequate exposure for the majority of rotator cuff surgery cases can be achieved by a deltoid-splitting incision at the acromioclavicular joint level. In major rotator cuff tears, cuff retraction generally occurs laterally, and an occasional posterior extension of the incision paralleling the scapular ridge at the infraspinatus fossa area may be indicated for adequate exposure. If supraspinatus retraction occurs proximally, the supraspinatus fossa is easily reached by resection of the distal end of the clavicle and extension of the incision over the supraspinatus fossa.

Rotator cuff tendinitis is often accompanied by adhesive capsulitis. If this occurs, a full manipulation of the shoulder before the surgical incision is made is an important premliminary procedure.

The preferred incision extends from the anterior edge of the acromioclavicular joint approximately 2 inches distally. If acromioclavicular osteoarthritis or the necessity to expose the supraspinatus or infraspinatus fossa is present, the incision is expanded posteriorly to the supraspinatus fossa or paralleling the scapular ridge on rare occasion. The decision to expand the incision is often made after preliminary exposure (Fig. 28-4).

The deltoid is easily split longitudinally, since the muscle is relatively thin and flat at this level. The subdeltoid bursa and coracoacromial ligament come into the view promptly. Normal bursa is protected and is incised only for exposure. Pathologic bursa is excised. An oblique incision in the coracoacromial ligament sufficient to expose the rotator cuff is utilized. *Caution:* Total release of the entire ligament may not be necessary for adequate exposure, and the oblique incision allows reconstitution of the ligament postoperatively.

Downward traction of the arm increases subacromial clearance allowing a palpat-

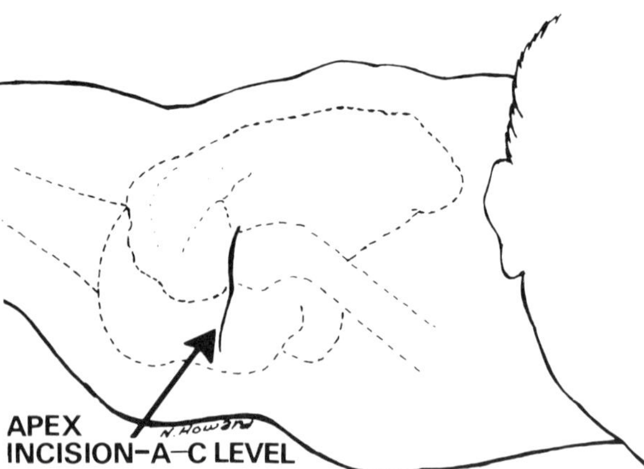

Fig. 28-4. Standard preliminary incision anterior to and at the level of the acromioclavicular joint. If resection of the distal end of the clavicle is necessary, the incision is expanded posteriorly toward the supraspinatus fossa as shown here.

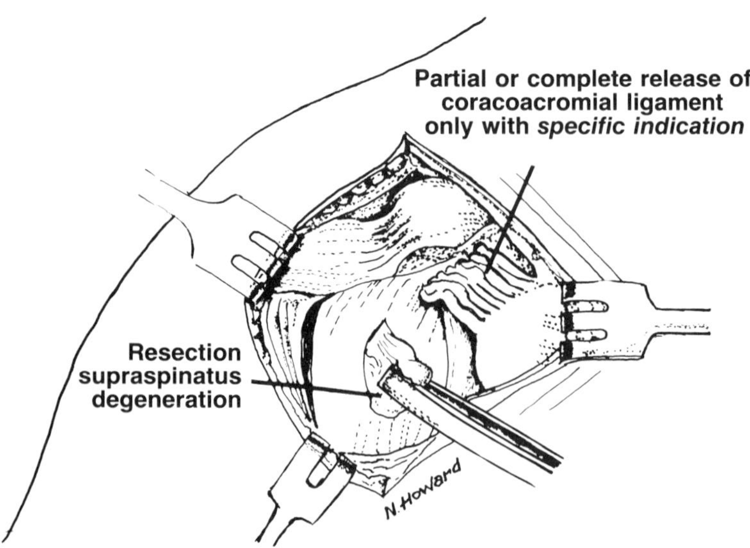

Fig. 28-5. Surgical technique. Release the coracoacromial ligament only with a specific indication. In my opinion the ligament is an important passive constraint to upward humeral migration. In this drawing there is a triangular release of the anterior edge only. Excise only the bursa that is pathologic. Remove pathologic changes in the cuff with a vertical ellipse, and repair the cuff as indicated.

ing finger to examine the subacromial space, the acromioclavicular joint, rotator cuff, and bicipital groove. If acromioclavicular osteoarthritis is present, or wide cuff exposure is needed, the skin incision is expanded to the posterior edge of the acromioclavicular joint, the acromioclavicular ligament is incised, and the metaphyseal flare of the distal end of the clavicle is removed by an oscillating saw. During bone removal a large periosteal elevator is placed over the supraspinatus tendon for protection. Visual inspection of the rotator cuff is easily attained by humeral rotation and abduction; thus the majority of the cuff can be inspected when the cuff is moved to the incision rather than expanding the incision to the cuff.

Inspection of the cuff may reveal a wide variety of pathologic changes from minimal erythema, changes in tissue density with edema, superficial erosion, partial flap tears, or full-thickness tears. The background pathologic condition in rotator cuff tendinitis is angiofibroblastic changes as noted in other tendinitis maladies[20,30] (elbow, patellar tendon, Achilles tendon, and plantar fascia). The major location of pathologic changes is in the supraspinatus tendon, but encroachment into the infraspinatus and biceps areas does occur. Even in the presence of full-thickness tears, however, it is unusual for the long head of the biceps to have any major pathologic change. This observation is also reported by Weaver.[34] This is in contradistinction to the report of Neviaser.[24]

In my observations, the majority of supraspinatus tears either partial or full thickness are vertical and not horizontal. This is fortunate because it allows elliptical vertical excision of pathologic tissue (that is, it allows rapid rehabilitation because abduction does not create undue tension on the anastomotic site). In those cases of pathologic tendon change without rupture (including calcific tendinitis) vertical elliptical excision with repair is always chosen. Since the biceps is a humeral head stabilizer, it is best to leave it undisturbed unless it is clearly symptomatic and major changes are present. In this instance, resection of pathologic changes is recommended. Total resection and distal bicipital groove attachment is reserved only if imminent rupture is anticipated or has occurred (Figs. 28-5 and 28-6).

The subacromial space is now inspected for possible compromise. It is conceivable, as Neer suggests, that the downward slope of the anterior acromion may be extreme by hereditary pattern and may thereby compromise the coracoacromial space, but there is no objective test to make this determination, and indiscriminate attack on the acromion in my opinion is unwarranted, since deltoid harm often results.

Subacromial pathologic change is not uncommon in the form of bony exostosis usually as a mirror image of clavicular alteration in acromioclavicular osteoarthritis. The isolated anterior acromial lesion as described by Neer is uncommon in my experience but does occur in long-standing problems associated with major upward humeral migration (most often noticed with full rotator cuff tear). If anterior subacromial exostoses are present (as found by palpation), they are easily removed by horizontal subacromial instrumentation (such as dental burrs, oscillating saw, or hand rasp). It is unnecessary to remove any deltoid from the anterior acromion with this

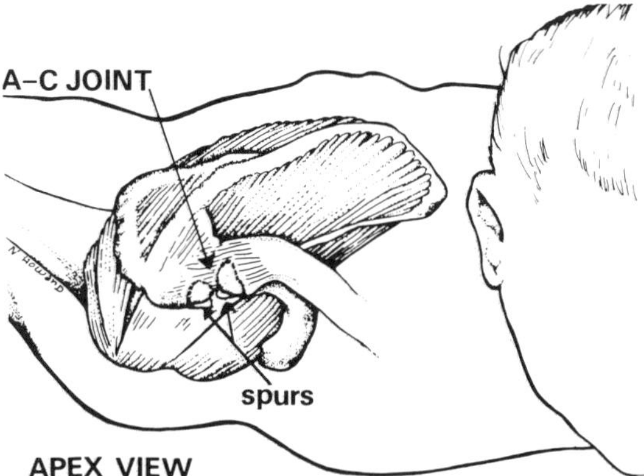

Fig. 28-6. Surgical technique. If acromioclavicular osteoarthritis is present or there is a need for wide exposure (usually with complete cuff tear), the metaphyseal flair of the distal clavicle is excised. Most acromial osteophytes reflect acromioclavicular osteoarthritis rather than the more uncommon anterior acromial lesion. Anterior acromioplasty is therefore unnecessary in most instances.

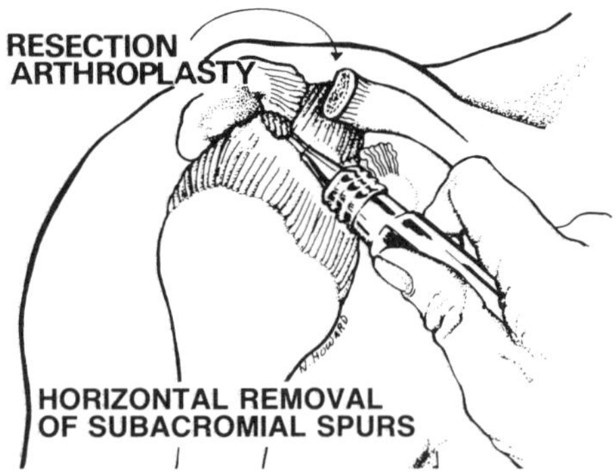

Fig. 28-7. Surgical technique. The more uncommon circumstance of subacromial anterior osteophytes being removed by subacromial approach thereby protects the deltoid origin on the acromion. This technique therefore allows one to avoid the traditional full-thickness acromioplasty.

technique. The full-thickness anterior acromioplasty is therefore unnecessary unless some rare extenuating circumstance is present (Fig. 28-7).

In those cases in which a major posterolateral cuff retraction occurs (unusual in competitive athletes but occasionally present in older recreational athletes), a secondary posterior expansion of the incision over the infraspinatus fossa by paralleling of the scapular ridge may help in mobilization. In a crisis situation, Neer has suggested a total anterior shift of the infraspinatus.[16]

If proximal retraction into the supraspinatus fossa occurs, resection of the distal end of the clavicle is necessary for maximum supraspinatus mobilization. If the retracted cuff cannot be returned to anatomic position, repair into the humeral head

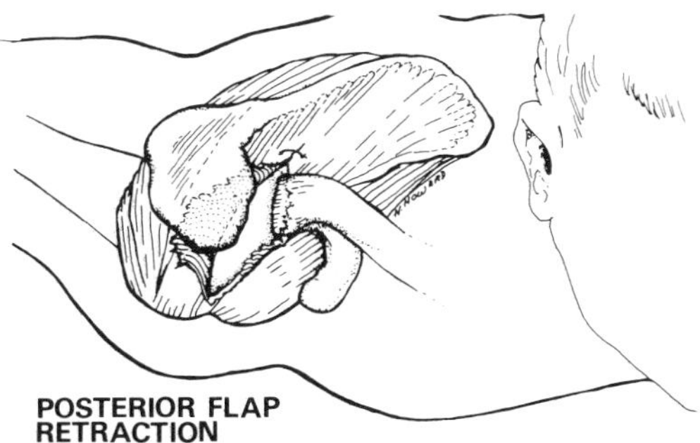

Fig. 28-8. Surgical technique. In those cases of full-thickness tear with retraction, the retraction is more likely to occur posterolaterally toward the infraspinatus fossa rather than proximally toward the supraspinatus fossa, since in most cases the tear is vertical and triangular rather than horizontal and transverse.

is indicated.[12] It is helpful to abduct the arm during this operative phase. In my view, however, the tension at the anastomatic site must not preclude the return of the arm to the patient's side at the time of surgery or the repair will most certainly be compromised during rehabilitation. In this regard, if it is necessary to maintain arm abduction in the immediate postoperative period, it is unlikely that the repair can be protected in the rehabilitative process. If resection of the acromioclavicular joint (distal end of the clavicle) is necessary, care is taken to protect the acromioclavicular ligament because repair of this structure is important in enhancing firm stabilization of the shoulder girdle to the distal end of the clavicle. The vertical spread of the deltoid is firmly closed along with the proximal closure of the acromioclavicular ligament. The subcutaneous and skin layers are closed in routine fashion (Fig. 28-8 to 28-10).

ROLE OF ARTHROSCOPY

Preliminary reports of the use of arthroscopic techniques in rotator cuff lesions have been made by Andrews[1] and others.[35] Since the spectrum of rotator cuff lesions is highly varied (including a high percentage of extra-articular changes), arthroscopy appears to be limited. Although intra-articular presentation of angiofibroblastic pathologic change may be amenable to arthroscopic resection, commonly associated extra-articular changes (subdeltoid bursa, acromioclavicular osteoarthritis, extra-articular cuff changes, subacromial exostosis) and lesions requiring repair seriously compromise the diagnostic accuracy and treatment capacity of the arthroscopic approach.

Andrews[1] has presented evidence that arthroscopy may have a more important role in intra-articular diagnostic problems including subluxation associated with labrum tears, loose bodies, and bicipital tendinitis in the areas of glenoid attachment. Further evaluation will be necessary for assessment of arthroscopic long-term value in these and other pathologic areas.

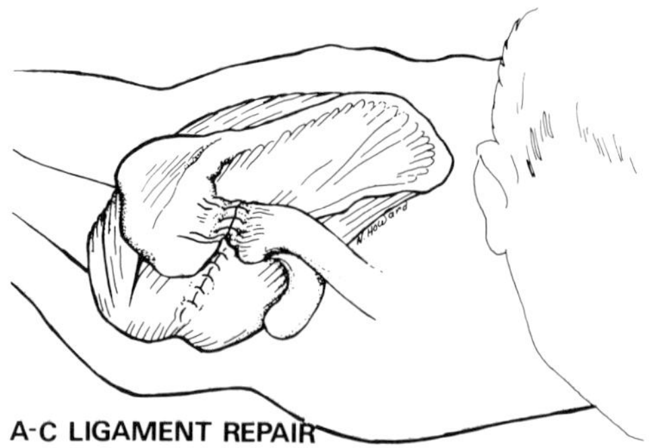

Fig. 28-9. Surgical technique for repair of the rotator cuff. If an acromioclavicular arthroplasty has been done, a firm repair of the acromioclavicular ligament enhances deltoid repair and postoperative rehabilitation. Many full-thickness cuff tears need only a sling for 2 to 3 weeks when care is taken not to harm normal tissues and firm vertical repairs are achieved.

POSTOPERATIVE CARE

Relaxed immobilization with a sling and swathe is utilized until healing adequate to tolerate mobility is achieved (usually 3 to 5 days). In the more standard athletic injury (which most commonly involves angiofibroblastic pathologic change or partial supraspinatus tear) vertical elliptical repair allows Codman's type of motion activity within a few days. Control of edema and pain are aided by early use of high-voltage electrical stimulation. A sling without swathe is utilized until patient comfort is equivalent with or without the sling (usually 2 to 3 weeks). Graduated resistance exercise in forward flexion can be started when 75% of motion is restored (usually 3 weeks). Progression of exercise is closely supervised, but activities such as easy swim strokes, gentle golf swing, and early tennis ground strokes can often be initiated at 6 to 8 weeks.

In full cuff tear repair with associated resection of the distal end of the clavicle, the rehabilitative progression is based upon the quality of tissue and security of the repair. A similar well-supervised rehabilitative progression as noted for partial tear is implemented in these instances as well.

RETURN TO SPORTS

The optimum success of rotator cuff surgery is full return to sports activity at the preinjury level. Total success as measured by this parameter is dependent on a variety of key factors.
1. Magnitude of injury
2. Quality of remaining tissues
3. Ultimate quality of repair
4. Maintenance of normalcy to uninjured tissues
5. Intrinsic biologic healing capacity

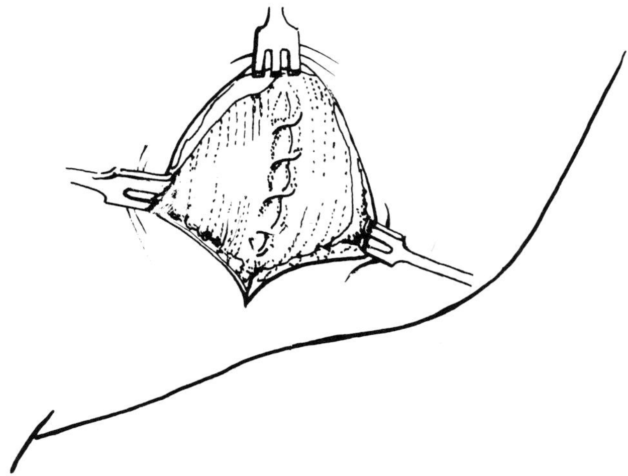

Fig. 28-10. Surgical technique for repair of the deltoid muscle. By avoiding the anterior acromioplasty, one can repair the deltoid easily. Since the acromial attachment is not harmed, rehabilitation is speeded and the danger of deltoid disruption is avoided.

6. Intensity of rehabilitative effort
7. Demands of the sport activity
8. Psychologic factors

Suffice it to say, when major injury occurs, competitive athletes in demanding sports such as swimming and baseball pitching face the greatest challenge in returning to high-level performance. The prognosis in this situation should always be guarded but with a favorable combination of factors, a high-level return on occasion will be achieved, especially if the tear is less than 1 cm as noted by Jobe.[9]

In contradistinction, the average recreational athlete can expect to return to sport activity at a reasonable level if satisfactory repair and adequate rehabilitation is achieved.

SHOULDER SUMMARY

The cause of shoulder tendinitis is a complex issue encompassing a variety of mechanical and biologic issues. Intrinsic tensile overload and subsequent muscle weakness and tendon pathologic alteration are likely primary factors. The impingement concept is more appropriately categorized as a secondary factor and occurs when rotator cuff weakness allows upward humeral migration. This distinction is important because it directs the treatment plan to the pathologic areas of the rotator cuff rather than the acromion.

The concept of controlling upward humeral migration by strengthening the rotator cuff muscles better explains the success of the conservative treatment plan in early tendinitis. Surgical techniques avoid full-thickness anterior acromioplasty, and the concept of coracoacromial ligament resection without specific indication is challenged.

REFERENCES

1. Andrews, J.: Shoulder arthroscopy. Presented at American Academy of Orthopaedic Surgeons: Instructional course lecture: Athletic upper extremity injuries, Jan. 1985, Las Vegas, Nevada.
2. Bateman, J.E.: The shoulder and neck, ed. 2, Philadelphia, 1978, W.B. Saunders Co.
3. Codman, E.A.: Complete rupture of the supra-spinatus tendon: operative treatment with report of 2 successful cases, Boston Med. Surg. J. **164:**708, 1911.
4. Codman, E.A.: The shoulder: rupture of the surpaspinatus tendon and other lesions in or about the subacromial bursa, Boston, 1934, Thomas Todd.
5. DePalma, A.F.: Surgery of the shoulder, ed. 2, Philadelphia, 1973, J.B. Lippincott Co.
6. Fowler, P.: Swimming injuries to the rotator cuff. Presented at American Academy of Orthopaedic Surgeons: Instructional course lecture: Athletic upper extremity injuries, Jan. 1985, Las Vegas, Nevada.
7. Hollingshead, W.H.: Anatomy for surgeons, vol. 3, The back and limbs, New York, 1958, Hoeber-Harper.
8. Inman, V.T., Saunders, J.B., and Abbott, L.C.: Observations on the function of the shoulder joint, J. Bone Joint Surg. **26A:**1, 1944.
9. Jobe, F.W., and Jobe, C.M.: Painful athletic injuries of the shoulder, Clin. Orthop. (173):117-124, 1983.
10. Lindblom, J., and Palmer, F.: Rupture of the tendon aponeurosis of the shoulder joint: the so-called supraspinatus rupture, Acta Chir. Scand. **82:**133, 1939.
11. McLaughlin, H.L.: Muscular and tendinous defects at the shoulder and their repair. In American Academy of Orthopaedic Surgeons: Lectures on reconstruction surgery of the extremities, Ann Arbor, 1944, J.W. Edwards.
12. McLaughlin, H.S.: Lesions of the musculotendinous cuff of the shoulder: the exposure and treatment of tears with retraction, J. Bone Joint Surg. **26A:**31, 1944.
13. Moseley, H.F.: Shoulder lesions, ed. 2, New York, 1953, Paul B. Hoeber, Inc.
14. Moseley, H.F., and Goldie, I.: The arterial pattern of the rotator cuff of the shoulder, J. Bone Joint Surg. **45B:**780, 1963.
15. Neer, C.S., II: Personal communication, 1984, Washington, D.C.
16. Neer, C.S., II: Anterior acromioplasty for the chronic impingement syndrome in the shoulder: a preliminary report, J. Bone Joint Surg. **54A:**41, 1972.
17. Neer, C.S., II: Impingement lesions, Clin. Orthop. (173):70, 1983.
18. Neer, C.S., II, and Marberry, T.A.: On the disadvantages of radial acromionectomy, J. Bone Joint Surg. **63A**(3):416, 1981.
19. Nirschl, R.P.: Swinging or throwing the shoulder pays, Physician and Sportsmedicine, no. 12, New York, Dec. 1974, McGraw-Hill, Inc.
20. Nirschl, R.P.: Arm care, Arlington, Va., 1983, Medical Sports Publishing.
21. Nirschl, R.P.: Athletic injuries to the elbow. Presented at American Academy of Orthopaedic Surgeons: Instructional course lecture: Athletic upper extremity injuries, Jan. 1985, Las Vegas, Nevada.
22. Nirschl, R.P.: Chapters 28 and 31 in Morrey, B.F., editor: The elbow and its disorders, Philadelphia, 1985, W.B. Saunders Co.
23. Nirschl, R.P., and Pettrone, F.P.: Tennis elbow: the surgical treatment of epicondylitis, J. Bone Joint Surg. **61A:**832, 1979.
24. Neviaser, T.J., Neviaser, R.J., and Neviaser, J.S.: Four-in-one arthroplasty for painful arch syndrome, Clin. Orthop. (163):107, 1982.
25. Perry, Jacqueline: Personal communication, 1985, Los Angeles, Calif.
26. Post, M., Jablom, J., Miller, H., and Singh, M.: Constrained total shoulder replacement: a critical review, Clin. Orthop. (144):135, 1979.
27. Post, M., Silver, R., and Singh, M.: Rotator cuff tear: diagnosis and treatment, Clin. Orthop. (173):78, 1983.

28. Rothman, R.H., and Parke, W.W.: The vascular anatomy of the rotator cuff, Clin. Orthop. (41):176, 1965.
29. Rathburn, J.B., and McNab, J.: The microvascular pattern of the rotator cuff, J. Bone Joint Surg. **52B:**540, 1970.
30. Stanish, W.D., and Curwin, S.: Tendinitis: its etiology and treatment, Lexington, Mass., 1984, The Collamore Press.
31. Saha, A.K.: The classic mechanism of shoulder movements and a plea for recognition of "zero position" of the glenohumeral joint, Clin. Orthop. (173):3, 1983.
32. Sarrafin, S.K.: Gross and functional anatomy of the shoulder, Clin. Orthop. (173):11, 1983.
33. Weiner, D.S., and MacNab, I.: Superior migration of the humeral head: a radiological aid in the diagnosis of tears of the rotator cuff, J. Bone Joint Surg. **52B:**524, 1970.
34. Weaver, J.K.: A systematic approach to the surgical treatment of chronic shoulder pain, Orthopaedics **7**(11):1697-1700, 1984.
35. Zarins, B.: Athletic injuries to the shoulder. In Eastern Orthopaedic Association: Instructional course lecture, Oct. 1983, Palm Beach, Florida.

29. Shoulder rehabilitation: rotator cuff tendinitis, strength training, and return to play

Janet Sobel

In embarking upon any rehabilitation program, we must first establish a basic framework of rehabilitation goals and a treatment plan. Whereas an adequate approach presumes an extensive knowledge of the anatomic and pathologic factors, a quality program involves in-depth consideration of the person's own needs and psyche and how he or she varies from the norm.

More commonly than not, the injury is attributable to deficits elsewhere; this is the ideal time to look for them and address ourselves to them. We can take advantage of this opportunity to get at those other aspects of the athlete, thus avoiding unnecessary stumbling blocks when he or she is ready to return to the sport. A common example in tennis is inadequate reconditioning from a prior injury resulting in decreased agility or poor trunk motion or decreased strength causing an overload on the shoulder structures to overcome these deficits. If these deficient areas are not addressed during the shoulder rehabilitation program, the athlete will be back again soon after return to play with yet another injury resulting from the improperly identified cause. The rehabilitation then must include maintaining the overall fitness level as well as overcoming deficits in aerobic and anaerobic capacity; coordination and agility; and strength, endurance, and flexibility of other body parts.
The basic tendinitis conservative treatment program includes the following:
Relief of pain and inflammation
Promotion of healing
Rehabilitation exercise
Conditioning exercise and maximization of overall fitness level
Sport-specific activities and protection from abusive overload for return to sport

"REST" PHASE: RELIEF OF PAIN AND INFLAMMATION

The duration of this period is highly variable, depending largely on the chronicity and severity of the tendinitis. Often the initial phase is very short lived, lasting 3 to 10

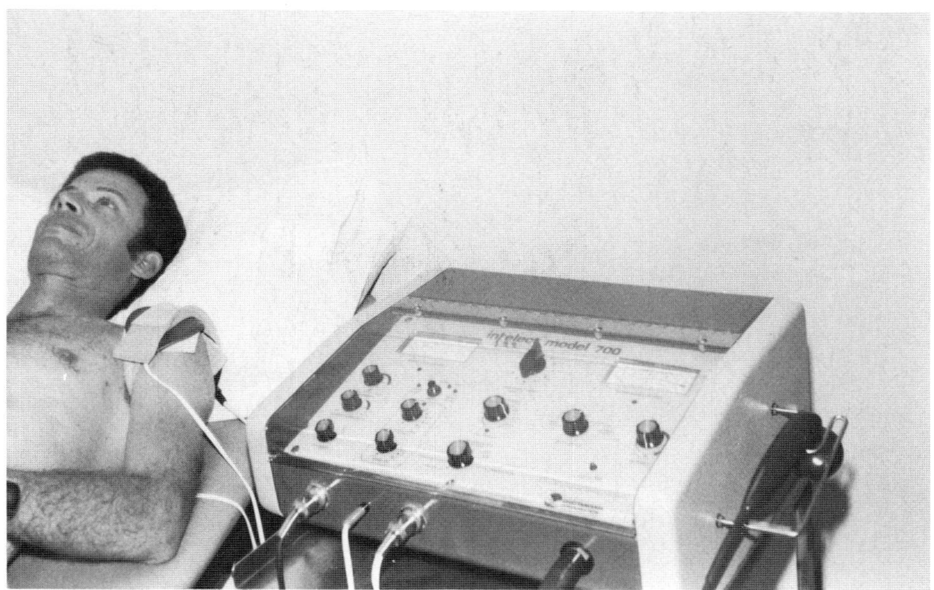

Fig. 29-1. High-voltage electrical stimulation for shoulder rotator cuff tendinitis.

days, but then it carries through the entire rehabilitation process. Rest is the backbone of this phase. Rest (in this context) means protection against abuse, not absence from activity. In fact, it is desirable to maintain as high an activity level as possible while avoiding those motions that are injurious to the rotator cuff. Absolute rest undoubtedly helps to eliminate the abuse, but it also initiates atrophy, it reduces the vascular supply to the area because of lack of demand, it is derogatory to the healing process, and it deconditions tissues.[4] It is important to note that although rest does address pain and inflammation, rest alone does not promote healing. All too often the athlete is misguided by the pain relief achieved by a period of rest, only to rediscover the pain immediately upon return to play. A period of rest must be followed by rehabilitative exercise to promote healing and avoid reinjury. Anti-inflammatory medications are often used in this phase along with the modalities of physical therapy. The modalities I find most effective in treating the shoulder are high-voltage electrical stimulation, moist heat, and ice. The usefulness of the high-voltage stimulators (Fig. 29-1) seems to be in their characteristic short pulse duration (thus creating a very comfortable stimulation) and high peak current (allowing deeper tissue penetration). It is currently believed, although not well supported with research data, that the combination of short pulse duration and high peak current enables the high-voltage stimulators to discriminatingly evoke sensory, motor, and pain responses. The use of electrical stimulation in our clinic is based on its theoretical effectiveness in pain reduction, enhancement of circulation, decrease of inflammation, and possibly promotion of soft-tissue healing.[1] As a general rule, four to six sessions over a 2 or 3-week period is a good indicator of the patient's response to this modality. Interestingly the

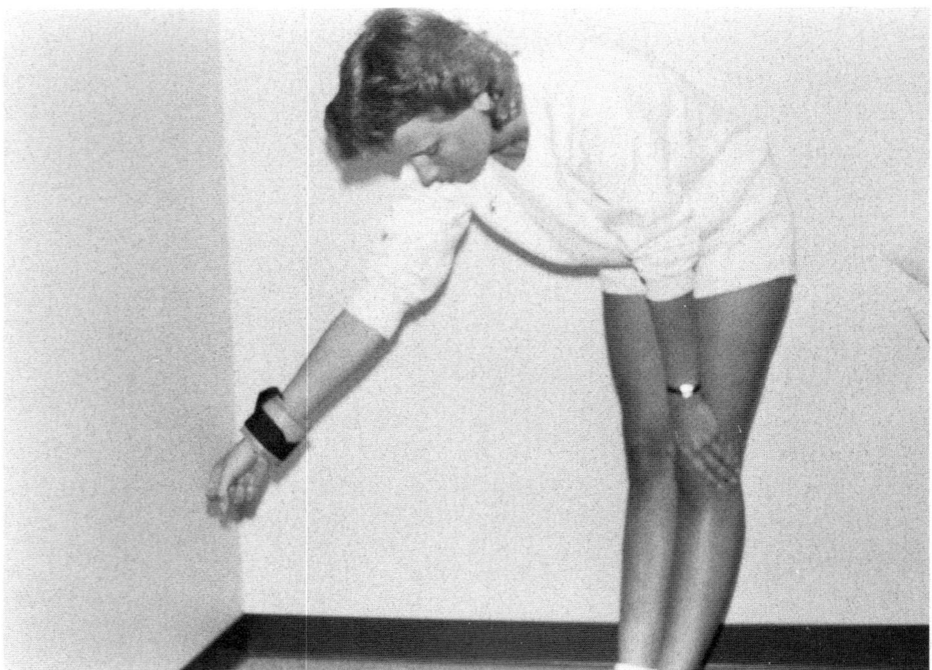

Fig. 29-2. Pendulum swings, in increasing arcs, diagonals, and cardinal planes. These also serve as an excellent presport warm-up.

patients I have treated who don't find it analgesic but find it more irritating usually do not respond well to the whole conservative effort. It is my belief that their tissue may have reached a pathologic stage beyond the reach of the conservative approach. Moist heat is routinely used with the electrical stimulation (1) to minimize the stiffness often experienced immediately after treatment and (2) as a method for warming up the area for exercise. Ultrasound is a form of deep heat, such that sound waves are absorbed by the tissues, producing heat. Absorption is greatest at tissue interfaces. Ultrasound has both thermal and nonthermal effects, caused by the vibration of molecules. Phonophoresis uses the ultrasound head to drive whole molecules of a medium (often steroids) percutaneously into the inflamed tissue. It should be noted that prolonged application of steroids may cause their failure under stress. I do not find ultrasound or phonophoresis a reliably effective modality in shoulder tendinitis and rarely use it in this context. Ice is essential throughout the rehabilitation program. In the early stages it offers a contrast effect after heat to help keep the inflammation down and for its analgesic effects. Later on, it is very effective after exercise to minimize the inflammatory response.

Rotator cuff tendinitis is unique in that the problem here is ultimately one of impingement and weakening but whose origin may be attributable to a wide variety of factors. The supraspinatus tendon is a flat, broad one. The shoulder stiffness that develops is from the capsule and subscapularis, not from the supraspinatus. Thus normal shoulder flexibility arcs do not further abuse the injured tendon (supraspinatus) so that stretching here should begin early. Pendulum swings and circles (Fig. 29-2), the PNF (proproceptive neuromuscular facilitation) diagonals of flexion–abduction–external rotation,[2] and external rotation stretching at different angles of flexion and of abduction are effective to stretch the anterior capsule and external rotators. Low-intensity exercise is initiated to the involved muscles, and at the same time adjacent muscle groups are worked more aggressively. The goals of these flexibility exercises are improved soft-tissue pliability and mobility, functional joint motion for everyday needs, a gain of even distribution of force loads, and enhanced blood supply and musculoskeletal nourishment.

Isometric exercises of all the muscle groups, using the other arm or a door frame for resistance, are started immediately at a submaximal intensity. These isometrics are worked in the muscles' shortened, middle, and lengthened positions as long as they do not cause tissue impingement or irritation. Gradually the patient works from submaximal to maximal contractions and from limited to full-range isometrics.

PHASES 2 AND 3: PROMOTE HEALING—REHABILITATIVE EXERCISE

The healing process is separate and distinct from the anti-inflammatory one, and ignorance of its necessity often results in a premature and unsuccessful attempt at sports return. To promote healing, we continue the effort to minimize abuse and inflammation (through electrical stimulation, ice, and protective activity) while superimposing rehabilitative exercise. This phase usually begins about 6 to 10 days after the initiation of treatment. Throughout this phase the patient is advised to avoid the painful arc of midrange abduction, horizontal adduction, and hyperextension. Rehabilitative exercise is low-intensity work with pain as its primary limiting factor. If the exercise reproduces the pain, the patient is advised to modify it by decreasing the repetitions, the resistance, or the range of motion, or all three. These exercises are performed daily, alternating Isoflex with isotonic programs. Isotonic resistance is generally greater in midrange, whereas Isoflex offers more end-range resistance so that the combination of the two is an effective one.

Isotonic exercises begin at a high number of repetitions with a 1-pound weight, which is incrementally increased to patient tolerance. The goals of exercise here are to reintroduce the injured part to activity, stimulate healing, maintain tone, and develop endurance without reinjury or excessive stress on injured tissue. The isotonic exercises include the PNF diagonals[2] (Fig. 29-3), supine internal rotation for the subscapularis (Fig. 29-4), and sidelying and prone external rotation for the infraspinatus and teres minor (Figs. 29-5 and 29-6). Heavy emphasis is placed on the external rotators because their weakness (as a rule) presents the shoulder's greatest muscle imbalance. The role of the supraspiratus in depressing the humeral head, thus resisting its vertical displacement, is critical to normal joint mechanics. The extent of this external rotator weakness is all the more noteworthy in view of the strength demands

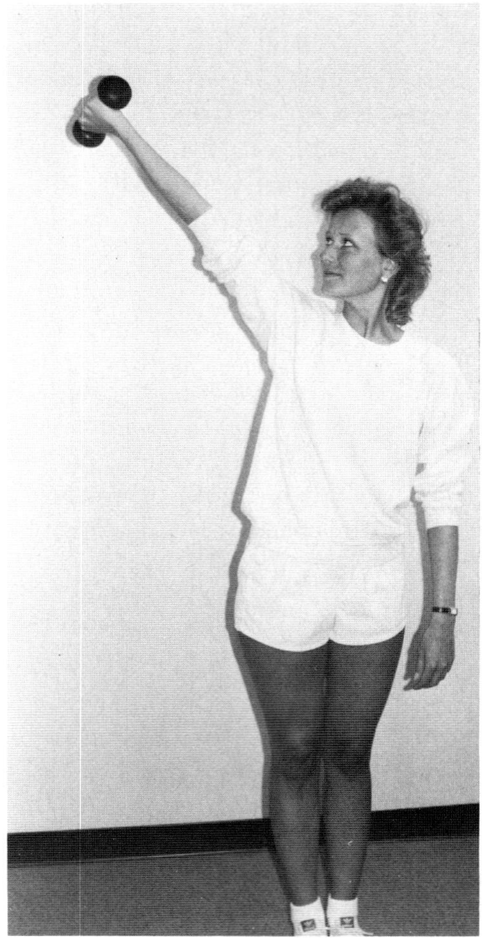

Fig. 29-3. Proprioceptive neuromuscular facilitation diagonals (PNF D_2) flexion:flexion–abduction–external rotation.

placed on these muscles in the racket and throwing sports. With rotator cuff tendinitis of even short duration, supraspinatus weakness on manual muscle testing is an almost predictable finding. An effective supraspinatus strengthening technique is seen in Fig. 29-7, where, once in the "empty can" position, the involved arm is elevated and then lowered. As the healing phase progresses, the exercises are carried out with higher weights for fewer repetitions.

Isoflex exercise[3] (Fig. 29-8) is with use of an elastic tension cord to supply increasing resistance through the range of motion. The patient determines the amount of tension by where he or she places the anchored end of the strap. The progression variables with the Isoflex are the range of motion, the rate of exercise, and the placement of the other end of the Isoflex for resistance. Once slow-motion repetitions are mastered, the repetitions are done at high speed for endurance and quickness training.

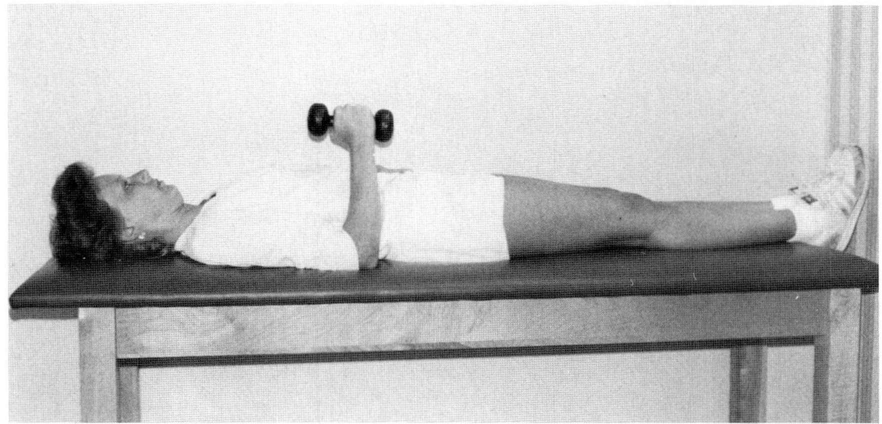

Fig. 29-4. Strengthening the subscapularis with supine internal rotation.

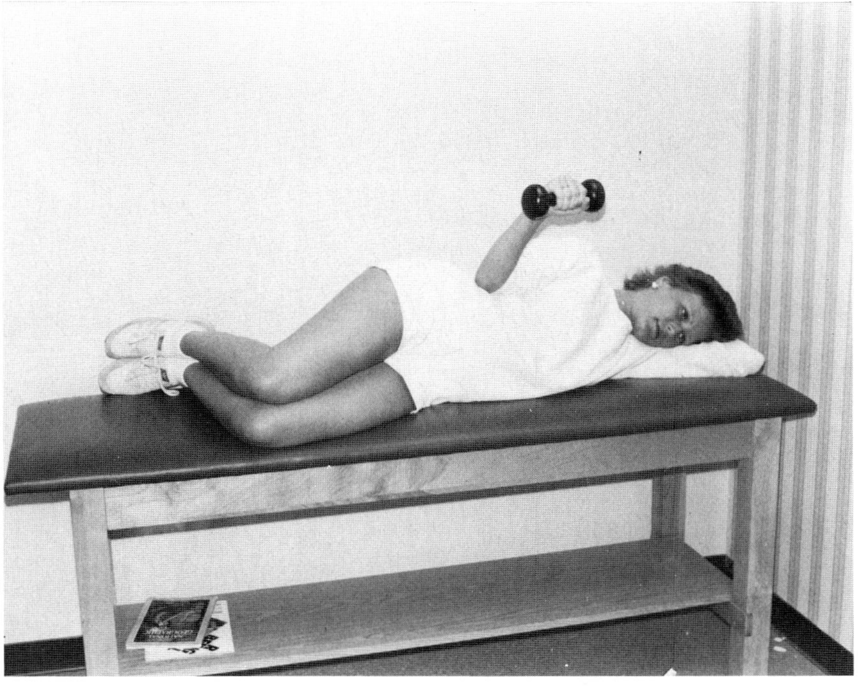

Fig. 29-5. Side-lying external rotation. This position with the arm along the side is most protective.

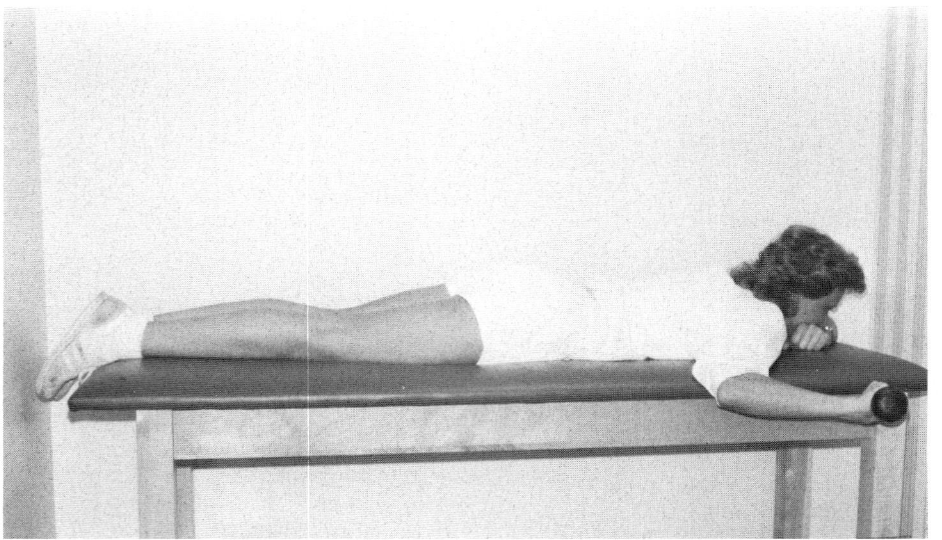

Fig. 29-6. External rotation strengthening prone. The shoulder and upper arm must be supported on a firm surface.

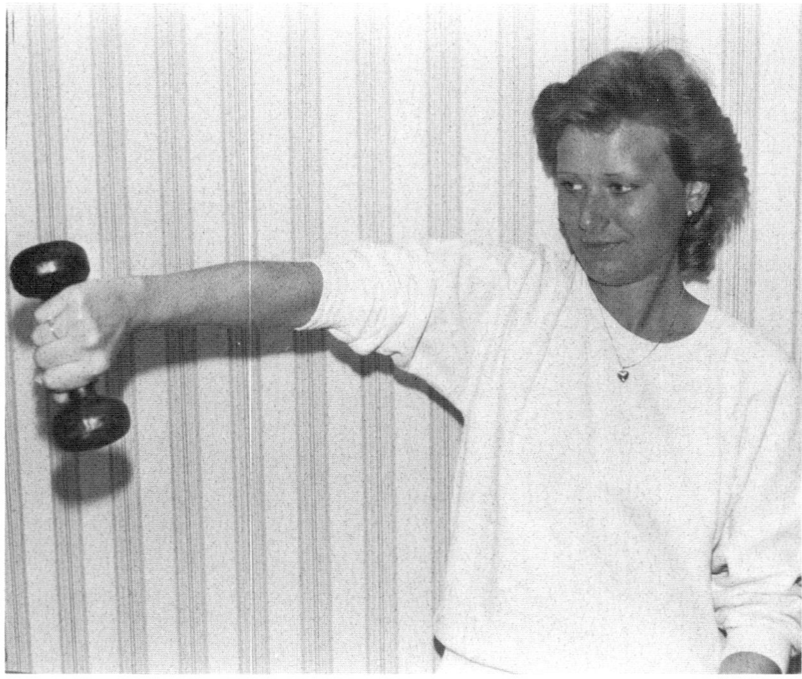

Fig. 29-7. The "empty can" for supraspinatus strengthening. Once in this position, the arm is slowly elevated and lowered approximately 30 degrees each way.

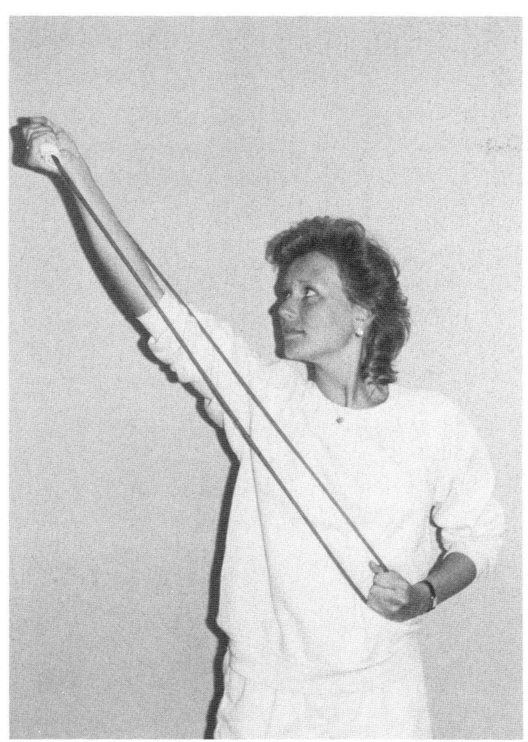

Fig. 29-8. D_2 flexion with the Isoflex. Resistance is monitored by placement of the anchoring hand.

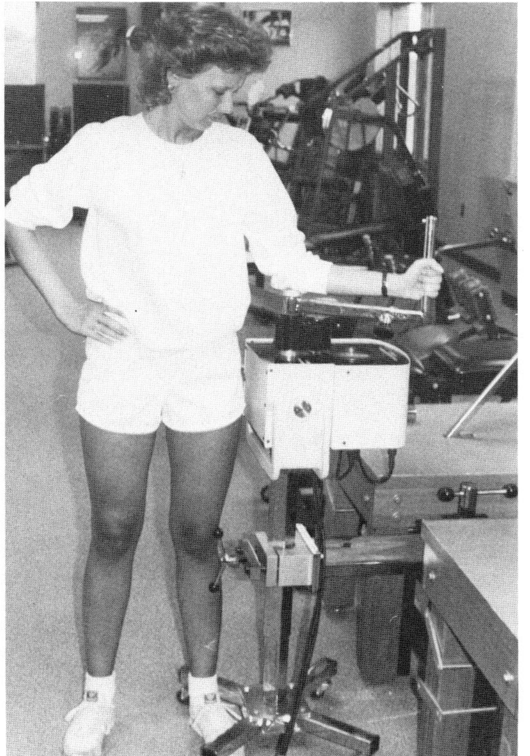

Fig. 29-9. Standing shoulder internal-external rotations on the Cybex.

Isokinetic exercise is started with standing rotations (Fig. 29-9) over a full range of speeds from 60 to 300 degrees per second. Short bouts initially progress to 50-second bouts at each speed as the program progresses. The isokinetic workouts later include PNF diagonals and blocked forward flexion. Isokinetics programs can be well-tailored to address sport-specific needs so that slow-speed, low-repetition, explosive-bouts, or high-speed endurance workouts are added as indicated.

Throughout rehabilitation, ice is essential after exercise. If any pain (other than muscle soreness) persists for more than 30 minutes after the workout, the exercise program needs to be modified.

PHASES 4 AND 5: RETURN TO SPORT

Once the injury is resolved, readiness for return to the sport is based on the following:

Full pain-free range of motion

Strength return within 10% of normal

Proper aerobic and anaerobic conditioning; full body conditioning for sport activity

Control of abuses[3]

Strength

Cybex strength testing involves three planes of motion: flexion-extension, abduction-adduction, and internal-external rotations. A normal-strength balance of these muscle groups is requisite: As a rule, we expect the adductors and extensors to be the strongest at all speeds; the flexors, internal rotators and abductors should have 60 to 75% of the extensor and adductor strength; the external rotators, to minimize injury potential, should be at least half the strength of the internal rotators' slow-speed output. Grip dynamometer testing is also performed, both with the elbow bent at the side and with the arm fully extended forward.

Proper conditioning

Once the injured part has regained its strength and flexibility, the sport-specific demands can be addressed. This involves emphasis on coordinated interaction of antagonistic and supporting muscle groups, performance training, and skill and speed drills. By this time, sport-specific fitness needs of all other body parts should have been met through full body workouts during the rehabilitation phases. Deficits elsewhere that may have set the stage for the injury should have been effectively addressed.

Control abuses by patient education

Our clinic places great emphasis on the athlete's full understanding of predisposing factors that caused the injury and how to control further abuses. He or she is taught that the shoulder canal is its tightest at about 90 degrees of abduction and that rotation in this position is most irritative to the rotator cuff. Shoulder motions well above and below the horizontal are far more protective of the rotator cuff. Sport technique or form modification may be necessary to avoid more abusive overload. A clear picture of the body's warning signals and when and how to respond to them puts the power to minimize the occurrence of severe injury in his control. The following guidelines are helpful:

Mild: Pain is usually benign if it presents as stiffness or soreness before or up to 24 hours after activity but is relieved by warm-up and absent during activity. This level of pain usually is self-limiting and gone within 1 or 2 days.

Significant: Stiffness or soreness that is not quieted by warm-up or activity. Although the pain persists through the activity, it does so mildly and in no way interferes with performance. Pain of this nature requires some activity modification and perhaps reintroduction of anti-inflammatory measures (ice, modalities, medication). If not attended to, this pain is likely to progress to harmful pain.

Harmful: The pain persists through the activity to the extent that it interferes with performance. It is particularly serious if it is not relieved by rest and the person is constantly aware of it. Medical attention is recommended here.[3]

Finally the athlete must recognize the importance of proper warm-up to increase body heat, and the techniques for specific shoulder warming before play (such as heat and massage) are instructed. The distinction is made between warm-up and flexibility: warm-up must precede flexibility exercises so that one can avoid unnecessary injury.

Progression variables

Full return to sport is best controlled by use of the variables of duration, frequency, and intensity of competition. By progressing these one by one, any causative injurious factors can be isolated and addressed. First, short bouts (about 20 minutes) of play involving nonstressful motions is progressed to longer play, alternating with progressing to motions that helped aggravate the shoulder. These are worked with in a well-controlled, noncompetitive environment. Finally, once full duration play involving all the motions is well tolerated, the intensity of competition is advanced. In this manner, full sports return is achieved with maximum protection against unidentifiable reinjury factors.

REFERENCES

1. Alon, G.: High voltage stimulation monograph, Chattanooga, Tenn., 1984, Chattanooga Corp.
2. Knott, M., and Voss, D.: Proprioceptive neuromuscular facilitation, New York, 1968, Harper & Row.
3. Nirschl, R.: Arm care, Arlington, Va., 1981, Medical Sports, Inc.
4. Nirschl, R.: Personal communication, 1984, Arlington, Va.

30. Supplemental exercise program for throwing, swimming, and gymnastics

Janet Sobel

Developing a supplemental exercise program for any sport must be, above all, a highly individualized procedure. No one sport fully meets all the fitness needs of any person. A supplemental program should overcome the imbalances imposed by the sport and should fill in the fitness gaps to create a fully conditioned, healthy athlete. Furthermore, each sport has specific supplemental needs for injury prevention and for maximum performance. Program development must also consider the person's own physical traits that predispose him to injury: age, hereditary factors and anatomic design, body proportion, and level of conditioning. The fundamentals of a quality program are as follows:

Risk factor analysis (cardiovascular and musculoskeletal)

Personal goals and interests

Current level of conditioning and activity

Injury and medical history

Hereditary factors and body proportion and alignment

Psychologic factors

GENERAL CONSIDERATIONS

A conditioning program to supplement any sport should include strength, flexibility, endurance, and cardiovascular and heat training. Such an exercise program is treated separately from a sport-training program that involves performance training, zeroing in on proper technique, skill, and coordination enhancement. This chapter addresses supplemental conditioning exercises.

Strength training

No one form of exercise can achieve all the strength training goals. A combination of several, some at different stages and some overlapping, is most effective. Maximal-effort multiangle isometrics are valuable, particularly in those areas where impingement or joint compressive forces are a problem, because strengthening can be accomplished without the part being moved through that area. Water exercises differ in

348

resistance from those with gravity and allow avoidance of the weight-bearing stresses. Elastic tension cord resistance (surgical tubing; IsoFlex) exercises the part with more resistance in the extremes of its motion range. Isotonics, on the other hand (dumbbells, barbells, weight machines), generally offer maximal strengthening effects in the midrange. Weight machines as a rule isolate muscle groups but are restricted to predetermined patterns of motion. With free weights, a wider variety of movements is available; thus free weights emphasize the coordinated interaction of muscles generally required in sports activities. Thus effective training for sports-specific demands should include free-standing equipment that can be modeled to meet varying needs.

Proprioceptive neuromuscular facilitation (PNF) is a technique of therapeutic exercise developed at the Kabat-Kaiser Institute (Vallejo, California), 1946-1951. It involves placing specific demands on the neuromuscular mechanism through stimulation of the proprioceptors in order to elicit a desired response. The spiral-diagonal movement patterns of facilitation are designed to work muscles from their fully lengthened state to their most shortened state. Three components of motion go into each diagonal pattern, and there are two diagonals for each major body part. Antagonistic movement patterns compose the two movements of each diagonal.[3] PNF can be used with free weight or tension cord resistance.

With both isotonics and elastic cord exercise, resistance is quite variable subject to leverage changes at different points in the range of motion. With isokinetic and hydraulic exercise, the speed is fixed, and the resistance accommodates automatically to the muscle tension developed by the exerciser. Its effectiveness is highly dependent on the exerciser's effort and motivational factors, but it has the potential to offer safe, dynamic maximal loading throughout the range of motion with resultant increased exercise efficiency. High-speed exercise allows for better joint lubrication and less joint compressive forces through the range; it can be effective to some extent for neuromuscular training nearing the higher speeds demanded by most sports. Currently available isokinetic devices do not offer eccentric loading, an important component in both strengthening and sport-specific exercise programs. Combining several forms of strength training then must be accomplished in any training program, but no form of strengthening will be effective unless it is done throughout a very flexible motion range. Throwing, swimming, and gymnastics place enormous demands on the part at its extremes of motion. Thus full-range strengthening into these extremes is essential for injury prevention and maximal sports performance. A quality program includes strengthening throughout a flexible range of motion.

Flexibility

In flexibility training, specific goals must be established based on the demands of the sport and of the activities of daily living. Without these goals, stretching can go on endlessly and harmfully or, on the other hand, can be undervalued and neglected because they become vague and seemingly purposeless. Flexibility exercises need only be done where functional deficits exist, based on individual evaluation. The goals of flexibility for sport are as follows:

1. *Injury prevention during sport participation.* All the motion demands the athlete may encounter during play must be met comfortably beforehand so that he or she does not get into an unmanageable position while playing. For example, poor flexibility and weakness in motion extremes often accounts for groin pulls in tennis.

2. *Good form.* A good example of this is seen in the tennis serve. If the player has inadequate shoulder flexion and external rotation, he or she is likely to compensate with a poor service motion at the shoulder ("tray position," where the arm is abducted to about 90 degrees), resulting in rotator cuff irritation and excessive elbow and forearm stresses. Equally as important as flexible motion is good strength throughout the motion extremes. As noted earlier, sports place enormous strength demands on a part in its extreme motion (such as the external rotators in throwing and serving and the abdominals and hip flexors in gymnastics), and inadequacy here is likely to show up as injury elsewhere.

3. *Overcome imbalances imposed by the sport.* Many sports and daily activities tend to tighten certain muscle groups. For example, hip flexor tightness is seen more often than not in most athletes (it is almost a rule in runners). Unless specific attention is paid to stretch these out, an imbalance around the hip will overstress the low back, hamstrings, and often the entire postural alignment when one is standing erect to try to overcome this forward pull.

4. *Less work effort by the antagonist.* When a muscle functions in sport, the less forces working against it, the better it will perform. Relief of its antagonistic muscle's tightness will decrease its work effort to overcome this resistance. For example, hamstring tightness is commonly found in chondromalacia of the patella. Many believe that this passive hamstring resistance increases the work effort and joint compressive forces of the quadriceps to overcome this impediment.

Flexibility training must be preceded by a full warm-up to avoid unnecessary injury during the stretching. The warm-up heats gelled ground substances interspersed between soft tissues, thus enhancing smooth lubricated tissue gliding.[4] Again, a distinct end point must be established because excessive stretching just invites lessened joint stability. A hyperflexible joint can be just as vulnerable to injury as a hypoflexible one can be. Key areas of deficit should be isolated and corrected.

In my experience, the most effective stretching techniques are as follows:

1. *Static stretch.* After warm-up, the part is brought to slight pain in a slow, smooth motion (no ballistics). Then ease back slightly, and hold the position for 20 to 30 seconds, coordinating deep breathing. Finally stretch a bit further and repeat the 20- to 30-second hold. We've found it more effective to stretch the larger muscle groups first.

2. *Dynamic stretch.* This is valuable in preparing for sports participation. The part is actively brought through the motion extremes in a flowing motion,

without the stresses of weight-bearing or impact. For example, taking a tennis racket several times rhythmically through the motions demanded in a match but without ball impact.

3. *PNF techniques.* The proprioceptive neuromuscular facilitation techniques are based on the principle of reciprocal inhibition, where the antagonist is relaxed (inhibited) during the agonist's work effort (facilitated). For example, "hold-relax" involves maximum resistance to an isometric contraction ("hold") followed by relaxation, and then the part is moved into more motion. "Contract-relax" involves isotonic contraction of the antagonist, allowing motion in rotation only against maximal resistance but no motion of the other components (flexion-abduction or extension-adduction). There follows a period of relaxation during which the part is moved into more range. These techniques are highly effective, especially when used with the PNF diagonals.[3]

Endurance

Swimming, gymnastics, and throwing sports require cardiovascular and muscular endurance to some extent. Muscular endurance training involves higher speed, mild resistance, full-range exercise with repetitions to fatigue. I have found it effective to work on endurance on alternate days with strength training.

Aerobics

Aerobic fitness is important for everyone but often overlooked in athletes. Many mistakenly assume that a good athlete is in good aerobic condition. In a recent study on the United States Pan-American Women's Gymnastics Team, with a bicycle ergometer and Cooper's 12-minute walk-run test, my group found several in the less than fair category.

SWIMMING

Swimming is probably the most benevolent sport of all at the recreational level, yet injuries are commonplace in the competitive swimmer. Unlike gymnastics and throwing, swimming is primarily an upper body sport in terms of its advantageous effects and injury potential. The swimmer's shoulder is subject to enormous stress because of the high repetition rate, the extremes of range used, and the sustained effort necessary for propulsion during the pull phase. As discussed by Richardson,[6] the swimming stroke is much like the acceleration phase of throwing, but in swimming the action has to be sustained. Because of the high repetitions, overload is unsurprising. To supplement the training program, then, all swimmers need a dry-land exercise program for strengthening, speed, endurance and flexibility.

Supplemental exercises for injury prevention and good form should include full-range strengthening of the latissimus dorsi, triceps, deltoids, shoulder internal and external rotators, wrist flexors, hip adductors, and ankle plantar flexors. Shoulder internal, external rotation, hyperflexion, and hyperextension flexibility work is important for good form and injury prevention. To overcome imbalances and inade-

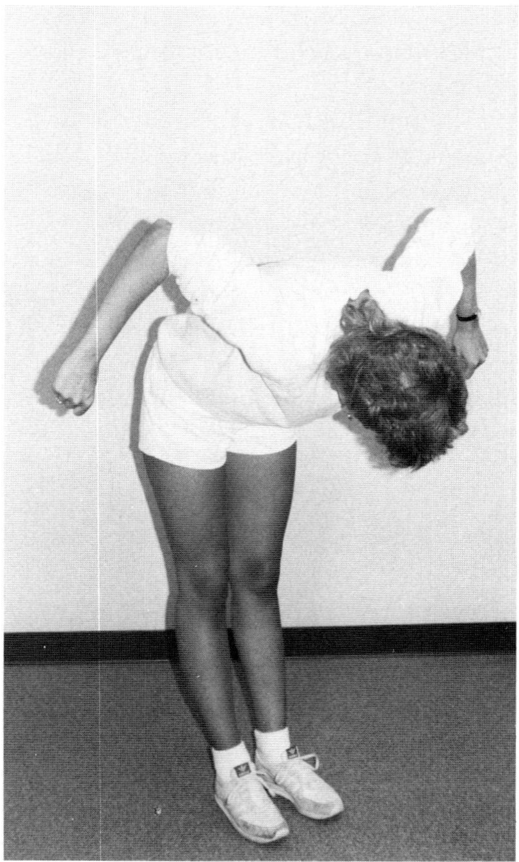

Fig. 30-1. Isometric posterior deltoid strengthening. Intensity can be made greater by a partner's resistance.

quacies of swimming, abdominal and leg strengthening with stretching of the low back and hip flexors and adductors should be included.

Isometrics are effective, especially against another person's manual resistance. For example, posterior deltoid strength is essential in order to get quick elbow exit during recovery. An effective isometric is bringing the shoulders to 90 degrees and hyperextending them intensely (Fig. 30-1). More resistance can be added by a trainer or partner. Nautilus machines offer the swimmer effective full-range strengthening, but caution must be taken against excessively high weights because extra bulk is undesirable.[1] IsoFlex, isokinetics, and hydraulics offer unilateral, full-range, high-speed workouts. Using these in PNF diagonals incorporates the coordinated interaction of muscle groups needed in each of the swimming strokes. Upper body cycling where the exerciser sits behind a bicycle and cycles with his arms is a valuable supplement to any swimming program (Fig. 30-2).

Emphasis on shoulder external rotator strengthening is fundamental to a quality

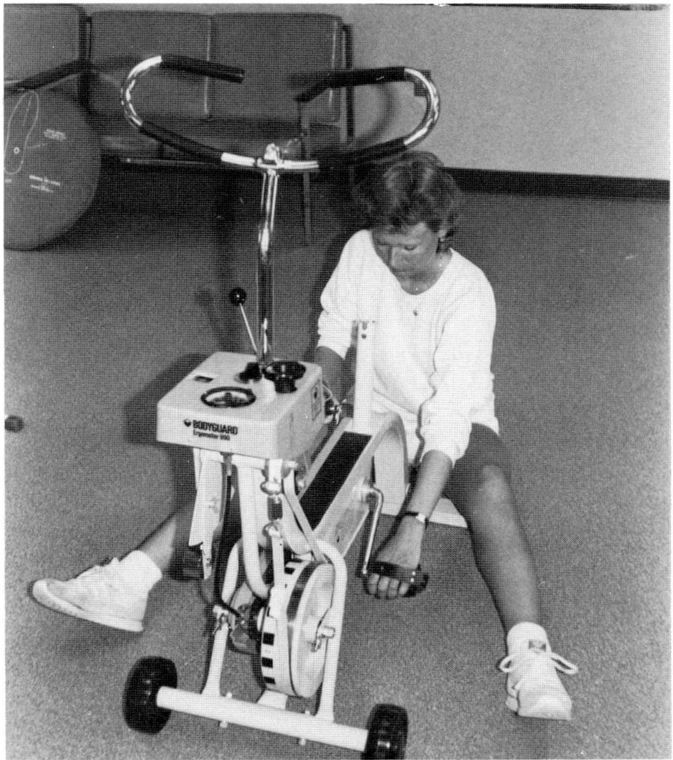

Fig. 30-2. Any stationary bicycle can be used for arm cycling.

supplemental program for any of these sports. Our Cybex studies show that the external rotators are as weak as 50% of internal rotators in peak torque produced at all speeds. This is the largest agonist-antagonist muscle imbalance in the upper body. External rotator strengthening with the arm at the side avoids repetitive irritation of the rotator cuff.

THROWING SPORTS

In the throwing sports, although most injuries are of the upper body, a great percentage of the power comes from the lower body and trunk. The body functions as a linked system whereby the force generated in the lower body is transferred through the kinetic chain to the ball.[2] Thus we need to emphasize hip and trunk strengthening.

Shoulder external rotator strengthening must include work at all angles of the range with particular attention to extreme abduction. Eccentric external rotator loading is critical to injury prevention because great demand is placed on the external rotators to decelerate in the follow-through phase.[6] Strengthening the biceps, wrist flexors, and the muscles around the medial elbow helps provide much-needed medial elbow support in the early phases of the throwing motion. In the acceleration phase, the latissimus and pectoralis major must quickly contract for powerful shoulder internal rotation.[5] Again, full-range strengthening is needed here. Effective biceps strengthening for throwing involves both concentric and eccentric loading. Supplemental lower body work should include abdominal and hip flexor strengthening to pull the body forward. All thigh and hip muscles should be strengthened throughout their full motion. Speed of movement and agility drills round out the supplemental exercise program for the throwing sports.

GYMNASTICS

Gymnastics is a unique sport in its demands on several body parts. The shoulder is challenged in stability (as in the handstand), mobility (uneven bars), power (rings), and endurance through sustaining quickly interacting compressive and distractive forces (parallel and uneven bars).[7] In fact, each of the joints undergoes an unusual combination of stresses.

A supplemental exercise program should include a two or three times a week workout with heavy weights and low repetitions for maximal strength gains. (Note: In young gymnasts, working against their own body weight is preferable to higher resistance from external weights). In the lower body, we found outstanding strength deficits in the hip adductors and in the ankle (ankle sprains are common to gymnasts). Alternate days with the strength training program should involve coordination and agility drills as well as dance to develop grace. Unfortunately, grace and elegance are often compromised because of emphasis on strengthening. Endurance training is effectively accomplished through 30-second sprints against elastic tubing resistance or just the athlete's own body weight.

Back problems are a serious threat to the gymnast. It has been my experience that emphasis is best placed on endurance of the low back muscles, rather than on maximum strengthening. High-repetition, full-range back extension against elastic tubing resistance has proved very effective. Abdominals too should be worked in similar manner. For ankle muscle endurance, coordination, and balance to minimize occurrence of sprains, the ankle balance board challenges the ankle in all directions through full motion (Fig. 30-3). Our test results with elite gymnasts showed an alarmingly short tolerance period to this, often only 10 to 15 seconds. Eccentric loading of the ankle plantar flexors is helpful to enhance performance in landings. At the same time, the dorsiflexors must not be overlooked because an imbalance here predisposes the gymnast to "shin-splint" pain. Hip clicks, another common problem , can often be averted by repeated internal and external hip rotation while one is in a sitting straight leg raise (Fig. 30-4).

Finally, wrist exercises should be included in a supplemental gymnastics program because injuries of the wrist are among the highest. Active wrist extension often measures in the 30- to 45-degree range for these athletes because of tendons' response to the weight-bearing stresses. This limited motion is unacceptable for competition, where the gymnast repeatedly hyperextends the wrists while bearing full body weight on them. Sitting wrist hyperflexion and hyperextension exercises then are in-

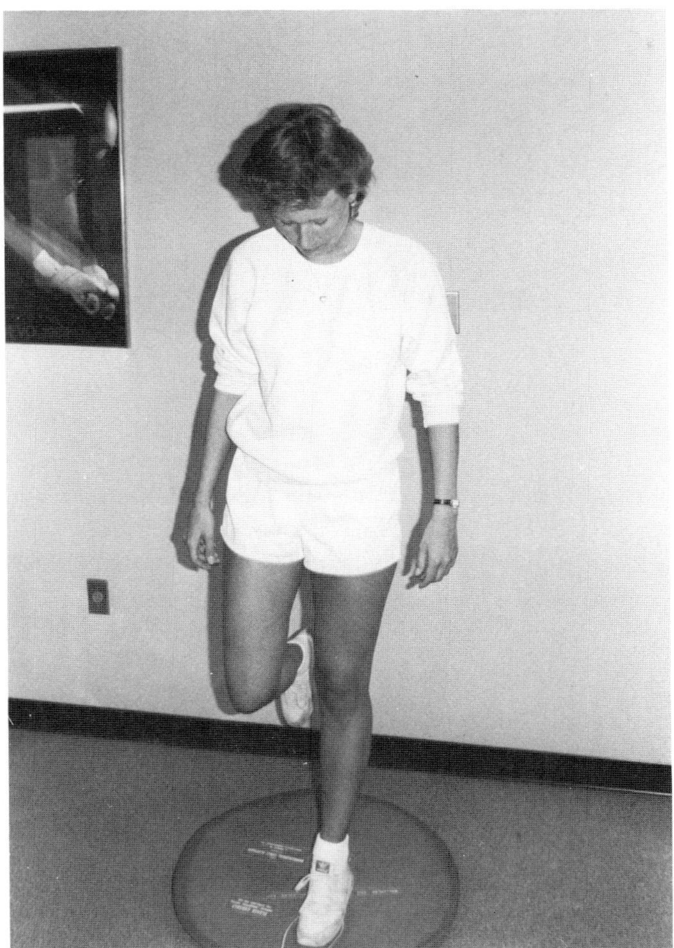

Fig. 30-3. The Biomechanical Ankle Platform System (Camp Therapy Products, Jackson, Michigan) for balance and muscle interaction. Challenge is added when the board is raised progressively higher off the floor (using larger ball underneath) or with weights on the board.

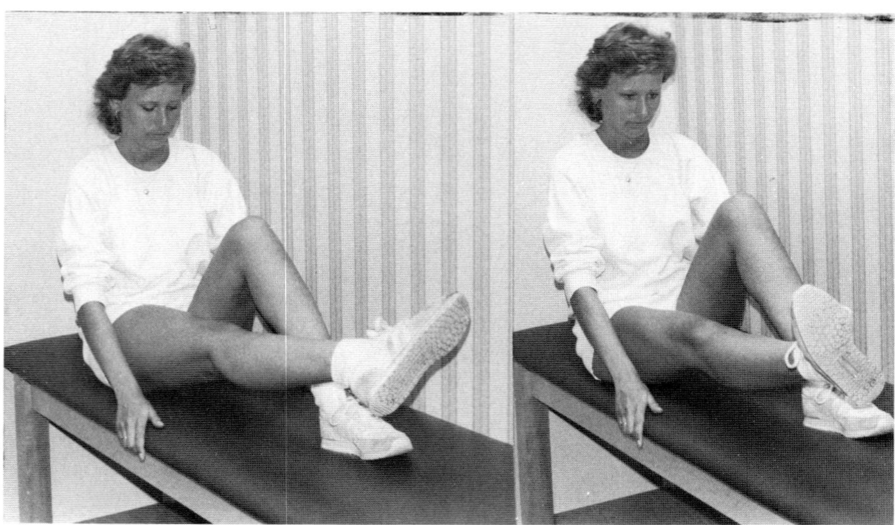

Fig. 30-4. In a sitting straight leg raise, the hip is internally and externally rotated. A good preventive exercise for hip clicks.

dicated. Other flexibility demands on the gymnast's body are overwhelming, and yet except for the wrist and the low back, this does not often present a problem for these athletes. Additional attention should be paid to wrist and low back flexibility.

The guidelines discussed in this chapter address common demands of each of the sports. A thorough evaluation of each athlete is prerequisite to developing the individualized program that will most benefit him or her.

REFERENCES

1. Counsilman, J.: The complete book of swimming, New York, 1983, Atheneum Publishers.
2. Groppel, Jack: Personal communication, 1984, Urbana, Ill.
3. Knott, M., and Voss, D.: Proprioceptive neuromuscular facilitation, New York, 1968, Harper & Row.
4. Nirschl, R.: Arm care, Arlington, Va., 1981, Medical Sports, Inc.
5. Perry, J.: Anatomy and biomechanics of the shoulder in throwing, swimming, gymnastics and tennis, Clinics in Sports Medicine, 2(2):247-270, July 1983, Philadelphia, W.B. Saunders Co.
6. Richardson, A.: Overuse syndromes in baseball, tennis, gymnastics and swimming, Clinics in Sports Medicine, 2(2):391-405, July 1983, Philadelphia, W.B. Saunders Co.
7. Tonry, D.: Sports illustrated women's gymnastics, New York, 1980, Lippincott & Crowell.

Other injuries

31. Gymnastic injuries: the Virginia experience

Edward Ricciardelli
Frank A. Pettrone

Participation in women's athletics has significantly increased since 1971. The popularity of female gymnastics, specifically, has reflected this growth with a 460% increase in participation just in the past 6 years. A major factor in this dramatic growth was worldwide exposure to the skills and grace of gymnasts such as Nadia Comenici, Olga Korbut, and the American Kathy Rigby during the Olympics of 1972 and 1976. By 1980, gymnastics had become the seventh most popular female sport. Attendant with this increased popularity, however, was a concomitant increase in the number of injuries.[5,6] The risks inherent in a sport that combines height, speed, and precision are obvious. It is surprising, however, to note that the injury rate in female gymnastics is double that of any other sport and, compared with all high school sports,[10] ranks behind only football, wrestling, and softball.[9] National Athletic Injury Illness Reporting System (NAIRS) data reported the average annual injury rate in women's collegiate gymnastics approximated that for collegiate football and ice hockey.[3]

The recent trend of concern within women's gymnastics is the increased frequency of significant injuries in 1977, the year after scoring changes were made more demanding. Such changes provided increased temptation for the athlete to attempt a higher risk routine before she had mastered it.

METHOD (Fig. 31-1)

To better understand the type, frequency, and predisposing features of gymnastic injuries, we performed a prospective analysis of club-level gymnastic injuries over a 7-month (one-season) period. I would like to present this data briefly and contrast it with other surveys in the literature and ultimately present conclusions for gymnastic safety. Questionnaires and flow sheets were sent to 32 private gymnastic clubs in Virginia. We received responses from 15 clubs with a total membership of 2558. Data on skill level (beginner to elite), student-to-instructor ratio, available safety equipment, and conditioning and warm-up exercises was collected in the questionnaire. In addition, flow sheets were completed for each club member. Data pertaining to

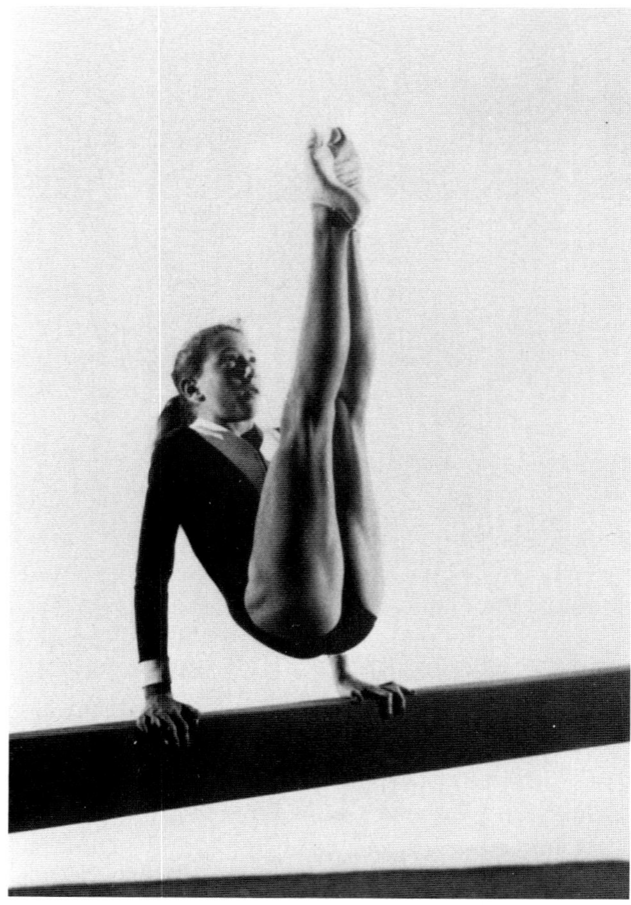

Fig. 31-1. The beauty, grace, and speed of gymnastics have contributed to its popularity.

physical characteristics, injuries sustained, and the event in which the injury occurred were elicited. For every gymnast who sustained an injury, additional information relating to setting (practice or competition), type of injury, and duration of disability was documented. Using the University of Virginia Academic Computer System, we assigned a 34-character code for each injured athlete. Injury was defined as any gymnastic-related incident that prevented participation by the gymnast in any part of a workout or competition. Analysis revealed the following:

1. Injuries occurred in 12 of the 15 participating clubs.
2. Sixty-two injuries occurred among the 542 competitive and 2016 noncompetitive level athletes.
3. Of the 62 injuries, 51 were acute and 11 chronic.
4. Only nine athletes sustained more than one injury over the season.

DATA

Our injury rate was 2.4 per 100 participant seasons, specifically 5.3 per 100 competitors (elite, advanced, intermediate) and 0.7 per 100 beginners. The distribution by ability level was for the elite, 1 injury; advanced, 5 injuries; intermediate, 23 injuries; and beginner, 15 injuries. There were 51 acute injuries—41 at practice (80%) and 10 at competition (20%). The event distribution of these 51 acute injuries were floor exercise 21, beam 13, vault 9, uneven parallel bars 6, and vault springboard 2. We were unable to find any statistically significant relationship (0.2655) between skill level and event.

The acute injuries (51) were 21 sprains (15 specified as ankle 11, knee 2, neck 1, and wrist 1), 16 fractures, 6 contusions, 4 dislocations, and 4 acute muscle strains.

There were 11 chronic injuries—5 sprains, 5 tendinitis, and 1 stress fracture.

We found that 19 injuries occurred at mount or dismount. The 16 dismount injuries occurred 6 in vault, 7 on beam, and 3 on unevens. The type of dismount injuries were 6 fractures (lower extremity and foot 3, upper extremity and hand 2, and neck 1), 4 sprains (ankle 3, and neck 1), 3 dislocations, 1 contusion, and 2 unspecified.

We were unable to find any correlation between skill level and type of injury (0.8096). There was also no correlation between type of injury and event (0.0943).

Thirty-three injuries occurred with learned moves, whereas 7 injuries occurred with new moves.

The duration of injury (disability) was less than 3 weeks in 44 (71%) and greater than 3 weeks in 18 (29%). Ten injuries (16%) lasted greater than 6 weeks. There was no correlation found between duration of injury and skill level (0.1553).

Spotters were present in 33 of the 51 injuries and not present in 18 of the 51 injuries.

Comparison of those clubs with the most injuries and those with no injuries

Two clubs had 32% of injuries	Three clubs had no injuries
Club 5: 7 injuries	*Clubs 3, 4, and 7*
Club 11: 13 injuries	

1. Safety equipment. There was no correlation found between the presence of safety equipment and injuries.

Club 5:	*Club 11:*	*Club 3:*	*Club 4:*	*Club 7:*
Mats	Mats	Mats	Mats	Mats
Spot belts	Belts	Bar pads	Hand belts	Belt
	Overhead belts			
	Bar pads			

2. Mats. There was no correlation found.

Club 5:	*Club 11:*
3 landing mats, 4 and 8 inches thick	7 landing mats, 8 inches thick
3 crash mats	

Club 3:	*Club 4:*	*Club 7:*
15 1½-inch base mats	13 1½-inch base mats	1 12-inch landing mat
1 4-inch landing mat	3 6-inch landing mats	4 4-inch basic mats
1 8-inch landing mat		

All landing mats should be 3¾ inches with a minimum size of 6 by 12 feet.

There were no specific deviations from NCAA, FIG, and USGF mat specifications found.

3. There was no correlation between conditioning exercises and injury rate.

Club 5:
Stretch (flexibility) / Running / Dance } 20 minutes

Club 11:
Stretch / Dance / Pull-ups / Leg lifts / Running } 45 minutes

Club 3:
Flexibility / Dance } 15 minutes

Club 4:
Flexibility / Strengthening } 15 minutes

Club 7:
Flexibility / Dance } 15 minutes

4. Duration of workout. There was a positive correlation between duration of workout and injury occurrence.

Club 5:
1 to 2 hours per week in class IV (beginners)
7.5 hours, 3 days/week to 9.5 hours, 4 days/week in classes I to III (competitors)

Club 11:
2½ hours, 3 or 4 days/week in class IV
4 hours, 5 or 6 days/week in classes III, II, and I

Club 3:
1½ to 2½ hours, 3 days/week

Club 4:
1 hour/week, class
1 to 1½ hours, 2 days/week, team

Club 7:
1 hour, 2 days/week, class
2 hours, 3 days/week, team

5. We investigated the student-instructor ratio but found no correlation to injuries.

Club 5:	*Club 11:*	*Club 3:*	*Club 4:*	*Club 7:*
8:1	7:1	8:1	6:1	10:1

6. All clubs stated that all participants had been exposed to safety instruction (how to fall, roll, and so on).

7. Size. There was a positive correlation between the size of the club and injury occurrence.

Club 5:	*Club 11:*	*Club 3:*	*Club 4:*	*Club 7:*
300	230	120	65	72

DISCUSSION

We reviewed the participation and injury rate in a representative sample of gymnasts in the commonwealth of Virginia over one season. The injury rate, for all skill levels, was 2.4 per 100 participant seasons, with a rate of 5 per 100 for competitors (intermediate, advanced, and elite) and 0.7 per 100 for noncompetitors. These percentages are consistently lower than those reported by Snook,[1] Garrick,[2] Weiker,[3] and Lowry.[4] However, each of these studies had a slightly different population. Snook looked at national-caliber college athletes; Garrick at high school, club, and college athletes; Weiker and Lowry at six and 14 private clubs respectively. The greater incidence of injuries in these studies reflects the increased competitive level of the participants. The majority of our population were noncompetitors, and one would anticipate a lower incidence of injuries among this group.

An explanation for our lower injury rate is the observation that practice and competition were less frequent in all but a few highly competitive clubs. Therefore a larger number of gymnasts participated less frequently and less intensely and hence sustained fewer injuries. The significantly higher injury rate among competitors versus noncompetitors is consistent with Lowry's study, which pointed out that noncompetitors have closer supervision, do additional spotting, spend less time in the gym, and hence have a lower risk of injury than competitors have.[4]

We demonstrated that more injuries occurred in the floor exercises (21) than in the beam (13) or vault (9). One would expect to see this difference, since the majority of practice time is spent on floor exercises. In our competitors we noted an increased number of injuries on the height events, that is, unevens and beam. In our noncompetitors, however, only three of 13 injuries occurred on the height events. This difference is suggestive of a greater degree of performance difficulty attempted by the competitor. The possibility of lowering the injury rate among advanced gymnasts by advancing to more difficult moves on a lower beam and with a slower progression warrants closer investigation.[3]

Another significant observation is related to the severity of injury occurring at dismount and on beam, vault, and uneven parallel bars. Of the 16 injuries, the most common was fracture (6). In addition, the only two neck injuries in the study (1 sprain and 1 fracture) also occurred at dismounts. Hunter's observation on the severity of injuries sustained at dismount parallel our findings.[7] She pointed out that present scoring systems call for a level of medium difficulty for dismount with points deducted for noncompliance. In addition, bonus points are scored for high-risk maneuvers. We would question the risk-to-benefit ratio of this system. Less difficult, safer dismounts could be substituted without detracting beauty or level of excellence from the core performance (Fig. 31-2).

Garrick made the observation that although competition involved only 0.4% of the gymnast's time it produced 5% of all injuries.[2] Our data likewise reveal that 20% of injuries occurred during competition. The intensity of the competition, that is, pressing for greater speed and power, and the execution of more hazardous and difficult maneuvers explain this disproportionate difference in percentage during competition.

Our most frequently observed injury was sprain (26), followed by fracture (17), tendinitis (9), contusion (6), and dislocation (4). Many studies have shown similar distributions.[1,2,8]

Most injuries occurring in our study resulted in a duration of disability of less than 3 weeks (71%). Weiker noted that 50% of elite gymnasts were out of practice for more than 15 days.[3] We could demonstrate no relationship between skill level and duration of disability.

An area of conflicting data from several studies is that of the correlation between the presence of spotters and injury rate. Weiker's data show that approximately 80% of all injuries occurred without spotting. We could not show this to be true. In our study, 33 of 51 (65%) occurred with spotting and 18 of 51 (35%) occurred without spotting. Our view, however, is that many injuries are prevented by the use of spotters and any data to suggest that spotting is of no value in preventing injury should be

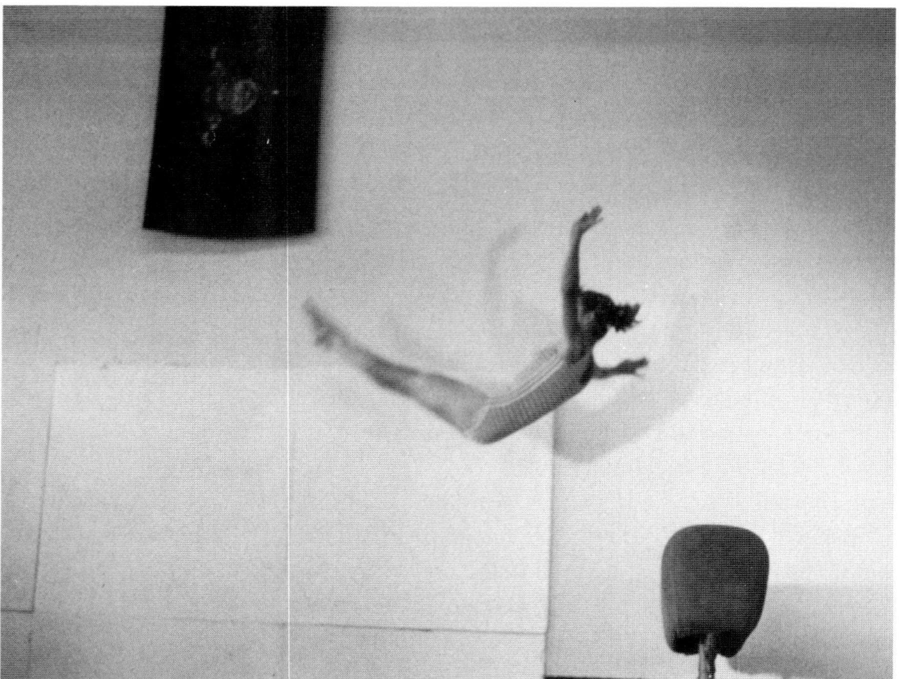

Fig. 31-2. Dismounts accounted for an increased severity of injury.

carefully questioned because most maneuvers are spotted in the gym.[3] The injury rate per unit time spent with spotters is lower than the same rate without spotters.

Another point of interest to coaches and physicians is the question of which safety features, conditioning programs, workout durations, and student-to-instructor ratios are most useful in preventing injury.[11] We compared the two clubs with the most injuries (20, 31%) to three clubs with no injuries. We found that there was no difference in the amount or type of safety equipment, mat number, or mat thickness. Likewise, conditioning programs, student-to-instructor ratios, and safety instruction were all comparable in the clubs with a high injury rate and those with no injuries. These findings are true across the board for all clubs in our study. Other studies[3,4] also found no correlation with student-to-instructor ratios or safety equipment with injury rate.[3,4] Lowry suggests that lower student-to-instructor ratios may mean greater pressure exerted on gymnasts by the instructor, such as more encouragement to attempt difficult skills, less time wasted in line, more time spent on performing with less time for recovery from fatigue. She also suggests that the presence of safety devices does not necessarily establish their use.[4]

We find that the duration and frequency of workouts in the clubs with high rates of injury were significantly greater than in those clubs with no injuries (20 to 30 hours per week versus 4 to 6 hours). We believe that fatigue plays a major role in the finding that those clubs practicing over 20 hours per week had a significantly higher injury rate.

I would like to delve into these three specific gymnastic injuries: spinal cord injury, spondylolysis, and elbow injury. I believe these three injuries highlight the dangers inherent in this graceful but demanding sport.

The National Athletic Injury Illness Reporting System (NAIRS) was organized in 1974 to carry out an analysis of data on injuries from all sports. Spinal cord injuries have received particular attention. Dr. Ken Clarke (1975) reported the survey results. The following were the permanent injuries recorded: death, quadriplegia, paraplegia, and hemiplegia. There were nine sports associated with spinal cord injury, and in only one, gymnastics, were females represented. Trampoline injuries dominated the statistics. Of the nine permanent spinal cord injuries among female gymnasts, five occurred on the trampoline. Fortunately, competition on the trampoline has been eliminated and a number of parent bodies, such as the American Academy of Pediatrics, has openly discouraged its usage (1977). There has been a definite drop in catastrophic gymnastic injuries from 1973 to 1978 (NAIRS reports), which is most likely attributable to attention to trampoline safety standards. In the United States today there are approximately 50 spinal cord injury cases per million persons per year. Seventy-six percent of these will render the victim paraplegic or quadriplegic. Vehicle accidents and falls each account for a third of these injuries. The remainder are seen in athletic injuries and missile wounds. The largest grouping of these catastrophic injuries was in the most highly skilled athletes. I will not discuss the physical examination and treatment of these injuries. Suffice it to say, gymnastics is a major source of cord injury, particularly in the female. Also in reporting gymnastic competition injuries, the neck and back were the third most frequently cited (19%), behind only below-knee and hip-to-knee injuries.

The low back is an area of the body most vulnerable to injury in the female gymnast (Fig. 31-3). Jackson first called our attention to the tremendous strains placed on the low back in gymnasts.[12] In a survey of 100 female competitive gymnasts (1976) he found an incidence of spondylolysis of 11%. This is in contrast to a general young white female incidence of 2.3%. Clinical and experimental data indicate that the basic lesion in spondylolysis is a fatigue fracture of the pars interarticularis. Observations of women gymnasts and analysis of movement reveal forces exerted at the lumbar spine that duplicate those found in the laboratory that cause spondylolysis. These movements include repetitive flexion and hyperextension during vaulting, dismounts, and flips. This excessive hyperextension posture with force loads transmitted to the lumbar spine must be implicated in the high frequency of spondylolysis in the gymnast.

The gymnast with spondylolysis will complain of low back pain associated with back bends, walkovers, and dismount. The pain is a dull ache, is noted coming out of the trick, and is often unilateral. This is often misinterpreted as a simple muscle strain. The most important physical finding is decreased straight leg raising. The examiner must be aware of the tremendous flexibility the gymnast possesses so that

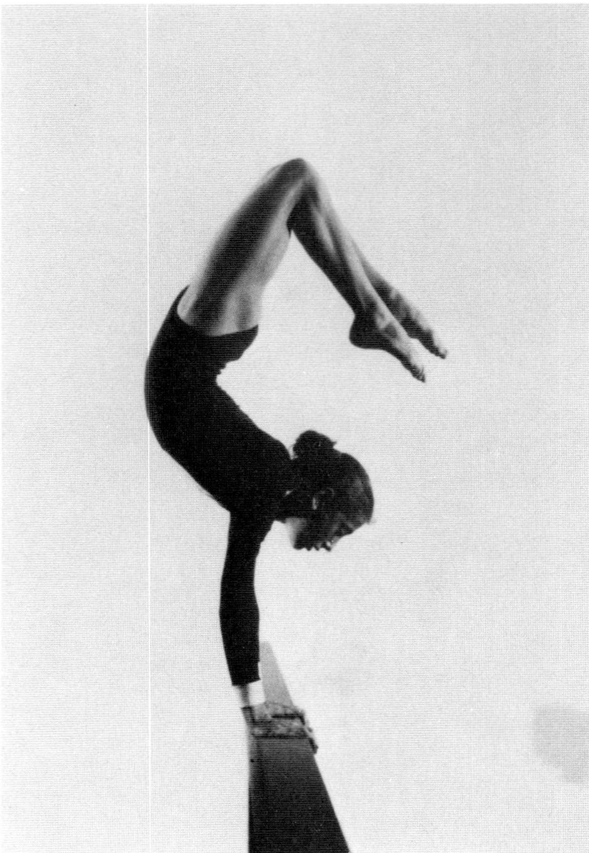

Fig. 31-3. Low back injuries are not uncommon. Flexibility and force loads account for this.

one should be suspicious when straight leg raising to less than 90 degrees is found. Other helpful signs are paravertebral spasm, scoliosis, and pain produced in the prone hyperextended position.

Plain roentgenograms may show a well-established bilateral pars interarticularis defect, unilateral findings, an attenuated pars, or unilateral sclerosis of the pedicle (Fig. 31-4). Often, however, the roentgenogram is normal. Bone scans are useful in this situation with increased uptake demonstrating the fatigue fracture. (Fig. 31-5).

Treatment should begin with rest, heat, and gentle stretching exercises. Muscle relaxants and the modalities of physical therapy are also useful. The athlete must not be allowed to return to practice until all pain has disappeared, full flexibility of the lumbar spine has returned, and strengthening exercises can be performed easily. Often a brace is useful for continued athletic participation. Cast treatment for the acute fracture may be used initially also. If the fracture does not heal, the athlete may still be allowed to return to practice provided that she has progressed satisfactorily

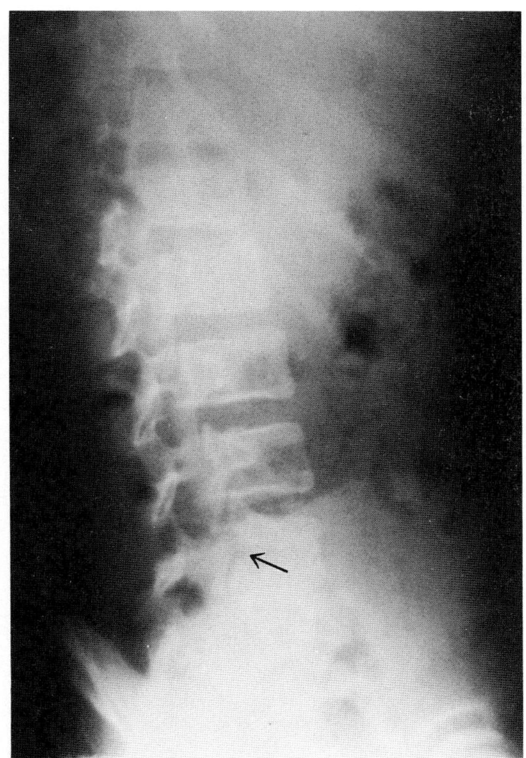

Fig. 31-4. Pars interarticularis defect.

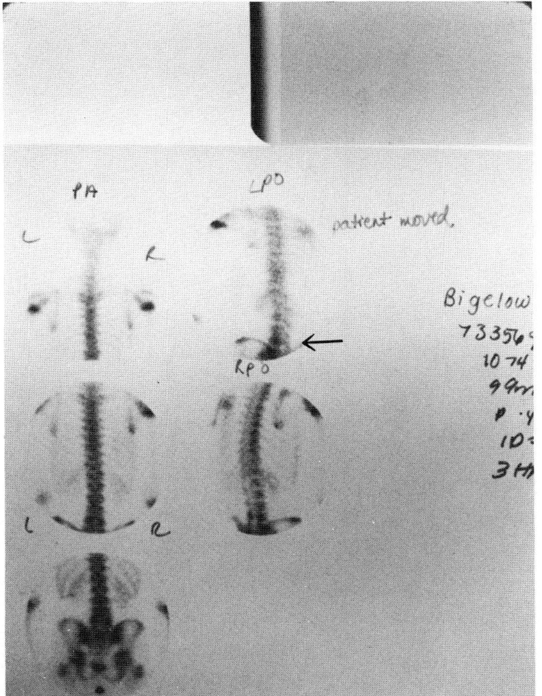

Fig. 31-5. Spondylolysis. Positive bone scan.

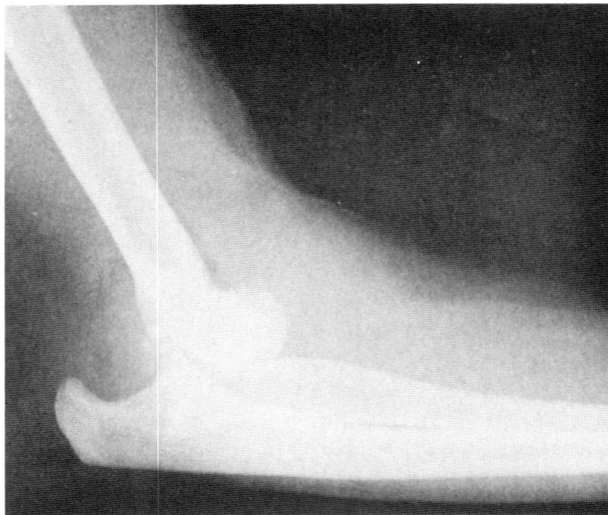

Fig. 31-6. Acute posterolateral elbow dislocation.

through the above rehabilitation process. Recurrent symptomatic episodes, however, predict a poorer prognosis for return to sports.

Gymnastics has become the women's power sport. The gymnasts convert the upper extremities to weight-bearing during tumbling, handstands, one-arm balance, vaults, and dismount maneuvers. Given the general ligamentous laxity of joints and the valgus carrying angle of the elbow in females, not surprisingly medial elbow injuries predominate. Numerous strains (stretch of the medial flexor muscle mass) and sprains (both wrist and elbow) occur. With further overload, subluxation and dislocation may occur. The most frequent direction of dislocation is posterolateral (Fig. 31-6). Prompt assessment usually allows reduction without difficulty. Postreduction roentgenograms (without overlying plaster) are essentials to ascertain that there are no fractures or fragments impinged within the joint. Immobilization for 2 weeks is recommended for a simple dislocation. Rehabilitation to restore motion and then strength is necessary before return to practice. The most frequent problem with dislocations is the slow restoration of full elbow motion. It is not unusual to take 6 months to regain full motion with an uneventful reduction and rehabilitation. However, full motion is not always obtained and permanent flexion contractures often ensue after dislocation. This can be disconcerting as well as physically and athletically limiting to the gymnast. An error of commission—forceful manipulation of the elbow—during early recovery is to be discouraged because the myositis ossificans that results can lead to even more stiffening of the joint. Surgical release of flexion contracture of the postdislocation elbow has been suggested, but its place in the competitive gymnast remains unclear. Persistent valgus instability is also a frequent consequence after dislocation, and it is disabling to the gymnast who needs a stable elbow-locked position in many maneuvers.

CONCLUSION

Several studies have acknowledged that female gymnastics is a hazardous sport.[1,4] To argue the varying incidence of injury in this sport is to ignore the fact that a significant risk of injury does exist. Our goals in this study were to highlight the caliber of the gymnast and the events that predict a higher risk of injury and to identify those factors that reduce that risk. We define a high-risk gymnast as one who is (1) performing at an advanced competitive level, (2) performing floor or beam exercises, and (3) practicing greater than 20 hours per week. Weiker has further cited the risk to be greater in low-weight gymnasts and greater during the second hour of workout.[3] Future studies should focus on specific maneuvers during which injuries occur, relationship of injuries to hours spent at practice, and identification of a male-to-female ratio of injuries.

We advocate the continued use of safety equipment to meet NCAA (National Collegiate Athletic Association) or USGF (United States Gymnastics Federation) specifications. The use of spotters whenever possible and adequate warm-up and conditioning programs are sound, logical approaches to the prevention of gymnastic injuries. We also recommend that weekly practice sessions be interrupted by "rest or light days" and that daily sessions include hourly rest periods.

It is our hope that with the continued study of gymnastic injuries, coaches and physicians can minimize the risk and maximize the beauty and excellence of gymnastics.

REFERENCES

1. Snook, G.: Injuries in women's gymnastics, Am. J. Sports Med. 7(4):242, 1979.
2. Garrick, J., and Requa, R.: Epidemiology of women's gymnastic injuries, Am. J. Sports Med. 8(4):261, 1980.
3. Weiker, G., and Ganim, R.: A prospective statistical analysis of gymnastic injuries on the club gymnastic level, USGF Technical J., p. 13, Dec. 1982.
4. Lowry, C.B., and Leveau, B.: A retrospective study of gymnastic injuries to competition and non-competition in private clubs, Am. J. Sports Med. 10(3):237, 1982.
5. Eisenberg, I., and Allen, W.C.: Injuries in women's varsity athletic program, Physician Sports Med. 6:112-120, 1978.
6. Haycock, C.E., and Gillette, J.V.: Susceptibility of women athletes to injury, J.A.M.A. 236:163-165, 1976.
7. Hunter, L.F., and Torgan, C.: Dismounts in gymnastics: should scoring be re-evaluated? Am. J. Sports Med. 11(4):208, 1983.
8. Clark, K.S., and Buckley, W.E.: Women's injuries in collegiate sports, Am. J. Sports Med. 8:187-191, 1980.
9. Garrick, J.G., and Requa, R.: Injuries in high school sports, Pediatrics 61:465-469, 1978.
10. Shaffer, T.E.: Summary in sports pages, Physician Sports Med. 2:23, 1974.
11. Wettstone, E., editor: Gymnastics safety manual, ed. 2, University Park, Pa., 1979, Pennsylvania State University Press.
12. Jackson, D.W., Wiltse, U., and Ciruncione, R.T.: Spondylolysis in the female gymnast, Clin. Orthop. (117):68-73, 1976.

Index

A

Abduction, overhead, method of demonstrating, 308

Acapulco cliff divers, cervical stress fractures in, 9

Acceleration, force, and mass, Newton's law of, 26-27

Acromioclavicular joint, 195-196
  injuries of, in athletes, 284-289
    classification of, 284-286
    surgery for, 288
    treatment of, 286-289
  and sternoclavicular joint, variations in, 194

Acromioplasty for shoulder tendinitis, 328-329

Action and reaction, Newton's law of, 27-28, 30

Adolescent elbow, 211-220
  capitellum of, 215, 216
  epicondyles of, 215, 216
  olecranon of, 214, 215
  radial head of, 214

Aerobic fitness, 351

Anatomy
  of forearm and hand, functional, 67-78
  of shoulder and elbow, functional, 193-210
  of wrist, biomechanical, 134-136

Angular momentum in racket sport stroke, 33-34

Archery gloves, 90, 92

Arm
  abductors of, 202
  adductors of, 202, 203
  flexors and extensors of, 200, 201, 202
  rotators of, 202, 203
    internal and external, 202, 204

Arteries
  of forearm and hand, 78
  of upper extremity, 209

Arthritis, monoarticular, and gout, 22-23
  case histories of, 22, 23

Arthroscopic anatomy of shoulder, 303-304

Arthroscopic examination of shoulder instability, 294

Arthroscopic technique for shoulder tendinitis, 333

Arthroscopy
  of elbow, 225, 228
    operative, 231
  of shoulder, 300-305
    history of, 300
    potential complications of, 304-305
    surgically amenable lesions for, 305
    technique of, 300-303

Articular fractures
  condylar, of distal interphalangeal joint, 143, 146, 147
  of distal radius, 96, 97, 98, 99-102

Artificial turf, wounds from, 89

Athletes
  adolescent, epiphyseal injuries of distal radius in, 103
  drug abuse among, 14
  medico-legal aspects of treating, 11-15
  peripheral nerve involvement among, 79, 81-85
  preadolescent, metaphyseal fractures of distal radius in, 103
  professional, with tennis elbow, 244-265
  throwing; *see* Pitching motion; Thrower's elbow; Throwing athlete

Athletic injuries; *see* Injuries

Axillary nerve, 208

B

Backstroke, mechanics for, 42, 43

Baseball pitching motion; *see* Pitching motion

Baseball players' gloves, 89, 92

Biceps, long head of, 6

Biomechanical application in upper extremity, 3-10

Biomechanical precursors to upper extremity trauma, 26-29

Biomechanics of elbow, 6-9

Blisters on weight lifter's and pitcher's hands, 87, 88

Bony injuries of elbow in throwing athlete, 221-232

Boutonnière deformity, splint for, 184, 185

Bowler's thumb, 84-85, 172, 173, 174, 175
Boxing gloves, 89
Brachial plexus, 208
Bracing and splinting of upper extremity, 182-189
Breach of confidence by physician, 13
Butterfly stroke, mechanics for, 39, 41, 43

C

Calluses on gymnast's hands, 87
Capener splint, 181, 182
Capitellum of adolescent elbow, 215, 216
  osteochondrosis of, 218
Carpal injuries, 122-133
  salvage procedure for, 133
Carpal tunnel, 71-73
Carpal tunnel syndrome, 174-176
  signs of, 175-176
  surgery for, 176
  symptoms of, 175
  tests for, 176
  treatment of, 176
Carpometacarpal joint injuries, 167-168
Carpus
  dislocations of
    lunate, 129-132
    other, 132
    perilunate, 127-129
  fractures of, 122-132
    other, 126
    scaphoid, 122-124
    transscaphoid perilunate, 125
Casts, silicone, 187, 189
  application of, 92, 93, 189
Catcher's mitt, 92
Cervical stress fractures in Acapulco cliff divers, 9
Childhood, sports in, social and psychological aspects of, 219
Clavicle
  anatomy of, 193
  fractures of, 279-282
    diaphyseal, 279
    lateral third of, 280-282
  use of, 6
"Clunk test" for diagnosis of labral tear, 317
Collateral ligament injuries
  of metacarpophalangeal joint, 160, 163-165, 166
  of proximal interphalangeal joint, 151, 152-154
Colles' fractures, 102
  malunited, 171
Compression of ulnar nerve, 177
Compression injuries, repeated, 85-86
Conditioning and warm-up in racket sports, 34-35
Condylar fractures, articular, 143, 146, 147
Coracoacromial arch, testing for impingement on, 309, 310

Coronary artery pain, 19-21
  case history of, 19
Cubital tunnel, 177-178
  signs of, 177-178
  surgery of, 178
  symptoms of, 177
  treatment of, 178
Curling gloves, 90, 92
Cybex strength testing, 346
Cyclists, ulnar nerve palsy in, 81
Cyclist's glove, 89, 90

D

Deltoid
  insertion of, 4, 6
  shape of, for power, 3, 5
Dermatone distribution in upper extremity, 208
Diaphyseal fractures
  distal third, 107-111
  and metaphyseal fractures, displaced, 96
Digit, motor function of, analysis of, 78
Digital joints, 73, 75
Digital perfusion, decreased, 85-86
Digits, trigger, 86
DIP joint; *see* Interphalangeal joint, distal
Dislocation
  of carpus
    lunate, 129-132
    other, 132
    perilunate, 127-129
  dorsal, of metacarpophalangeal joint, 154, 157-160, 161-162
  palmar, of proximal interphalangeal joint, 151, 154, 155-156
  of shoulder, anterior
    after surgical repair, treatment of, 298
    primary, treatment of, 297
    recurrent, treatment of, 297-298
    rehabilitation of, 298
  and subluxation, anterior, of shoulder, 290-299
    incidence of, in sports, 290
    mechanism of, 291
Dissociation of wrist
  lunotriquetral, 136, 138-139
  scapholunate, 136, 137
Drug abuse among athletes, 14

E

Elbow, 205-209
  adolescent, 211-220
    capitellum of, 215, 216
    epicondyles of, 215, 216
    olecranon of, 214, 215
    radial head of, 214
    roentgenologic evaluation of, 213

Elbow—cont'd
  arthroscopy of, 225-228
  biomechanics of, 6-9
  bony injuries of, in throwing athlete, 221
    classification of, 223-224
  injuries of, in gymnasts, 368
  Little League, 217-219
  maladies of, other, 264
  motor function of, factors involved in, 207
  movements of, 206
  and shoulder, 191-356
    functional anatomy of, 193-210
  skeleton of, 205-206
  stability of, 7, 225-226
  tennis; *see* Tennis elbow
  thrower's
    diagnosis of, 225-228
    lateral compression injuries of, 228
    medial stress injuries of, 228
    treatment of, 228-231
    vagaries of, 214-216
  valgus extension overload of, 229
Entrapment neuropathies, proximal, of median
    nerve, 176-180
Entrapment syndromes, 79
Entrapments of forearm and wrist, peripheral
    nerve injuries and, 174-181
Epicondylar growth plate, medial, delayed clo-
    sure of, 218
Epicondyle, medial, avulsion of, in Little League
    elbow, 218
Epicondyles of adolescent elbow, 215, 216
Epicondylitis; *see* Tennis elbow
Epiphyseal injuries
  of distal radius, 103-106
    in adolescent athlete, 103
  of metacarpophalangeal joint, 165, 167
Epiphyseal plate fracture of distal phalanx, 115
  treatment of, 116
Epiphyseal plate injuries, Salter-Harris classifica-
    tion of, 98, 99
Examination, physical
  preparticipation, 14
  for upper extremity pain, 18-19
Exercise aids, 187, 188
Exercise program, supplemental, for throwing,
    swimming, and gymnastics, 348-356
  endurance training in, 351
  flexibility training in, 349-351
  general considerations in, 348-351
  strength training in, 348-349
Extensor carpi ulnaris tendon, recurrent disloca-
    tion of, 120
Extensor hood mechanism of fingers, 69, 70-71
  at proximal interphalangeal joint, 70-71

Extensor intersection syndrome, 172
Extensor mechanism over metacarpal head, 117-
    120
  split, 118-120
  tooth wound of, 118
Extensor retinaculum, 67-68
Extensor tendon(s)
  and flexor tendons, injuries of, 114-121
  of hand 69-71
    and wrist, tendinitis of, 86
  injuries of, at proximal interphalangeal joint,
    116-117
  split in, 119-120
Extensor tendon avulsion, pathosis of, 115

F

Fencer's gauntlet, 89
Finger(s)
  extensor hood mechanism of, 69, 70
  flexor tendon mechanism in, 75
  ring avulsion of, 80
  and wrist motions, 72-73
Finger splints, 184-187
Flexibility training, exercise program for, 349-351
Flexor carpi radialis, 71-72
Flexor carpi ulnaris, 71-72
  tendon mechanism of, lesions of, 120
Flexor digitorum profundus, 73
  avulsion of, 116-117
    late, 117
Flexor digitorum superficialis, 73
Flexor and extensor tendons, injuries of, 114-121
Flexor pulleys and sheath, 73
Flexor tendon mechanism in finger, 75
Football players, protective devices for, 92
Football players' gloves, 89, 90, 91
Force
  accommodation of, through warm-ups, 28-29
  ground reaction, 30-32
    tennis stroke and, 30-32
  mass, and acceleration, Newton's law of, 26-27
Forces, joint, continuity of, 32-33
Forearm
  cultaneous nerves of, 209
  fractures of, 109, 111
  functional anatomy of, 67-78
  hand, and wrist, 65-189
    arteries of, 78
    nerves of, 78
  plated
    criteria for management of, 111
    refracture of, 111
  pronators and supinators of, 206, 207
  and wrist, entrapments of, peripheral nerve in-
    juries and, 174-181

Fracture(s)
  articular
    condylar, 143, 146, 147
    of distal radius, 96, 97, 98, 99-102
  of bone, reduction of, by muscle, 8
  of carpus, 122-132
  cervical stress, in Acapulco cliff divers, 9
  of clavicle, 279-282
    diaphyseal, 279
    lateral third of, 280-282
  Colles', 102
  diaphyseal
    distal third, 107-111
    and metaphyseal, displaced, 96
  of distal ends of radius and ulna, 95-112
    roentgenographic analysis of, 95-99
  epiphyseal plate, treatment of, 116
  forearm, 109, 111
  hamate, 81, 82, 126
  of humerus, proximal, 266-279
    four-part, 270, 273, 274
    head-splitting, 274-279
    three-part, 267-270, 271-272
    two-part, 266-267, 268-269
  from karate, 87
  mallet, 142-143, 144-146
  metaphyseal, of distal radius, 102-103
    of preadolescent athlete, 103
  nightstick, 108-109, 110
  open, 109, 111
  of proximal humerus, clavicle, and scapula,
    266-283
  of radius, 107-108
  of scaphoid, 122-124
  of scapula, 282-283
    body and neck of, 282-283
    glenoid of, 282
  Smith's, 102
  of triquetrum, 126
  of ulna, 108-109, 110
Fracture-dislocations
  dorsal, of proximal interphalangeal joint, 147-
    151
  transscaphoid perilunate, 125
Freestyle swimming stroke, mechanics of, 39, 40

G

Galeazzi equivalent lesions, 103, 104, 105, 107-
    108
Ganglion of wrist, 172
Glenohumeral joint, 196, 197, 200
  instability of, classifications of, 290-291
  rotation of, confirming, 319, 320
  subluxation and dislocations of, 290-299
    diagnosis of, 291-295

Glenohumeral joint—cont'd
  subluxation and dislocations of—cont'd
    mechanisms of, 291
Gloves and protective devices for hands, 89-93
Good samaritan law, 13
Gout and monoarticular arthritis, 22-23
  case histories of, 22, 23
Grip, precision and power, 75
Growth center appearance in upper extremity,
    212
Guyon's canal, injury to, 81, 82
Gymnastic injuries, 359-369
  analysis of, 361-369
  dismount, 363, 364
  elbow, 368
  floor exercise, 363
  low back, 365, 366
  spinal cord, 365
Gymnastics
  supplemental exercise program for, 354-355
  throwing, and swimming, supplemental exer-
    cise program for, 348-356
Gymnasts
  hands of
    calluses on, 87
    protection for, 87
  with spondylolysis, 365-366, 367

H

Hamate fractures, 81, 82, 126
Hand(s)
  cross sections through, 74
  dorsal skin and compartments of, 67
  extensor tendons of, 69-71
  forearm, and wrist, 65-189
  functional anatomy of, 67-78
  gloves and protective devices for, 89-93
  of gymnasts, 87
    calluses on, 87
    protection for, 87
  interossei muscles of, 69
  joint injuries of, complex, 142-169
  lumbrical muscles of, 70
  palmar skin and compartments of, 71
  skeleton of, 73
  skin of, 87-89
  soft-tissue injuries to, 79-94
  tendinitis of, 86
  transverse fibers of, 69
  vascular problems of, 85-86
Hand splints, static versus dynamic, 182-183
Handball glove, 89
Hollis's swan neck and boutonnière splints, 185

Humerus
 anatomy of, 193
 latissimus dorsi insert on, 4, 7
 proximal, fractures of, 266-279
  four-part, 270, 273, 274
  head-splitting, 274-279
  three-part, 267-270, 271-272
  two-part, 266-267, 268-269
 and scapula, relationship between relative motion of, 3
Hunting gloves, 92
Hypothenar hammer syndrome, 85
Hypothyroidism, 24-25
 case history of, 24

I

Impingement syndrome in competitive swimmer, 37-38
Inertia
 moment of, 28
 Newton's law of, 26
Injuries
 of acromioclavicular joint in athletes, 284-289
  classification of, 284-286
  surgery for, 288
  treatment of, 286-289
 bony, of elbow in throwing athlete, 221-232
  classification of, 223-224
 carpal, 122-133
  salvage procedure for, 133
 of collateral ligaments
  of metacarpophalangeal joint, 160, 163-165, 166
  of proximal interphalangeal joint, 151, 152-154
 compression, repeated, 85-86
 epiphyseal
  of distal radius, 103-106
  of metacarpophalangeal joint, 165, 167
 epiphyseal plate, 98, 99
 extensor tendon, at proximal interphalangeal joint, 116-117
 flexor and extensor tendon, 114-121
 gymnastic; *see* Gymnastic injuries
 interosseous nerve, 84
 joint
  carpometacarpal, 167-168
  distal interphalangeal, 142-147
  glenohumeral, 290-299
  of hand, complex, 142-169
  from karate, 87
  metacarpophalangeal, 154-167
  proximal interphalangeal, 147-154, 155-156
 ligament, wrist, 134-141
 miscellaneous, 170-173

Injuries—cont'd
 nerve, 174-176
  median, 83
  peripheral, and entrapments of forearm and wrist, 174-181
  radial, 84
  ulnar, 81
 role of torque in, 28
 soft-tissue, of hand, 79-94
 thrower's elbow, 225-231
 upper extremity
  general principles of, 1-63
  proper racket sports mechanics to avoid, 30-35
Instability
 of distal ulna, 139-140
 of shoulder
  arthroscopic examination of, 294
  classifications of, 290-291
  diagnosis of, 291-295
  examination of, 291-294, 295
  pathosis of, 295-296
Interossei muscles of hand, 69
Interosseous nerve, anterior, injury to, 84
Interphalangeal joints, 75
 distal
  articular condylar fractures of, 143, 146, 147
  fracture subluxation of, 115
  injuries of, 142-147
  mallet fractures of, 142-143, 144-146
 proximal
  collateral ligament injuries of, 151, 152-154
  dorsal fracture-dislocations of, 147-151
  extensor tendon injuries at, 116-117
  injuries of, 147-154, 155-156
  palmar dislocations of, 151, 154, 155-156
Isoflex exercise
 for shoulder tendinitis, 341, 342, 345
 for tennis elbow, 249
Isokinetic exercise
 for shoulder tendinitis, 345, 346
 for tennis elbow, 249, 250
Isometric exercise for tennis elbow, 248, 249
Isotonic exercise
 for shoulder tendinitis, 341-342
 for tennis elbow, 248, 249

J

Joint(s)
 acromioclavicular, 195-196
  injuries of, in athletes, 284-289
 carpometacarpal, injuries of, 167-168
 digital, 73, 75
 distal interphalangeal
  fracture subluxation of, 115

Joint(s)—cont'd
  distal interphalangeal—cont'd
    injuries of, 142-147
  elbow, valgus extension overload of, 229
  glenohumeral, 196, 197, 200
    instability of, classifications of, 290-291
  of hand, injuries of, 142-169
    from karate, 87
  interphalangeal, 75
  metacarpophalangeal, 73, 75
    dorsal dislocation of, 154, 157-160, 161-162
    injuries of, 154-167
  proximal interphalangeal
    extensor tendon injuries at, 116-117
    injuries of, 147-154, 155-156
    palmar dislocations of, 151, 154, 155-156
  shoulder, 193-196, 200-205
    arthroscopic anatomy of, 303-304
  sternoclavicular, 193-195
    anatomy of, 194
  wrist, 75-78
Joint forces, continuity of, 32-33

K

Karate, 86-87
  tenosynovitis from, 87
Kienböck's disease, 171

L

Lacrosse glove, 89
Latissimus dorsi insert on humerus, 4, 7
Ligaments
  collateral, injuries of
    of metacarpophalangeal joint, 160, 163-165,
      166
    of proximal interphalangeal joint, 151, 152-
      154
  of wrist, 76, 77, 78
    injuries of, 134-141
Limb-girdle motion, 198-200
Linear momentum in racket sport stroke, 33-34
Little League elbow, 217-219
  incidence of, 219
Low back injuries in gymnasts, 365, 366
Lumbrical muscles of hand, 70
Lunate dislocations of carpus, 129-132
Lunotriquetral dissociation of wrist, 136, 138-139
Lymphatics of upper extremity, 210

M

Mallet deformity, 114-116
  splints for, 184
  treatment of, 115-116
Mallet fractures, 142-143, 144-146

Mass, force, and acceleration, Newton's law of,
  26-27
Median nerve, 209
  injury to, 83
  proximal entrapment neuropathies of, 176-180
Medico-legal aspects of treating athletes, 11-15
Mesenchymal syndrome in tennis elbow, 255
Metacarpal head, extensor mechanism over, 117-
  120
  split, 118-120
  tooth wound of, 118
Metacarpophalangeal joint
  dorsal dislocation of, 154, 157-160, 161-162
  injuries of, 154-167
    collateral ligament, 160, 163-165, 166
    epiphyseal, 165, 167
Metaphyseal fractures of distal radius, 102-103
  and diaphyseal fractures, displaced, 96
  of preadolescent athlete, 103
Momentum in racket sport stroke
  angular, 33-34
  linear, 33-34
Motion, Newton's laws of, 26-28
Motor function of digit, analysis of, 78
Muscle strain as cause of shoulder pain, 43, 45
Muscles
  reduction of bone fracture by, 8
  of shoulder, 196-197
    extrinsic, 196-197
    intrinsic, 197
Musculocutaneous nerve, 209

N

National Athletic Injury Illness Reporting System, 365
Negligence, legal definition of, 12-13
Nerves
  of forearm and hand, 78
  injuries of, 174-176
  peripheral, problems of, 79, 81-85
  of upper limb, 206, 208-209
Neuropathies, proximal entrapment, of median
  nerve, 176
Newton's laws of motion, 26-28
Nightstick fractures, 108-109, 110

O

Olecranon
  of adolescent elbow, 214
  of thrower's elbow, débridement of, 230
Osteochondritis dissecans in Little League elbow,
  218
Osteochondrosis of radial head and capitellum of
  Little League elbow, 218

Overuse syndrome in competitive swimmer, 37-38
  treatment of, 45

P

Pain
  coronary artery, 19-21
  upper extremity
    local causes of, 17
    medical aspects of, 16-25
    medical causes of, 16-17
    muscle strain as cause of, 43, 45
    as part of generalized disorder, 17-18
    physical examination for, 18-19
    referred from internal organs, 18
    referred from local structures, 17
Palmar dislocations of proximal interphalangeal
    joint, 151, 154, 155-156
Panner's disease, 228
Pectoralis major insertion on humerus,
    4, 7
Perilunate dislocations of carpus, 127-129
Peripheral nerve injuries and entrapments of
    forearm and wrist, 174-181
Peripheral nerve problems, 79, 81-85
Physeal closure in upper extremity, 212, 213
Physical examination
  preparticipation, 14
  for upper extremity pain, 18-19
Physician
  breach of confidence by, 13
  obligation of, in treatment, 11
  team
    future of, 14-15
    role of, 12
    standard of care for, 12-13
PIP; *see* Interphalangeal joint, proximal
Pitcher's hands, blister formation on,
    87, 88
Pitching motion, 59-63
  acceleration phase of, 61-62, 222-223
  biomechanics of, 221-222
  cocking phase in, 59, 60, 222
  deceleration in, 223
  follow-through phase of, 62-63, 223
  phases of, 59
  stresses in, 225-226
  windup in, 59, 60, 222
Platform tennis mitten or sock, 89, 92
Pleural effusion, 21-22
  case history of, 21
Polymyalgia rheumatica, 23-24
  case history of, 23
Power
  definition of, 3

Power—cont'd
  shape of deltoid for, 3
Precision and power grip, 75
Preparticipation examination, 14
Pronator syndrome, 83-84
Pulleys, flexor, and sheath, 73

R

"Racket player's pisiform," 120
Racket sport mechanics, to avoid upper extremity
    injury
  improper, 34-35
  proper, 30-35
Racket sport stroke, angular and linear momen-
    tum in, 33-34
Racket sports, need for warm-up and condition-
    ing in, 34-35
Radial artery, arteriovenous fistula of, 85
Radial head of adolescent elbow, 214
  osteochondrosis of, 218
Radial nerve, 208
Radial nerve compression syndromes, 84
Radial nerve injuries, 84
Radial tunnel, anatomy of, 179
Radial tunnel syndrome, 179-180
  signs of, 180
  surgery of, 180
  symptoms of, 179-180
Radioulnar congruity, measurement of, 98
Radioulnar joint, distal, stable, preservation of,
    98
Radius, distal
  articular fractures of, 96, 97, 98, 99-102
    reduction of, 101-102
  epiphyseal injuries of, 103-106
    in adolescent athlete, 103
  fractures of, 107-108
  metaphyseal fractures of, 102-103
    in preadolescent athlete, 103
  and ulna, distal, fractures of, 95-112
    roentgenographic analysis of, 95-99
Rehabilitation of shoulder, 338-347
  exercises for, 341-346
    Isoflex, 342, 345
    isokinetic, 345, 346
    isotonic, 341-342, 343-344
Rehabilitative exercise for tennis elbow, 247, 249
Ring avulsion of finger, 80
Rotator cuff, origin of, 4, 6
Rotator cuff tendinitis; *see* Shoulder tendinitis

S

Safety-pin splint, 185, 187
Sagittal band mechanism, longitudinal split in,
    119

Salter-Harris classification of epiphyseal plate injuries, 98, 99
Scaphoid, fracture of, 122-124
Scapholunate dissociation of wrist, 136, 137
Scapula
  anatomy of, 193
  depressors of, 198, 199
  downward rotators of, 200, 201
  elevators of, 198, 199
  fractures of, 282-283
    body and neck of, 282-283
    glenoid of, 282
  and humerus, relationship between relative motion of, 3
  as movable platform, 3, 5
  protractors and retractors of, 198
  shape of, 4
  upward rotators of, 200
Scapulothoracic joint, fixing of, 6
Serratus anterior muscle, checking for weakness in, 310, 312
Sheath and flexor pulleys, 73
Shoulder
  adduction of, horizontal, checking, 313, 314
  arthroscopic anatomy of, 303-304
  arthroscopy of, 300-305
    history of, 300
    potential complications of, 304-305
    surgically amenable lesions for, 305
    technique of, 300-303
  biceps tendon of, testing, 315, 317
  dislocations of, anterior, 297-298
    after surgical repair, treatment of, 297
    primary, treatment of, 297
    recurrent, treatment of, 297-298
    rehabilitation of, 298
  and elbow, 191-356
    functional anatomy of, 193-210
  examination and diagnosis of, in throwing athlete, 306-321
  functions of, 198-205
  instability of
    arthroscopic examination of, 294
    diagnosis of, 291-295
    examination of, 291-294, 295
    incidence of, 290
    mechanism of, 291
    pathosis of, 295-296
    posterior, assessing, 315, 316
    in swimmers, treatment of, 45
  muscles of, 196-197
    anterior, palpation of, 318-319
    extrinsic, 196-197
    intrinsic, 197

Shoulder—cont'd
  muscles of—cont'd
    posterior, examination of, 309-310, 311
  rehabilitation of, 338-347
  rotation of
    internal, measuring, 310, 312
    observing, 313
  skeleton of, 193
  stability of, anterior, testing for, 309, 311
  subluxation of, anterior
    and dislocation of, 290-299
    nonoperative treatment of, 296
    surgical treatment of, 296-297
    testing, 313, 314
  skeleton of, 193
  thrower's, injury of
    additional diagnostic procedures for, 320
    history of, 307
    physical examination and diagnosis of, 307-320
  use of, in sports, 3-6
  and wrist, factors involved in motor function of, 205
Shoulder joints, 193-196, 200-205
Shoulder pain, muscle strain as cause of, 43, 45
Shoulder stress in sports, 37, 38
Shoulder tendinitis, 322-337
  high-voltage electrical stimulation for, 339-340
  pathoetiology of, 322-324
  postoperative care of, 334
  rehabilitative exercise for, 341-346
    Cybex strength testing after, 346
    Isoflex, 342, 345
    isokinetic, 345, 346
    isotonic, 341-342, 343-344
  relief of pain and inflammation in, 338-341
  return to sports after, 334-335, 346-347
    progression variables for, 347
    proper conditioning for, 346
  role of arthroscopy in, 333
  signs and symptoms of, 324-326
  treatment of
    with acromioplasty, 328-329
    conservative, 326-328
    surgical, 328, 329-333
Silicone cast, 187, 189
  application of, 92, 93, 189
Skateboard glove, 90
Skeleton, immature, 211-212, 213
Ski gloves, 89, 91
Skin
  dorsal, and compartments of hand, 67
  of hands, 87-89
  palmar, and compartments of hand, 71

Soccer goalie's glove, 89
Soft-tissue injuries to hand, 79-94
Spinal cord injuries in gymnasts, 365
Splinting
    and bracing of upper extremity, 182-189
    principles of, 183-184
Splints
    finger, 184-187
    hand, static versus dynamic, 182-183
Spondylolysis in gymnasts, 365-366, 367
Sports in childhood, social and psychologic aspects of, 219
Sternoclavicular joint, 193-195
    and acromioclavicular joint, variations in, 194
    anatomy of, 194
Strength training, 348-349
Subluxation, anterior
    and dislocation of shoulder, 290-299
        incidence of, in sports, 290
        mechanism of, 291
        treatment of
            nonoperative, 296
            surgical, 296-297
Supraspinatus, testing for strength of, 309
Swan-neck deformity, splint for, 184, 185
Swimmer, competitive, impingement syndrome in, 37-38
    treatment of, 45
Swimming
    competitive
        clinical considerations in, 37-38
        training considerations in, 36-37
    supplemental exercises for, 351-353
    throwing, and gymnastics, supplemental exercise program for, 348-356
    upper extremity in, 36-46
Swimming stroke mechanisms, 39-45
    for backstroke, 42, 43
    for butterfly, 39, 41, 43
    for freestyle, 39, 40

T

Team physician
    future of, 14-15
    role of, 12
    standard of care for, 12-13
Tendinitis
    of extensor tendons of wrist and hand, 86
    shoulder; *see* Shoulder tendinitis
Tennis
    overexertion in, 58
    serve in, 49-52
    warm-up for, 56
Tennis elbow
    alteration of force transmission in, 238, 241-242

Tennis elbow—cont'd
    alteration of playing technique with, 252-253
    change to proper equipment with, 253-254
    control of abusive force overload in, 251-254
    control of inflammation in, 247
    counterforce bracing in, 251-252
    effect of ability and playing time on, 234
    epidemiology and conservative treatment of, 233-265
    equipment modification for, 241
    etiology of, 234
    evaluation of patient with, 235-236
    high-voltage electrical stimulation for, 249-250
    improvement of strength and flexibility of muscles in, 238, 239, 240, 241
    incidence of, 233
    lateral, surgical technique for, 257-259
    management of, 236-238
    medial, surgical technique for, 260-262
    mesenchymal syndrome in, 255
    pathologic change in tendon in, 254
    pathology of, 235, 244-245
    posterior, surgical technique for, 262-263
    postoperative care of, 263
    promotion of healing in, 247
    rehabilitative exercises for, 247, 249
    relation of age and sex to, 233-234
    sign and symptoms of, 245-247
    surgical indications for, 254-255
    surgical pathology of, 256-257
    surgical treatment of, 255-264
        basic concepts for, 257
        historical review of, 255-256
        results of, 263-264
        technique for, 257-259
    surgery and rehabilitation of professional athlete with, 244-265
    treatment of, 247-254
Tennis racket, choosing proper, 52-55, 253-254
Tennis stroke, 47-58
    beginning of, 30-32
    complete shoulder turn in, 47, 49
    follow-through swing in, 47, 50, 51
    preparing for, 47, 50
    production of, 47-48
Tenosynovitis from karate, 87
Thoracic nerve, 209
Thoracic outlet syndrome in swimmers, 45
Thrombosis of ulnar artery, 81, 83
Thrower's elbow
    diagnosis of, 225-228
    lateral compression injuries of, 228
    medial stress injuries of, 228
    treatment of, 228-231

Throwing
  supplemental exercises for, 353-354
  swimming, and gymnastics, supplemental exercise program for, 348-356
Throwing athlete
  bony injuries of elbow in, 221-232
  shoulder examination and diagnosis in, 306-321
  shoulder injury to
    additional diagnostic procedures for, 320
    history of, 307
    physical examination and diagnosis of, 307-320
Throwing motion; *see* Pitching motion
Tooth wound of extensor mechanism of metacarpal head, 118
Torque, role of, in injury, 28
Traction apophysitis in Little League elbow, 218
Transscaphoid perilunate fracture-dislocation, 125
Transverse fibers of hand, 69
Trauma, upper extremity, biomechanical precursors to, 26-29
Trigger digits, 86
Triquetrum, fracture of, 126

U

Ulna
  distal, instability of, 139-140
  fractures of, 108-109, 110
  and radius, fractures of distal ends of, 95-112
    roentgenographic analysis of, 95-99
Ulnar artery, thrombosis of, 81, 83
Ulnar nerve, 209
  compression of, 177
  injury of, 81
    to cyclist, 81
Ulnar tunnel, anatomic relations of structures within, 178
Ulnar tunnel syndrome, 178-179
Ulnar variance, 98
Upper extremity
  arteries of, 209
  biomechanical applications in, 3-10
  complex functional anatomy of, 9
  dermatome distribution in, 208
  growth center appearance in, 212
  lymphatics of, 210
  nerves of, 206, 208-209
  physeal closure in, 212, 213
  protection of, 8-9
  splinting and bracing of, 182-189

Upper extremity—cont'd
  in swimming, 36-46
  veins of, 210
  vessels of, 209-210
Upper extremity injuries in athletes
  general principles of, 1-63
  racket sport mechanics to avoid
    improper, 34-35
    proper, 30-35
Upper extremity pain
  local causes of, 17
  medical aspects of, 16-25
  medical causes of, 16-17
  as part of generalized disorder, 17-18
  physical examination for, 18-19
  referred from internal organs, 18
  referred from local structures, 17
  in swimmers, treatment of, 45
Upper extremity trauma, biomechanical precursors to, 26-29

V

Valgus extension overload of elbow joint, 229
Vascular problems of hand, 85-86
Veins of upper extremity, 210

W

Warm-ups
  accommodation of force through, 28-29
  and conditioning, need for in racket sports, 34-35
Weight lifter's hands, blister formation on, 87, 88
Wheelchair racer's glove, 89
Wrist
  anatomy of, 134-136
  dissociation of
    lunotriquetral, 136, 138-139
    scapholunate, 136, 137
  and forearm, peripheral nerve injuries and entrapments of, 174-181
  ganglion of, 172
  hand, and forearm, 65-189
  ligaments of, 76, 77, 78
    injuries of, 134-141
  and shoulder, factors involved in motor function of, 205
  tendinitis of, 86
Wrist and finger motions, 72-73
Wrist joints, 75-78